Current Clinical Neurology

Series editor

Daniel Tarsy, MD
Department of Neurology
Beth Israel Deaconness Hospital
Boston, MA
USA

More information about this series at http://www.springer.com/series/7630

Alireza Minagar • J. Steven Alexander

Editors

Inflammatory Disorders of the Nervous System

Pathogenesis, Immunology, and Clinical Management

Second Edition

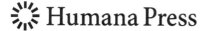 Humana Press

Editors
Alireza Minagar, MD
Department of Neurology
LSU Health Sciences Center
Shreveport, LA
USA

J. Steven Alexander, PhD
Department of Molecular and Cellular
Physiology
LSU Health Sciences Center
Shreveport, LA
USA

Current Clinical Neurology
ISBN 978-3-319-84595-1   ISBN 978-3-319-51220-4   (eBook)
DOI 10.1007/978-3-319-51220-4

Printed on acid-free paper

This Humana Press imprint is published by Springer Nature
The registered company is Springer International Publishing AG
The registered company address is: Gewerbestrasse 11, 6330 Cham, Switzerland

Series Editor Introduction

As stated in my introduction to *Inflammatory Disorders of the Nervous System*, published in 2005, the role of the inflammatory response in the pathophysiology of certain nervous system disorders had been known for quite some time. However, not unexpectedly, since that volume was published, the field has grown very rapidly. The creation of new journals such as the *Journal of Neuroinflammation* and *Neuroimmunology and Neuroinflammation* speaks to the enormous growth of the field. It is therefore timely that in an effort to update the field, Dr. Minagar and Dr. Alexander have produced a second edition of their book, *Inflammatory Disorders of the Nervous System: Pathogenesis, Immunology, and Clinical Management*. Although there is some overlap of topics which have been updated from the first volume, several are new and were not addressed in the first edition. These include HIV infection, autoimmune encephalitis including paraneoplastic and nonneoplastic disorders, Guillain-Barre syndrome, chronic inflammatory demyelinating polyneuropathy, myasthenia gravis, inflammatory myopathies, and the role of veins in neurodegenerative disease. The editors have recruited a number of new experts in the field who provide new information concerning the basic mechanisms of these disorders as well as new clinical information regarding their diagnosis and treatment. As stated in my introduction to the first edition, it may possibly still be appropriate to state that a balance may exist between useful and protective and possibly damaging effects of various neuroinflammatory mechanisms. The extent to which neuroinflammation is a primary cause or a more passive bystander in the pathophysiology of certain neurologic disorders may turn out to vary considerably among the various conditions considered here.

Boston, MA, USA

Daniel Tarsy, MD

Preface

Many, if not all, diseases of the central and peripheral nervous systems exhibit neuroinflammation which plays a central even initiating role in the pathogenesis of these conditions. Only by meticulously exploring the mechanisms and key events in neuroinflammatory disturbances can clinicians advance diagnosis and treatment of these maladies. In this, our second edition of *Inflammatory Disorders of the Nervous System: Pathogenesis, Immunology, and Clinical Management*, we have collected, updated, and extended our understanding of the developing descriptions of these conditions from the perspective of clinical and basic neuroscientists. Owing to many recent scientific and technical developments, our general understanding, paradigms, and approaches towards neuroinflammation have changed again, and with them greater refinement of novel biologic immunotherapies making these often lifelong and progressive maladies more manageable; cures for some may be in sight.

Our second edition encompasses the most up-to-date research findings in the rapidly evolving and expanding arena of neuroinflammation establishing it as a separate domain within the field of neuroscience. The chapters in this collection underscore how an improved realization of these conditions as inflammatory phenomena may be most rapidly and safely translated to the clinic. We hope that the next generation of clinicians and basic scientists will benefit and become enthusiastically inspired to apply, develop, and expand on the collected findings presented in this edition.

We would like to acknowledge and thank the group of diverse and international teams of physicians and scientists who contributed to make this volume timely, despite their active clinical and academic duties. The editors of this edition would also like to thank and acknowledge the patient discipline of our editorial colleagues at Springer Inc. including Mr. Karthikeyan Gurunathan and Gregory Sutorius without whose superior guidance and organization this volume would not have been possible. We, the editors, would like to thank you, the readers for studying this volume and hope that our contribution will again help to drive this field forward and make the neurologic conditions described here only a part of future clinical history.

Shreveport, LA, USA

Alireza Minagar, MD
J. Steven Alexander, PhD

Contents

List of Contributors

R. Aachi, MD Department of Neurology, LSU Health Sciences Center, Shreveport, LA, USA

Y.S. Ahn, MD University of Miami, Department of Medicine (Wallace H. Coulter Platelet Laboratory), Miami, FL, USA

C. Beggs, PhD Buffalo Neuroimaging Analysis Center, Department of Neurology, School of Medicine and Biomedical Sciences, University at Buffalo, Buffalo, NY, USA

Institute for Sport, Physical Activity and Leisure, Carnegie Faculty, Leeds Beckett University, Leeds, UK

S.C. Beh, MD Department of Neurology and Neurotherapeutics, Multiple Sclerosis and Neuroimmunology Program, University of Texas Southwestern School of Medicine, Dallas, TX, USA

C. Cajavilca, MD Department of Neurology, LSU Health Sciences Center, Shreveport, LA, USA

O.Y. Chernyshev, MD, PhD Department of Neurology, LSU Health Sciences Center, Shreveport, LA, USA

D. Davis, MD Department of Neurology, LSU Health Sciences Center, Shreveport, LA, USA

R. El-Khoury, MD Department of Neurology, Tulane University School of Medicine, New Orleans, LA, USA

J.D. Engand, MD Department of Neurology, LSUHSC School of Medicine, New Orleans, LA, USA

M. Fowler, MD Departments of Pathology, LSU Health Sciences Center, Shreveport, LA, USA

E.M. Frohman, MD, PhD Department of Neurology and Neurotherapeutics, University of Texas Southwestern School of Medicine, Dallas, TX, USA

Department of Ophthalmology, University of Texas Southwestern School of Medicine, Dallas, TX, USA

T.C. Frohman, PA-C Department of Neurology and Neurotherapeutics, University of Texas Southwestern School of Medicine, Dallas, TX, USA

E. Gonzalez-Toledo, MD, PhD Department of Neurology, LSU Health Sciences Center, Shreveport, LA, USA

Departments of Radiology, LSU Health Sciences Center, Shreveport, LA, USA

E. Grebenciucova University of Chicago Medical Center, Department of Neurology, Chicago, IL, USA

L.L. Horstman, BS Department of Medicine (Wallace H. Coulter Platelet Laboratory), University of Miami, Miami, FL, USA

O. Hussein, MD Department of Neurology, LSU Health Sciences Center, Shreveport, LA, USA

W. Jy, PhD Department of Medicine (Wallace H. Coulter Platelet Laboratory), University of Miami, Miami, FL, USA

B.P. Kelley, BS Department of Neurology, Tulane University School of Medicine, New Orleans, LA, USA

R.E. Kelley, MD Department of Neurology, Tulane University School of Medicine, New Orleans, LA, USA

A.A. Lizarraga, MD Miller School of Medicine, University of Miami, Miami, USA

A. Minagar, MD Departments of Neurology, LSU Health Sciences Center, Shreveport, LA, USA

J. McGee, DHEd, MSHS Department of Neurology, LSU Health Sciences Center, Shreveport, LA, USA

R.M. Paddison Department of Neurology, LSUHSC School of Medicine, New Orleans, LA, USA

K. Rezania, MD Department of Neurology, University of Chicago Medical Center, Chicago, IL, USA

W. Richeh, MD Department of Neurology, LSUHSC School of Medicine, New Orleans, LA, USA

Shannon Clinic, Brain and Spine Institute, San Angelo, Texas, USA

R.N. Schwendimann, MD Department of Neurology, LSU Health Sciences Center, Shreveport, LA, USA

W.A. Sheremata, MD, FRCPC, FACP, FAAN Miller School of Medicine, University of Miami, Miami, FL, USA

J. Steven Alexander, PhD Department of Molecular and Cellular Physiology, LSU Health Sciences Center, Shreveport, LA, USA

Departments of Neurology, LSU Health Sciences Center, Shreveport, LA, USA

J. Winny Yun, BS Department of Molecular and Cellular Physiology, LSU Health Sciences Center, Shreveport, LA, USA

R. Zand, MD Department of Neurology, University of Tennesse, Geisinger Health System, Danville, PA, USA

Emerging Roles of Endothelial Cells in Multiple Sclerosis Pathophysiology and Therapy

1

J. Winny Yun, Alireza Minagar, and J. Steven Alexander

Introduction

Normal BBB Anatomy and Physiology

The internal milieu of the brain is isolated from solutes and cells in the bloodstream, creating an immunologically and pharmacologically "privileged" compartment owing to the BBB. The BBB is a highly organized and strictly regulated multicellular system, creating physical, chemical, and metabolic barriers, which has at its heart the CEC. These closely apposed cells are integrated functionally and metabolically with pericytes, astrocytes, and neurons to regulate blood flow and exchange of materials via transporters, pores, and channels normally protecting the brain with disturbances during acute and chronic inflammatory responses.

J.W. Yun, BS
Department of Molecular and Cellular Physiology, LSU Health Sciences Center,
1501 Kings Highway, Shreveport, LA 71130, USA

A. Minagar, MD
Departments of Neurology, LSU Health Sciences Center,
1501 Kings Highway, Shreveport, LA 71130, USA

J.S. Alexander, PhD (✉)
Department of Molecular and Cellular Physiology, LSU Health Sciences Center,
1501 Kings Highway, Shreveport, LA 71130, USA

Departments of Neurology, LSU Health Sciences Center,
1501 Kings Highway, Shreveport, LA 71130, USA
e-mail: jalexa@lsuhsc.edu

© Springer International Publishing AG 2017
A. Minagar, J.S. Alexander (eds.), *Inflammatory Disorders of the Nervous System*, Current Clinical Neurology, DOI 10.1007/978-3-319-51220-4_1

Transport Across the BBB

The BBB prevents the passive entry of water, charged solutes, soluble mediators (including circulating neurotransmitters), proteins (immunoglobulins, cytokines, chemokines), and immune cells in the peripheral circulation into the CNS, protecting it from unintended immune activation and excitotoxic stress. BBB homeostasis is a prerequisite for normal neuron functioning; neurons are extremely sensitive to fluctuations in parenchymal ionic strength ($Ca2^+$, Na^+, K^+). Although limited immune cell exchange across the BBB is normal, a low continuous level of immune cell surveillance protects the brain against viral (e.g., JC virus) reactivation and is a consequence of BBB immune suppression and MS therapy.

Among the cells forming the BBB, CEC lines the intimal surface of larger cerebral vessels and are the major component of brain capillaries. The highly specialized CEC establishes physical barriers against the exchange of solutes, ions, and formed blood elements. Trans-BBB exchange of immune cells can take place *transcellularly* (penetrating the endothelial cytoplasm) or at inter-CEC junctions (paracellularly) as is found in most other endothelia [1]. The "decision" for immune cells to either pathway reflects the level of expression and context for presentation of intercellular adhesion molecule-1 (ICAM-1) [1]. The ICAM-1 cytoplasmic domain appears to be absolutely required for Rho-mediated signaling, which leads to cytoskeletal rearrangements necessary for T cell penetration of the CEC [2]. Gorina et al. (2014) have suggested that both neutrophil "crawling" mediated by ICAM-1 and ICAM-2 are necessary events leading to BBB extravasation [3]. von Wedel-Parlow and colleagues have suggested that neutrophils can pass across BBB endothelium transcellularly without disturbing the junctional barrier [4], although perturbations in tight and adherens junction binding and organization can increase extravasation at this route as well [5, 6]. Consequently, both tight and adherens junctional organization as well as adhesion molecule expression can influence trans-BBB immune cell exchange.

This BBB restriction to cells and solute exchange is achieved by cooperative interactions between tight junctions (TJs) and adherens junctions (AJs) between apposed endothelial cells. These interactions allow the BBB to create an electrically resistive barrier of up to 1500 ohms/cm^2 (known as "gate" function). The lateral sealing of apical and basolateral membrane domains ("fence" function) [7, 8] segregates luminal and abluminal adhesion molecules, transporter and matrix binding, and cell contact domains. BBB establishment and development depend on several paracrine signals from astrocytes and glia to the endothelium; neurons may also indirectly influence BBB. Astrocyte-derived brain-derived neurotrophic factor (BDNF) [9], platelet-derived growth factor-β (PDGF-BB), pericyte-derived transforming growth factor-β (TGF-β), GDNF, bFGF, IL-6, and steroids [10, 11] all contribute to the establishment and organization of the BBB [11, 12]. PDGF-β stabilizes BBB phenotype by recruiting pericytes to the BBB [13]. Pericytes in turn continuously release TGF-β, which establishes and induces the BBB by inducing transcription of claudin-5, an important component of TJ [11]. The actual physical barrier of the BBB occurs at the molecular level of the tight junctions, which is supported by adherens junctions, between adjacent BECs, which is regulated by these factors. Although pericyte TGF-β may help to establish BBB, ischemic pericyte release of VEGF-A can also trigger vascular leakage [14], illustrating the complexity of the "support" cells, which are able to both enhance and disintegrate the BBB. Astrocytes significantly upregulate VEGF expression during MS [15], which in turn downregulates claudin-5 and occludin levels by activating p38 mitogen-activated protein kinase (MAPK) [16]. Astrocytes are instrumental in MS neuroinflammation, not only due to the release of factors that disrupt the BBB but also because the loss of its polarity can also cause BBB dysfunction. Loss of polarized expression of aquaporin 4 (AQP4) in the astrocytic foot processes is seen in an animal model of MS, experimental allergic encephalomyelitis (EAE) [17]. Loss of astrocytic polarity suggests that the polarized secretion of various astrocytic-derived factors (e.g., sonic hedgehog (Hh)) is also compromised in experimental and clinical MS. Astrocytes secrete Hh and bind Hh receptors expressed on BBB endothelial cells to promote BBB formation and integrity [18]. Hh is upregulated in active demyelinating lesions and is correlated with increased Hh receptor expression in BBB endothelial cells, indicating a possible compensatory mechanism to promote BBB repair.

Adherens Junctions in BBB

AJ forms continuous band-like structures along apposed cells known as "adhesion belts," holding adjacent cells together. During embryonic development, AJs initiate cell-cell contacts, and throughout life they maintain TJs (and hence the BBB). Although endothelial cells express several calcium-dependent adhesion molecules (cadherins), vascular endothelial cadherin (VE-cadherin), also referred to as cadherin-5, is considered to be specific to endothelial cells. VE-cadherin is one of the first endothelial cell-specific markers expressed during embryonic development [19] and establishes the basic organization of endothelial AJs to regulate permeability [20]. It interacts with actin cytoskeleton and intermediate filament vimentin via its cytoplasmic domain to create the endothelial-specific "complexus AJ" [21]. This interaction is not direct but rather occurs via association with linker proteins α-, β-, x- and p120 catenins. AJ complexes also interact with various proteins, but in endothelial cells they bind to and interact with endothelial-specific proteins, such as platelet adhesion molecule-1 (PECAM-1) and vascular endothelial growth factor receptor-2 (VEGFR-2), regulating the organization of AJ and barrier function [22]. PECAM-1 contributes to endothelial barrier function and also helps accelerate and restore barrier integrity upon disturbances [23]. In EAE, PECAM-1 deficiency elevates cellular infiltration into sites of inflammation suggesting that PECAM-1 negatively regulates leukocyte diapedesis. This is concurrent with increased vascular permeability in the CNS, which occurs during EAE [24]. Another important BBB cadherin is cadherin-10 which is expressed specifically in BBB endothelial cells but not in other BECs or in non-CNS cells [25], demonstrating the specificity of cadherin-10 as a barrier-forming AJ protein of the BBB.

Tight Junctions in BBB

The TJs are multiprotein complexes between brain microvascular endothelial cells providing closely approaching intercellular connections. TJs are the major complex forming the BBB and are the most important structure underlying the normal physiology of the BBB. TJs in the BBB consist of several proteins, which include occludin, [26], claudin-1, claudin-3, claudin-5, claudin-10, and claudin-12, and junctional adhesion molecules (JAM-A, JAM-B, and JAM-C). Furthermore, there are important cytoplasmic scaffolding proteins that link TJs to cortical actin filaments such as zonula occludens (ZO)-linker proteins 1 and 2 (ZO-3 is not expressed by BECs) [7, 27]. Loss of claudin-3 in BBB TJ in EAE [28], in which BBB integrity is compromised, suggests an important role of claudin-3 in maintaining BBB TJ integrity. Claudin-3 is also distinctly localized to TJ in hCMEC/D3 cells, which are widely used as an in vitro model of human BBB [29]. Occludin and claudin-5 and claudin-11 are "tetraspan" transmembrane proteins (four transmembrane helices and two extracellular loops) known as myelin and lymphocyte protein (MAL) and related proteins for vesicle trafficking and membrane link (MARVEL) domain. The second extracellular loop of occludin contains the LYHY motif, which mediates occludin's role in cell-cell adhesion contributing to barrier function [30] as well as leukocyte emigration [5]. Activated immune cells also express occludin in some cases – which may permit them to link with occludin of BECs of BBB – ultimately allowing passage of these immune cells across tight junctions [31]. These proteins interact with various proteins on the cytoplasmic side of the membrane. For example, the extended C-terminus is essential for occludin dimerization as well as its interaction with ZO-1. These domains also interact with various kinases such as protein kinase C isoforms, tyrosine kinases, and phosphoinositol 3 kinase (PI3 kinase) as well as tyrosine phosphatases [32]. The reversible phosphorylation state of occludin and claudin as well as the abundance of these proteins is understood to be a key aspect of barrier function controlling the organization and barrier of endothelial tight junctions [33–36]. Another family of proteins localized in endothelial TJ is the JAMs. All three JAMs (JAM-A, JAM-B, and JAM-C) may be involved in leukocyte migration – for example, JAM-A mediates T cell migration by binding to LFA-1 [37]. TJ protein mutations or elimination leads to the breakdown of BBB and is functionally linked with some neurological disorders including band-like calcification with simplified gyration and polymicrogyria (BLC-PMG) [38]. Lastly, the tricellular and bicellular junctions in CEC appear to contain different components, with lipolysis-stimulated lipoprotein receptor (LSR)/angulin-1 recently defined as a tricellular tight junction protein contributing to the formation of the BBB [39].

Other Junctional Components

Although tight and adherens junctions are important components of the BBB, integrins also contribute to CEC integrity. Although alpha V integrin deficiency does not impair pericyte-endothelial interactions, it does disturb endothelial and nervous system parenchymal connections leading to BBB failure [40]. Additionally, connexons between endothelial cells (containing connexin 43) modulate calcium and BBB organization [41], and astrocyte connexin 43 modulates endothelial immune activation and enhances immune cell emigration.

Cerebral Endothelial Junctional Disorganization in MS

MS has a strong association with BBB dysfunction as well as loss of structural integrity [42], both of which together reflect several levels of BEC dysfunction (Fig. 1.1). Immunofluorescence staining of postmortem MS brain samples revealed an abnormal TJ molecule distribution, including occludin, JAM-A, and ZO-1, which correlated with patterns of serum protein leakage in active lesions [43]. This suggests that TJ disruption strongly contributes to BBB dysfunction seen in MS. Disintegration of the BBB by degradation and downregulation of TJ and AJ appear to play central roles in relapsing-remitting, primary progressive, and secondary progressive MS. The critical role TJ plays in BBB maintenance has been

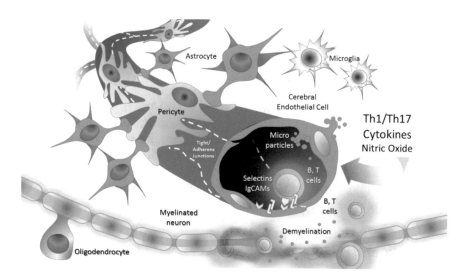

Fig. 1.1 Are cerebral endothelial cell and vascular dysfunction contributing to MS pathophysiology? The barrier maintained by CEC involves several junctional complexes, which are supported and regulated by pericytes, astrocytes, and neurons. During inflammatory conditions, CEC monolayers express and present selectins and several IgCAMs to become hyper-adhesive and permit extravasation of blood-borne tracers. Activated CEC is less effective at excluding immune cells from trans-BBB penetration. These inflammatory stimuli may include cytokines, altered NO production, viruses, trauma, etc. Once activated, endothelial cells may progress toward apoptosis and may also shed membrane fragments called "microparticles" which are both mediators and markers of CEC injury in MS

demonstrated using EAE model of MS. Inducible endothelial-specific expression of claudin-1 alleviated clinical symptoms of EAE by preventing BBB leakiness [44]. However, ectopic claudin-1 expression did not affect immune cell trafficking into the CNS, which suggests that BBB TJs may be critical structures regulating BBB solute exchange but not immune cell diapedesis. Nonetheless, immune cell migration may amplify BBB TJ pathology as is illustrated by the loss of claudin-3 and claudin-5 as mentioned above [28]. We have demonstrated that serum from MS patients in relapse (known to contain higher levels of inflammatory cytokines) diminishes occludin and VE-cadherin expression in cultured brain endothelial cells [45]. More recently, Shimizu and colleagues have also described barrier disturbances in response to serum from RRMS and SPMS [46]. During MS flares, Th1 cytokine levels increase in the CNS interstitium as well as in the circulation. We have demonstrated that endothelial cell exposure with inflammatory mediators or calcium chelation initiates the reversible internalization (endocytosis) of classical and VE-cadherins from inter-endothelial junctions by a PKC [33, 47, 48]. Among these, IFN-γ in particular may directly modulate BBB function by suppressing the expression of TJ and AJ components [45] as well as triggering internalization of TJ proteins (e.g., occludin, JAM-A) [49]. In addition, inflammatory cytokines can also indirectly influence the BBB function by disturbing the adventitial cells that can stabilize and enhance BBB [50].

Disruptions of cell-cell contact and communication resulting from breakdown of intercellular junctions not only lead to a decline in barrier function but can also cause endothelial apoptosis through the extrinsic pathway [51]. Although TJ disruption is sometimes regarded as a consequence of apoptosis, mislocalization of claudins that also leads to occludin disruption (and hence of TJ) can activate caspases and eventually promote cell death [52]. The association of the two events is influenced by interferon-β1b (Betaseron), which has been shown to protect endothelial cells from apoptosis in vitro [53] and while at the same time preserving junctional integrity [45]. Interestingly, despite diverse pathways for immune cell passage across the intact CEC monolayer, tricellular junctions containing LSR are down-regulated during EAE and may increase the penetration of immune cells at tricellular junctions [39], possibly consistent with a preference for the paracellular route when junctions are less well organized (as may exist in MS).

Metabolic and Hypoxic Disturbances of CNS in MS

The use of T1-weighted MRI with gadolinium contrast as a diagnostic tool for MS relapse suggests that BBB disruption is a key feature of MS and causes leakage of the contrast agent at perivascular cuffs in the brain. The effectiveness of MS therapies and whether they improve BBB function can be seen by whether they relieve lesions since the number, size, and intensity of these lesions reflect BBB failure and disease severity. White matter lesions in MS are characterized by oligodendrogliopathy (apoptosis and regression of oligodendrocytes) and can be exacerbated by metabolic disturbances [54]. For example, ischemic stress can also intensify the injury that results from the proinflammatory cytokines present in MS. This stress may be especially important in MS etiology because BECs are sensitive not only to metabolic stress but also to ischemic stress that disrupt barrier function, promote microparticle (MP) release [55], and induce endothelial cell adhesion molecule (ECAM) expression. MS involves intense neuroinflammation; this inflammation can cause vasoconstriction, limited perfusion resulting from edema, thrombosis, and activation of macrophages or glial cells, ultimately leading to tissue hypoxia. In addition, ischemic stress can occur even in the presence of adequate oxygen: toxic metabolite accumulation can interfere with mitochondrial ATP production, leading to ischemic stress despite oxygenation [54]. Such metabolites include glutamate, oxidants, and peroxynitrite, which can cause excitotoxicity in CNS neurons. Excitotoxicity and oxidative stress mediate neuronal loss characteristic of neurodegenerative diseases including MS [56]. Glutamate can indirectly contribute to oxidant generation as well, which is suggested to cause barrier disturbances in stroke and possibly in MS [57, 58]. Glutamate-dependent stress is exacerbated in MS due to glutamate accumulation that results from increased levels of proinflammatory cytokines in the CNS that impair glial clearance of glutamate [59].

Endothelial Energy Metabolism

Glucose is the major source of energy in neurons. Therefore, it is not surprising that glucose transporter-1 (GLUT1) is one of the most abundant proteins and the solute carrier which is most enriched in the BBB [60]. Under hypoxic conditions (such as that provoked by inflammation in MS), GLUT1 expression can increase in a hypoxia-inducible factor 1-alpha (HIF-1)-dependent manner. This may involve prostanoid signals originating from either hypoxic astrocytes [61] or pericytes [62] and may represent a type of metabolic "switch." Reductions in GLUT1 expression intensify CNS stress and are frequently observed in Alzheimer's disease (AD) [63]. Decreased GLUT1 expression and function exacerbate neurovascular degeneration in MS, because of disastrous effects on BBB integrity [64]. Several endothelial functions are compromised by defects in energy homeostasis during MS exacerbations including depressed endothelial barrier function, increased endothelial apoptosis, expression of ECAMs, and conversion into a prothrombotic phenotype, all of which increase disease activity.

Endothelial Microparticles

Even under normal physiological conditions, individuals and endothelial cells continuously shed small, cell membrane-enclosed vesicles, carrying many cytoplasmic as well as surface markers, especially adhesion molecules deprived from "parent" or originating cells. These particles (diameters in the range of 0.1–1 µm) can be found either freely circulating in plasma bound to other blood components and are known as "endothelial microparticles" (EMPs). In addition to these many protein biomarkers that indicate their origin, microparticles (MPs) also exhibit phosphatidylserine (PS) on the outer leaflets of their plasma membrane. PS exposed on the surface of EMP binds to annexin V and describes "apoptotic endothelial microparticles" [55]. Because of this, characteristic MPs were once thought to represent "apoptotic bodies." However, MPs are now accepted to be a separate population of secreted vesicles. There has been increased research interest in deducing the function of MP release, whether it is adaptive and protective or damaging to the endothelial cells, and it still remains unclear. However, MPs may be a double-edged sword: although MP release is associated with various pathologies, inhibition of cellular MP release is associated with cell detachment and death [65]. When exposed to metabolic and inflammatory stress, such as in MS, endothelial cells release significantly more MPs, indicating the potential application of MPs as diagnostic marker and indices of disease severity and indicators of therapeutic response [66]. However, MPs are not only a marker (or a consequence) of MS but also pathological factors, contributing to the initiation and progression of disease activity [139]. Elevation in MP release is associated with a decline in BBB function and correlates with increase in leukocyte infiltration [67]. We found that blood-circulating MPs are not homogeneous but consist of several different species that show different patterns of release depending on disease states [68]. Although various EMPs, including CD31+ and CD54+ EMPs (EMP^{CD31+} and EMP^{CD54+}), are high in active MS and decrease during therapy, EMP^{CD146+} did not show such correlation [66]. EMPs are also not the only type of MPs present in the blood. MPs can also be derived from other cells including platelets, erythrocytes, and leukocytes [55]. Platelet MPs (PMPs), which can activate thrombosis, are also elevated in MS and contribute to vascular injury [69], and such increased EMP can elevate extravasation of immune cells across the BBB by promoting monocyte adhesion and migration contributing to the pathogenesis of MS [70, 71].

Endothelial Targets in MS Therapy

Interferon-β

Interferon-β family members, especially interferon-β1b (Betaseron), exhibit multiple mechanistic effects that protect the endothelium in MS. Interferon-β1b decreases the transendothelial migration of monocytes by inhibiting complex formation between monocytes and EMPs [70]. An MS clinical trial has shown decreased T1-weighted gadolinium-enhanced brain lesions and decreased serum MMP-9 by using interferon-β1a plus doxycycline, an anti-inflammatory broad-spectrum MMP inhibitor, combination therapy. Additionally, MS serum induces leukocyte extravasation *in vitro*. Taken together, this suggests that MMPs play an important role in MS pathophysiology. We reported an elevated level of MMP-8 and MMP-9 in RRMS serum [72], and others have similarly reported elevated levels of MMP-9 in RRMS, PPMS, and SPMS [73]. However, reports of elevated MMP-2 levels in PPMS and SPMS and MMP-9 polymorphisms showed no correlation with disability [73]. Although neutrophils are not commonly believed to contribute to MS pathology, some phases may be mediated at least in part by neutrophils [74]. MMP-8 is associated with neutrophils [75], and CXCR2+ neutrophils may contribute to the oligodendrocyte pathology seen in the cuprizone MS model. Neutrophils from MS patients display an "active" phenotype, which is typically characterized by reduced apoptosis and increased tissue persistence; increased levels of toll-like receptor-2 (TLR-2), formyl peptide receptor (fMLP receptor), interleukin-8 receptor (IL-8R), and cluster of differentiation 43 (CD43); as well as increased granule and superoxide release [76, 77] making them more longer-lasting cellular mediators of inflammation. Occludin is susceptible to proteolysis by MMPs [78, 79], which degrade and disintegrate TJ architecture required for BBB function. Cytokines such as TNF-α and IL-1-β are known to induce MMP synthesis in several cell types within the BBB [80]. Additionally hypoxia, which contributes to MS and Alzheimer's pathogenesis, can activate pro-forms of MMP to active enzymes which can degrade occludin in TJs [81]. Therefore, MMP activity represents a potential therapeutic target for interferon-β in MS treatment. MMPs also directly target and degrade interferon-β. The use of minocycline, a potent MMP inhibitor, has anti-inflammatory effects that help to maintain interferon-β at therapeutic levels [82].

Chemokines

Chemokines are inflammatory mediators and are a subtype of cytokines that are secreted as chemoattractants, directing the migration of various cells interacting with endothelial cells during inflammation. Serum CXCL10 level is elevated in MS and correlates with T2-weighted MRI lesions. CXCL10 is also increased by IFN-β-1a or IFN-β-1b after 36 h. Levels of CCL2 and CXCL9 were also elevated during MS relapses. Levels of CCL4 and CCL5 were variable and appeared to depend on patient gender and on other forms of therapy [83]. Chemokines, such as MCP-1, contribute to monocyte extravasation across the BBB in MS [84]. Extracellular matrix metalloproteinase inducer (EMMPRIN/CD147) is a chemokine, which supports immune cell trafficking across the endothelium in MS as well as in the EAE model. EMMPRIN is also linked with increased MMP-9 activity and thus may contribute to MS pathogenesis [85, 86]. CXCL13 levels also increase in relapsing MS [87]. This is actually potentially beneficial as it can contribute to neural precursor cell recruitment across the BBB [88]. CXCL13 appears to be an important biomarker of MS (whose presence reflects the BBB's attempt to repair MS injury) rather than a cause that contributes to pathology; MS therapy does not decrease CXCL13 levels.

Paradoxically, levels of inflammatory but also anti-inflammatory cytokines increase above baseline in inflamed MS lesions and include IFN-γ, IL-2, IL-1β, TNF-α, IL-4, IL-10, IL-12/23, and IL-13 [72, 89]. Many of these cytokines can directly modulate endothelial barrier function and change surface activation properties. Plasma and CNS concentrations of TNF-α, IL-1β, receptor activator of NF-kB ligand (RANKL), and C-reactive protein (CRP) are elevated in MS, particularly during flares [90]. IL-1β upregulation in the CNS contributes to BBB dysfunction by inducing nuclear translocation of β-catenin in CECs to repress claudin-5 expression [91]. Although IL-12/23 is elevated in MS, the IL-12/23 blocking antibody, ustekinumab, has so far shown no benefit in MS therapy [92]. IL-12 suppresses VEGFR-3 expression in brain endothelial cells [93], and VEGFR-3 levels correlate with endothelial dysfunction [94] suggesting that VEGFR-3 may contribute to normal endothelial function and are dysregulated in MS, potentially implicating this lymphatic marker in MS.

Endothelial Cells Represent Important Targets in MS

"Statins" are anti-cholesteremic hydroxymethylglutaryl-CoA (HMG-CoA) reductase inhibitors that may potentially be therapeutic in MS, based on their' ability to regulate immune responses and "stabilize" the endothelium, exerting neuroprotective effects [95–97]. Statins have been an attractive candidate for treating MS because of their various immunomodulatory and neurotrophic effects [98]. Statins have demonstrated therapeutic benefit in disease severity in mouse models of MS as well as in clinical trials. By slowing down cholesterol production (by inhibiting HMG-CoA), they lower serum lipids/cholesterol [99] which appears to track with MS outcomes. Statins also exert potent anti-inflammatory effects by suppressing T cells and by maintaining endothelial nitric oxide (NO) output [97, 100, 101]. Importantly, statins downregulate matrix metalloproteinase-9 (MMP-9) expression and activity, thereby protecting the CNS against macrophage penetration into the CNS (which contributes to MS pathogenesis) [102, 103]. The immunomodulatory effects of β-sitosterol and simvastatin were recently compared in a clinical study. This study revealed that simvastatin suppresses the release of both TNF-α and IL-10 from peripheral blood mononuclear cells (PBMC) in MS patients in a dose-dependent manner; healthy controls showed no changes [103]. However, an observational clinical study reported that statins, although well tolerated and safe, were not effective at reducing MS disease progression or relapse when used alone [97]. Consequently, the use of statins in adjunctive therapy, with interferon-β in particular, has been intensively studied with equivocal results. One study reported a significant reduction in both the number and volume of MS lesions, while another reported the opposite showing an increase in the rate of relapse and increased appearance of new lesions [97]. Hence, these studies did not provide conclusive evidence for statin use in MS therapy. As such, the ultimate benefits of statins in treatment of MS patients are difficult to determine. However, since statins confer beneficial effects on endothelial function by helping nitric oxide (NO) production and reducing inflammation [100, 101], they are definitely not contraindicated in MS. The use of statins should be considered when deciding on adjuvant therapy to help restore endothelial function in MS patients.

Natalizumab (Tysabri™)

Tysabri™, an anti-α4 integrin humanized monoclonal antibody, is used in MS and ulcerative colitis [104]. In MS it is used to manage patients with highly active relapsing MS (first line) and those with RRMS unresponsive to beta-interferon therapy [105]. Early on in its clinical use, natalizumab was discovered to have an associated risk for progressive multifocal leukoencephalopathy (PML) reflecting immunosuppression and reactivation of JC virus in the CNS. This caused a temporary halt in its use, but it has now returned to the forefront of MS treatment [105]. Natalizumab effectively blocks binding of α4β1 integrin (VLA-4) and α4β7 integrin (lymphocyte Peyer's patch adhesion molecule, LPAM) to VCAM-1 and MAdCAM-1, respectively, on cytokine-activated brain endothelial cells [106]. Both α4β1 and α4β7 bind fibronectin, and additionally α4β7 binds fibrinogen [107], possibly involved in immune cell motility in the parenchyma. Endothelial cells express VCAM-1 and MAdCAM-1 when activated by cytokines, and natalizumab antagonizes lymphocyte-endothelium binding in MS treatment. The reactivation of JC virus and PML development in some MS patients receiving Tysabri™ seems to be a relatively delayed event. Therefore, healthy BBB may be continuously penetrated by immune cells that express α4 integrin and depend on these integrins for appropriate immune surveillance [108].

Tecfidera

One of the most recently approved drugs for treating MS is dimethyl fumarate (DMF), known commercially as Tecfidera (Biogen). DMF is a fumaric acid derivative originally used as a sensitizing agent to increase hypoxic tumor cell response to radiation, which has now been applied in the setting of MS. DMF, is a highly potent inhibitor of the transcription factor NF-kB [109]. By interfering with NF-kB-dependent mobilization of endothelial cell adhesion molecules, cytokines, and cytokine responses, DMF can block several essential CEC responses to inflammatory cytokines which support the BBB penetration of inflammatory immune cells [110, 111]. While highly effective, Tecfidera also has some clinical limitations associated with immune suppression (as has been described for Tysabri™/natalizumab) [112]. As of the time of this writing, several cases of PML have been reported in individuals using Tecfidera (four cases as of November 2015), and the use of this agent may need to be further supervised.

Fingolimod

Fingolimod (Gilenya), a sphingosine-1-phosphate modulator, has been described as accomplishing its beneficial immune effects in MS by sequestering inflammatory lymphocytes in lymph nodes and minimizing their crossing of the BBB. Nishihara et al. have reported that fingolimod also has a direct effect on claudin-5 (but apparently does not alter occludin), potentially stabilizing tight junctions against the influence of elevated inflammatory cytokines [113].

Cytokines and Chemokines in Endothelial Pathogenesis of MS

Th1, Th2, and Th17 cytokines have all been implicated in neuroinflammation and may influence brain EC functions in MS. Tumor necrosis factor-alpha (TNF-α) is one of the cytokines best investigated in the pathogenesis of MS, as well as with interferon gamma (IFN-γ). Both TNF-α and IFN-γ are overexpressed in MS and may increase endothelial activation and impair BBB junctional integrity [114, 115]. Indeed, MR measures have revealed a surge in TNF-α levels along with a decrease in anti-inflammatory cytokines (e.g. IL-10 and TGF-β) before MS relapses and inflammatory flares [116]. Of these anti-inflammatory cytokines, IL-10 has been reported to prevent MAdCAM-1 induction and junctional disruption [5, 117]. TNF-α is produced mainly by activated macrophages, but several cells in the CNS/BBB may also contribute. TNF-α is a major immunomodulatory cytokine involved in many inflammatory diseases including AD [118], inflammatory bowel disease (IBD) [119], and MS [120]. The role of TNF-α in MS is complex with anti-TNF-α actually intensifying disease in some cases [121]. Anti-TNF-α therapy is not widely used in MS therapy, although TNF-α mRNA transcript levels have been reported to be significantly increased in active MS lesions compared to inactive ones [122].

Another study revealed abundant expression of ADAM metallopeptidase domain 17 (ADAM17) within MS lesions. [123] ADAM17 is a member of ADAM protein family of disintegrins and metalloproteases and is also known as tumor necrosis factor-alpha-converting enzyme (TACE), due to its role in cleavage of TNF-α at cell surface. The elevated levels of these proinflammatory cytokines may promote and amplify MS neuroinflammation. Proinflammatory cytokines activate macrophages by upregulating the expression of major histocompatibility complex II (MHC-II) and endothelial adhesion molecules as well as on glial cells, to further recruit Th1 immune cells. This ultimately results in an even greater demyelination [124]. Paradoxically, TNF-α inhibition has actually been reported to result in the induction of demyelination of the CNS and worsening of MS [125, 126].

Another cytokine that has received much attention regarding MS pathogenesis is IFN-γ, which is involved in MS pathogenesis and in EAE. IFN-γ is a dimeric soluble cytokine type 2 interferon and was originally described as a macrophage-activating factor [127–129]. Since then, many targets including endothelial cells have been described. IFN-γ is crucial for both innate and adaptive immunity against viral and intracellular bacterial infections. It also plays an important role in tumor control and can cause autoimmune disease if expression is abnormally increased. IFN-γ is involved in a feed-forward loop, where Th1 immune cells produce IFN-γ that increases Th1 cells by differentiating CD4+ cells into Th1 cells. This positive cascade occurs concurrently with the decrease of differentiation into Th2 cell. IFN-γ production is also reported to occur before clinical MS relapses [130, 131]. Elevated IFN-γ levels correlate with inflammation within the CNS in MS [132]. A pilot study of 18 MS patients helped to understand IFN-γ's role in MS pathogenesis [133, 134]. Patients were treated with recombinant IFN-γ to assess toxicity and dosage responses. IFN-γ was given intravenously to three treatment groups. The group receiving "low dose" was given 1 microgram, "intermediate" was given 30 micrograms, and "high dose" was administered 1000 micrograms twice a week for 4 weeks. Although IFN-γ was not detected in the CSF, levels in the serum correlated with administration. Interestingly, during this study, relapse rate significantly increased with seven patients experiencing relapses. Circulating monocyte bearing class II surface antigens also significantly increased, from which the investigators concluded that IFN-γ intravenous administration to MS patients has a significant and negative impact on cellular immunity associated with elevated MS relapse rates. The investigators therefore recommended a study of specific inhibitors of IFN-γ production or action, on immune cells as a treatment of MS.

An intriguing conclusion from murine-based MS models however is that interferon-γ may be beneficial in these models [135, 136]. Studies in EAE suggest that IFN-γ blockade intensified disease severity with poorer survival; these studies may reflect strain (JJL/J)-dependent effects. Conversely, the addition of IFN-γ delayed the initiation of EAE. Thus, while EAE is an excellent model of some MS processes, not all pathomechanisms may be recapitulated by all MS models.

Abnormal Flow and MS Pathophysiology

While still early in its understanding, abnormal flow and pressure pulsations may also lead to disturbances in vascular endothelial functioning which may contribute to MS pathogenesis and progression as well as forms of vascular dementias. Because MS is associated with increased vessel stiffness [137], there may be a decreased Windkessel component within several vascular components, which lead to an abnormal and potentially inappropriate communication of pressure waves into smaller branches of the brain vasculature than would normally be seen in healthy individuals. Such abnormal pressure phenomena could change endothelial barrier function and endothelial activation, coagulation, and interactions with support cells necessary to maintain barrier and other vascular characteristics. In the setting of chronic neurovascular diseases and other chronic inflammatory phenomena, inflammatory cytokines may impair smooth muscle contractility to dysregulate autoregulation; in the face of hypertension, combined with altered vessel distensibility, autoregulatory failure could also provoke microbleeds. The extent to which this is communicated to the venous side of the circulation is unclear, but could contribute to perivascular stress and venous cuffing as well as Dawson's fingers. In the setting of Alzheimer's disease, amyloid-beta may cooperate to provoke similar forms of vascular stress.

Conclusions

While MS is most widely known as an immune-mediated neurodegenerative condition within the human CNS which shows extensive myelin sheath damage and oligodendrocyte injury, these events may occur after or secondary to BBB disturbances which reveal these previously sequestered epitopes to elements of the immune system. Viral and oligodendrocyte protein (MOG, MAG, and PLP) exposure models may recapitulate phases of MS which "break" this barrier and expose BBB antigens normally concealed from the immune system. The progressive, remitting, and relapsing vascular injuries of MS can be observed in contrast enhancing lesions, which are often vascularly associated, appearing, and often resolving. Excessive activation of the CNS microvasculature therefore may support excessive immune cell penetration of the CNS which can lead to repeated waves of immune cell penetration into the CNS with destruction of brain tissue seen in MS. Because suppression of endothelial adhesion molecules and their leukocyte counter-receptors now represents a main approach to MS therapy, future research into additional endothelial contributions may provide novel methods to prevent initiation and block persistence, stimulation, and penetration of immune cells into the MS-inflamed brain.

References

1. Abadier M, Haghayegh Jahromi N, Cardoso Alves L, Boscacci R, Vestweber D, Barnum S, et al. Cell surface levels of endothelial ICAM-1 influence the transcellular or paracellular T-cell diapedesis across the blood-brain barrier. Eur J Immunol. 2015;45(4):1043–58. Epub 2014/12/30. doi:10.1002/eji.201445125. PubMed PMID: 25545837.
2. Lyck R, Reiss Y, Gerwin N, Greenwood J, Adamson P, Engelhardt B. T-cell interaction with ICAM-1/ICAM-2 double-deficient brain endothelium in vitro: the cytoplasmic tail of endothelial ICAM-1 is necessary for transendothelial migration of T cells. Blood. 2003;102(10):3675–83. Epub 2003/08/02. doi:10.1182/blood-2003-02-0358. PubMed PMID: 12893765.
3. Gorina R, Lyck R, Vestweber D, Engelhardt B. *beta*2 integrin-mediated crawling on endothelial ICAM-1 and ICAM-2 is a prerequisite for transcellular neutrophil diapedesis across the inflamed blood-brain barrier. J Immunol (Baltimore, Md : 1950). 2014;192(1):324–37. Epub 2013/11/22. doi:10.4049/jimmunol.1300858. PubMed PMID: 24259506.
4. von Wedel-Parlow M, Schrot S, Lemmen J, Treeratanapiboon L, Wegener J, Galla HJ. Neutrophils cross the BBB primarily on transcellular pathways: an in vitro study. Brain Res. 2011;1367:62–76. Epub 2010/09/30. doi:10.1016/j.brainres.2010.09.076. PubMed PMID: 20875807.
5. Oshima T, Blaschuk O, Gour B, Symonds M, Elrod JW, Sasaki M, et al. Tight junction peptide antagonists enhance neutrophil trans-endothelial chemotaxis. Life Sci. 2003;73(13):1729–40. Epub 2003/07/24. PubMed PMID: 12875904.
6. Gotsch U, Borges E, Bosse R, Boggemeyer E, Simon M, Mossmann H, et al. VE-cadherin antibody accelerates neutrophil recruitment in vivo. J Cell Sci. 1997;110(Pt 5):583–8. Epub 1997/03/01. PubMed PMID: 9092940.
7. Redzic Z. Molecular biology of the blood-brain and the blood-cerebrospinal fluid barriers: similarities and differences. Fluids Barriers CNS. 2011;8(1):3. Epub 2011/02/26. doi:10.1186/2045-8118-8-3. PubMed PMID: 21349151; PubMed Central PMCID: PMCPMC3045361.
8. Engelhardt B. Neuroscience. Blood-brain barrier differentiation. Science. 2011;334(6063):1652–3. Epub 2011/12/24. doi:10.1126/science.1216853. PubMed PMID: 22194564.
9. Fulmer CG, VonDran MW, Stillman AA, Huang Y, Hempstead BL, Dreyfus CF. Astrocyte-derived BDNF supports myelin protein synthesis after cuprizone-induced demyelination. J Neurosci Off J Soc Neurosci. 2014;34(24):8186–96. Epub 2014/06/13. doi:10.1523/jneurosci.4267-13.2014. PubMed PMID: 24920623; PubMed Central PMCID: PMCPMC4051974.

10. Abbott NJ. Astrocyte-endothelial interactions and blood-brain barrier permeability. J Anat. 2002;200(6):629–38. Epub 2002/08/07. PubMed PMID: 12162730; PubMed Central PMCID: PMCPMC1570746.

11. Dohgu S, Takata F, Yamauchi A, Nakagawa S, Egawa T, Naito M, et al. Brain pericytes contribute to the induction and up-regulation of blood-brain barrier functions through transforming growth factor-beta production. Brain Res. 2005;1038(2):208–15. Epub 2005/03/11. doi:10.1016/j.brainres.2005.01.027. PubMed PMID: 15757636.

12. Shimizu F, Sano Y, Saito K, Abe MA, Maeda T, Haruki H, et al. Pericyte-derived glial cell line-derived neurotrophic factor increase the expression of claudin-5 in the blood-brain barrier and the blood-nerve barrier. Neurochem Res. 2012;37(2):401–9. Epub 2011/10/18. doi:10.1007/s11064-011-0626-8. PubMed PMID: 22002662.

13. Armulik A, Genove G, Mae M, Nisancioglu MH, Wallgard E, Niaudet C, et al. Pericytes regulate the blood-brain barrier. Nature. 2010;468(7323):557–61. Epub 2010/10/15. doi:10.1038/nature09522. PubMed PMID: 20944627.

14. Bai Y, Zhu X, Chao J, Zhang Y, Qian C, Li P, et al. Pericytes contribute to the disruption of the cerebral endothelial barrier via increasing VEGF expression: implications for stroke. PloS One. 2015;10(4):e0124362. Epub 2015/04/18. doi:10.1371/journal.pone.0124362. PubMed PMID: 25884837; PubMed Central PMCID: PMCPMC4401453.

15. Argaw AT, Asp L, Zhang J, Navrazhina K, Pham T, Mariani JN, et al. Astrocyte-derived VEGF-A drives blood-brain barrier disruption in CNS inflammatory disease. J Clin Invest. 2012;122(7):2454–68. Epub 2012/06/02. doi:10.1172/jci60842. PubMed PMID: 22653056; PubMed Central PMCID: PMCPMC3386814.

16. Hudson N, Powner MB, Sarker MH, Burgoyne T, Campbell M, Ockrim ZK, et al. Differential apicobasal VEGF signaling at vascular blood-neural barriers. Dev Cell. 2014;30(5):541–52. Epub 2014/09/02. doi:10.1016/j.devcel.2014.06.027. PubMed PMID: 25175707; PubMed Central PMCID: PMCPMC4160345.

17. Wolburg-Buchholz K, Mack AF, Steiner E, Pfeiffer F, Engelhardt B, Wolburg H. Loss of astrocyte polarity marks blood-brain barrier impairment during experimental autoimmune encephalomyelitis. Acta Neuropathol. 2009;118(2):219–33. Epub 2009/06/18. doi:10.1007/s00401-009-0558-4. PubMed PMID: 19533155.

18. Alvarez JI, Dodelet-Devillers A, Kebir H, Ifergan I, Fabre PJ, Terouz S, et al. The Hedgehog pathway promotes blood-brain barrier integrity and CNS immune quiescence. Science. 2011;334(6063):1727–31. Epub 2011/12/07. doi:10.1126/science.1206936. PubMed PMID: 22144466.

19. Breier G, Breviario F, Caveda L, Berthier R, Schnurch H, Gotsch U, et al. Molecular cloning and expression of murine vascular endothelial-cadherin in early stage development of cardiovascular system. Blood. 1996;87(2):630–41. Epub 1996/01/15. PubMed PMID: 8555485.

20. Corada M, Mariotti M, Thurston G, Smith K, Kunkel R, Brockhaus M, et al. Vascular endothelial-cadherin is an important determinant of microvascular integrity in vivo. Proc Natl Acad Sci U S A. 1999;96(17):9815–20. Epub 1999/08/18. PubMed PMID: 10449777; PubMed Central PMCID: PMCPMC22293.

21. Dejana E, Zanetti A, Del Maschio A. Adhesive proteins at endothelial cell-to-cell junctions and leukocyte extravasation. Haemostasis. 1996;26(Suppl 4):210–9. Epub 1996/10/01. PubMed PMID: 8979126.

22. Kevil CG, Payne DK, Mire E, Alexander JS. Vascular permeability factor/vascular endothelial cell growth factor-mediated permeability occurs through disorganization of endothelial junctional proteins. J Biol Chem. 1998;273(24):15099–103. Epub 1998/06/17. PubMed PMID: 9614120.

23. Privratsky JR, Newman PJ. PECAM-1: regulator of endothelial junctional integrity. Cell Tissue Res. 2014;355(3):607–19. Epub 2014/01/18. doi:10.1007/s00441-013-1779-3. PubMed PMID: 24435645; PubMed Central PMCID: PMCPMC3975704.

24. Graesser D, Solowiej A, Bruckner M, Osterweil E, Juedes A, Davis S, et al. Altered vascular permeability and early onset of experimental autoimmune encephalomyelitis in PECAM-1-deficient mice. J Clin Invest. 2002;109(3):383–92. Epub 2002/02/06. doi:10.1172/jci13595. PubMed PMID: 11827998; PubMed Central PMCID: PMCPMC150854.

25. Williams SG, Connelly DT, Jackson M, Bennett A, Albouaini K, Todd DM. Does treatment with ACE inhibitors or angiotensin II receptor antagonists prevent atrial fibrillation after dual chamber pacemaker implantation? Europace. 2005;7(6):554–9. doi:10.1016/j. eupc.2005.06.003. PubMed PMID: WOS:000233324000008.
26. Furuse M, Hirase T, Itoh M, Nagafuchi A, Yonemura S, Tsukita S. Occludin: a novel integral membrane protein localizing at tight junctions. J Cell Biol. 1993;123(6 Pt 2):1777–88. Epub 1993/12/01. PubMed PMID: 8276896; PubMed Central PMCID: PMCPMC2290891.
27. Wilhelm I, Fazakas C, Krizbai IA. In vitro models of the blood-brain barrier. Acta Neurobiol Exp. 2011;71(1):113–28. Epub 2011/04/19. PubMed PMID: 21499332.
28. Wolburg H, Wolburg-Buchholz K, Kraus J, Rascher-Eggstein G, Liebner S, Hamm S, et al. Localization of claudin-3 in tight junctions of the blood-brain barrier is selectively lost during experimental autoimmune encephalomyelitis and human glioblastoma multiforme. Acta Neuropathol. 2003;105(6):586–92. Epub 2003/05/08. doi:10.1007/s00401-003-0688-z. PubMed PMID: 12734665.
29. Schrade A, Sade H, Couraud PO, Romero IA, Weksler BB, Niewoehner J. Expression and localization of claudins-3 and -12 in transformed human brain endothelium. Fluids Barriers CNS. 2012;9:6. Epub 2012/03/01. doi:10.1186/2045-8118-9-6. PubMed PMID: 22373538; PubMed Central PMCID: PMCPMC3305566.
30. Blaschuk OW, Oshima T, Gour BJ, Symonds JM, Park JH, Kevil CG, et al. Identification of an occludin cell adhesion recognition sequence. Inflammation. 2002;26(4):193–8. Epub 2002/08/20. PubMed PMID: 12184633.
31. Alexander JS, Dayton T, Davis C, Hill S, Jackson TH, Blaschuk O, et al. Activated T-lymphocytes express occludin, a component of tight junctions. Inflammation. 1998;22(6):573–82. Epub 1998/11/24. PubMed PMID: 9824772.
32. Gonzalez-Mariscal L, Betanzos A, Nava P, Jaramillo BE. Tight junction proteins. Prog Biophys Mol Biol. 2003;81(1):1–44. Epub 2002/12/12. PubMed PMID: 12475568.
33. Alexander JS, Alexander BC, Eppihimer LA, Goodyear N, Haque R, Davis CP, et al. Inflammatory mediators induce sequestration of VE-cadherin in cultured human endothelial cells. Inflammation. 2000;24(2):99–113. Epub 2000/03/16. PubMed PMID: 10718113.
34. Kevil CG, Okayama N, Trocha SD, Kalogeris TJ, Coe LL, Specian RD, et al. Expression of zonula occludens and adherens junctional proteins in human venous and arterial endothelial cells: role of occludin in endothelial solute barriers. Microcirculation (New York, NY : 1994). 1998;5(2–3):197–210. Epub 1998/10/28. PubMed PMID: 9789260.
35. Kevil CG, Oshima T, Alexander B, Coe LL, Alexander JS. H(2)O(2)-mediated permeability: role of MAPK and occludin. Am J Physiol Cell Physiol. 2000;279(1):C21–30. Epub 2000/07/18. PubMed PMID: 10898713.
36. Kevil CG, Oshima T, Alexander JS. The role of p38 MAP kinase in hydrogen peroxide mediated endothelial solute permeability. Endothelium J Endothelial Cell Res. 2001;8(2):107–16. Epub 2001/09/27. PubMed PMID: 11572474.
37. Ostermann G, Weber KS, Zernecke A, Schroder A, Weber C. JAM-1 is a ligand of the beta(2) integrin LFA-1 involved in transendothelial migration of leukocytes. Nat Immunol. 2002;3(2):151–8. Epub 2002/01/29. doi:10.1038/ni755. PubMed PMID: 11812992.
38. O'Driscoll MC, Daly SB, Urquhart JE, Black GC, Pilz DT, Brockmann K, et al. Recessive mutations in the gene encoding the tight junction protein occludin cause band-like calcification with simplified gyration and polymicrogyria. Am J Hum Genet. 2010;87(3):354–64. Epub 2010/08/24. doi:10.1016/j.ajhg.2010.07.012. PubMed PMID: 20727516; PubMed Central PMCID: PMCPMC2933344.
39. Sohet F, Lin C, Munji RN, Lee SY, Ruderisch N, Soung A, et al. LSR/angulin-1 is a tricellular tight junction protein involved in blood-brain barrier formation. J Cell Biol. 2015;208(6):703–11. Epub 2015/03/11. doi:10.1083/jcb.201410131. PubMed PMID: 25753034; PubMed Central PMCID: PMCPMC4362448.
40. McCarty JH, Monahan-Earley RA, Brown LF, Keller M, Gerhardt H, Rubin K, et al. Defective associations between blood vessels and brain parenchyma lead to cerebral hemorrhage in

mice lacking alphav integrins. Mol Cell Biol. 2002;22(21):7667–77. Epub 2002/10/09. PubMed PMID: 12370313; PubMed Central PMCID: PMCPMC135679.

41. Kaneko Y, Tachikawa M, Akaogi R, Fujimoto K, Ishibashi M, Uchida Y, et al. Contribution of pannexin 1 and connexin 43 hemichannels to extracellular calcium-dependent transport dynamics in human blood-brain barrier endothelial cells. J Pharmacol Exp Ther. 2015;353(1):192–200. Epub 2015/02/12. doi:10.1124/jpet.114.220210. PubMed PMID: 25670633.

42. Minagar A, Alexander JS. Blood-brain barrier disruption in multiple sclerosis. Mult Scler (Houndmills, Basingstoke, England). 2003;9(6):540–9. Epub 2003/12/11. PubMed PMID: 14664465.

43. Kirk J, Plumb J, Mirakhur M, McQuaid S. Tight junctional abnormality in multiple sclerosis white matter affects all calibres of vessel and is associated with blood-brain barrier leakage and active demyelination. J Pathol. 2003;201(2):319–27. Epub 2003/10/01. doi:10.1002/path.1434. PubMed PMID: 14517850.

44. Pfeiffer F, Schafer J, Lyck R, Makrides V, Brunner S, Schaeren-Wiemers N, et al. Claudin-1 induced sealing of blood-brain barrier tight junctions ameliorates chronic experimental autoimmune encephalomyelitis. Acta Neuropathol. 2011;122(5):601–14. Epub 2011/10/11. doi:10.1007/s00401-011-0883-2. PubMed PMID: 21983942; PubMed Central PMCID: PMCPMC3207130.

45. Minagar A, Long A, Ma T, Jackson TH, Kelley RE, Ostanin DV, et al. Interferon (IFN)-beta 1a and IFN-beta 1b block IFN-gamma-induced disintegration of endothelial junction integrity and barrier. Endothelium J Endothelial Cell Res. 2003;10(6):299–307. Epub 2004/01/27. PubMed PMID: 14741845.

46. Shimizu F, Tasaki A, Sano Y, Ju M, Nishihara H, Oishi M, et al. Sera from remitting and secondary progressive multiple sclerosis patients disrupt the blood-brain barrier. PloS One. 2014;9(3):e92872. Epub 2014/04/02. doi:10.1371/journal.pone.0092872. PubMed PMID: 24686948; PubMed Central PMCID: PMCPMC3970956.

47. Kevil CG, Ohno N, Gute DC, Okayama N, Robinson SA, Chaney E, et al. Role of cadherin internalization in hydrogen peroxide-mediated endothelial permeability. Free Radic Biol Med. 1998;24(6):1015–22. Epub 1998/06/02. PubMed PMID: 9607613.

48. Alexander JS, Jackson SA, Chaney E, Kevil CG, Haselton FR. The role of cadherin endocytosis in endothelial barrier regulation: involvement of protein kinase C and actin-cadherin interactions. Inflammation. 1998;22(4):419–33. Epub 1998/07/24. PubMed PMID: 9675612.

49. Bruewer M, Utech M, Ivanov AI, Hopkins AM, Parkos CA, Nusrat A. Interferon-gamma induces internalization of epithelial tight junction proteins via a macropinocytosis-like process. FASEB J Off Publ Fed Am Soc Exp Biol. 2005;19(8):923–33. Epub 2005/06/01. doi:10.1096/fj.04-3260com. PubMed PMID: 15923402.

50. Chaitanya GV, Cromer WE, Wells SR, Jennings MH, Couraud PO, Romero IA, et al. Gliovascular and cytokine interactions modulate brain endothelial barrier in vitro. J Neuroinflammation. 2011;8:162. Epub 2011/11/25. doi:10.1186/1742-2094-8-162. PubMed PMID: 22112345; PubMed Central PMCID: PMCPMC3248576.

51. Beeman NE, Baumgartner HK, Webb PG, Schaack JB, Neville MC. Disruption of occludin function in polarized epithelial cells activates the extrinsic pathway of apoptosis leading to cell extrusion without loss of transepithelial resistance. BMC Cell Biol. 2009;10:85. Epub 2009/12/17. doi:10.1186/1471-2121-10-85. PubMed PMID: 20003227; PubMed Central PMCID: PMCPMC2796999.

52. Beeman N, Webb PG, Baumgartner HK. Occludin is required for apoptosis when claudin-claudin interactions are disrupted. Cell Death Dis. 2012;3:e273. Epub 2012/03/01. doi:10.1038/cddis.2012.14. PubMed PMID: 22361748; PubMed Central PMCID: PMCPMC3288343.

53. Haghjooy Javanmard S, Saadatnia MM, Homayouni VV, Nikoogoftar MM, Maghzi AH, Etemadifar M, et al. Interferon-beta-1b protects against multiple sclerosis-induced endothelial cells apoptosis. Front Biosci (Elite edition). 2012;4:1368–74. Epub 2011/12/29. PubMed PMID: 22201961.

54. Lassmann H. Hypoxia-like tissue injury as a component of multiple sclerosis lesions. J Neurol Sci. 2003;206(2):187–91. Epub 2003/02/01. PubMed PMID: 12559509.
55. Horstman LL, Jy W, Bidot CJ, Nordberg ML, Minagar A, Alexander JS, et al. Potential roles of cell-derived microparticles in ischemic brain disease. Neurol Res. 2009;31(8):799–806. Epub 2009/09/03. doi:10.1179/016164109x12445505689526. PubMed PMID: 19723448.
56. Gonsette RE. Oxidative stress and excitotoxicity: a therapeutic issue in multiple sclerosis? Mult Scler (Houndmills, Basingstoke, England). 2008;14(1):22–34. Epub 2007/09/21. doi:10.1177/1352458507080111. PubMed PMID: 17881394.
57. Sharp CD, Hines I, Houghton J, Warren A, Jackson THt, Jawahar A, et al. Glutamate causes a loss in human cerebral endothelial barrier integrity through activation of NMDA receptor. Am J Physiol Heart Circ Physiol. 2003;285(6):H2592–8. Epub 2003/08/02. doi:10.1152/ajpheart.00520.2003. PubMed PMID: 12893641.
58. Sharp CD, Houghton J, Elrod JW, Warren A, Jackson THt, Jawahar A, et al. N-methyl-D-aspartate receptor activation in human cerebral endothelium promotes intracellular oxidant stress. Am J Physiol Heart Circ Physiol. 2005;288(4):H1893–9. Epub 2004/12/04. doi:10.1152/ajpheart.01110.2003. PubMed PMID: 15576430.
59. Tilleux S, Hermans E. Neuroinflammation and regulation of glial glutamate uptake in neurological disorders. J Neurosci Res. 2007;85(10):2059–70. Epub 2007/05/15. doi:10.1002/jnr.21325. PubMed PMID: 17497670.
60. Enerson BE, Drewes LR. The rat blood-brain barrier transcriptome. J Cereb Blood Flow Metab Off J Int Soc Cereb Blood Flow Metab. 2006;26(7):959–73. Epub 2005/11/25. doi:10.1038/sj.jcbfm.9600249. PubMed PMID: 16306934.
61. Regina A, Morchoisne S, Borson ND, McCall AL, Drewes LR, Roux F. Factor(s) released by glucose-deprived astrocytes enhance glucose transporter expression and activity in rat brain endothelial cells. Biochim Biophys Acta. 2001;1540(3):233–42. Epub 2001/10/05. PubMed PMID: 11583818.
62. Dore-Duffy P, Balabanov R, Beaumont T, Katar M. The CNS pericyte response to low oxygen: early synthesis of cyclopentenone prostaglandins of the J-series. Microvasc Res. 2005;69(1–2):79–88. Epub 2005/03/31. doi:10.1016/j.mvr.2004.11.004. PubMed PMID: 15797264.
63. Mooradian AD, Chung HC, Shah GN. GLUT-1 expression in the cerebra of patients with Alzheimer's disease. Neurobiol Aging. 1997;18(5):469–74. Epub 1997/12/09. PubMed PMID: 9390772.
64. Zheng PP, Romme E, van der Spek PJ, Dirven CM, Willemsen R, Kros JM. Glut1/SLC2A1 is crucial for the development of the blood-brain barrier in vivo. Ann Neurol. 2010;68(6):835–44. Epub 2011/01/05. doi:10.1002/ana.22318. PubMed PMID: 21194153.
65. Abid Hussein MN, Boing AN, Sturk A, Hau CM, Nieuwland R. Inhibition of microparticle release triggers endothelial cell apoptosis and detachment. Thromb Haemost. 2007;98(5):1096–107. Epub 2007/11/15. PubMed PMID: 18000616.
66. Lowery-Nordberg M, Eaton E, Gonzalez-Toledo E, Harris MK, Chalamidas K, McGee-Brown J, et al. The effects of high dose interferon-beta1a on plasma microparticles: correlation with MRI parameters. J Neuroinflammation. 2011;8:43. Epub 2011/05/11. doi:10.1186/1742-2094-8-43. PubMed PMID: 21554694; PubMed Central PMCID: PMCPMC3120694.
67. Marcos-Ramiro B, Oliva Nacarino P, Serrano-Pertierra E, Blanco-Gelaz MA, Weksler BB, Romero IA, et al. Microparticles in multiple sclerosis and clinically isolated syndrome: effect on endothelial barrier function. BMC Neurosci. 2014;15:110. Epub 2014/09/23. doi:10.1186/1471-2202-15-110. PubMed PMID: 25242463; PubMed Central PMCID: PMCPMC4261570.
68. Alexander JS, Chervenak R, Weinstock-Guttman B, Tsunoda I, Ramanathan M, Martinez N, et al. Blood circulating microparticle species in relapsing-remitting and secondary progressive multiple sclerosis. A case-control, cross sectional study with conventional MRI and advanced iron content imaging outcomes. J Neurol Sci. 2015;355(1–2):84–9. Epub

2015/06/16. doi:10.1016/j.jns.2015.05.027. PubMed PMID: 26073484; PubMed Central PMCID: PMCPMC4550483.

69. Sheremata WA, Jy W, Horstman LL, Ahn YS, Alexander JS, Minagar A. Evidence of platelet activation in multiple sclerosis. J Neuroinflammation. 2008;5:27. Epub 2008/07/01. doi:10.1186/1742-2094-5-27. PubMed PMID: 18588683; PubMed Central PMCID: PMCPMC2474601.

70. Jimenez J, Jy W, Mauro LM, Horstman LL, Ahn ER, Ahn YS, et al. Elevated endothelial microparticle-monocyte complexes induced by multiple sclerosis plasma and the inhibitory effects of interferon-beta 1b on release of endothelial microparticles, formation and transendothelial migration of monocyte-endothelial microparticle complexes. Mult Scler (Houndmills, Basingstoke, England). 2005;11(3):310–5. Epub 2005/06/17. PubMed PMID: 15957513.

71. Minagar A, Alexander JS, Schwendimann RN, Kelley RE, Gonzalez-Toledo E, Jimenez JJ, et al. Combination therapy with interferon beta-1a and doxycycline in multiple sclerosis: an open-label trial. Arch Neurol. 2008;65(2):199–204. Epub 2007/12/12. doi:10.1001/archneurol.2007.41. PubMed PMID: 18071030.

72. Alexander JS, Harris MK, Wells SR, Mills G, Chalamidas K, Ganta VC, et al. Alterations in serum MMP-8, MMP-9, IL-12p40 and IL-23 in multiple sclerosis patients treated with interferon-beta1b. Mult Scler (Houndmills, Basingstoke, England). 2010;16(7):801–9. Epub 2010/07/14. doi:10.1177/1352458510370791. PubMed PMID: 20621951.

73. Benesova Y, Vasku A, Stourac P, Hladikova M, Beranek M, Kadanka Z, et al. Matrix metalloproteinase-9 and matrix metalloproteinase-2 gene polymorphisms in multiple sclerosis. J Neuroimmunol. 2008;205(1–2):105–9. Epub 2008/10/07. doi:10.1016/j.jneuroim.2008.08.007. PubMed PMID: 18835646.

74. Liu L, Belkadi A, Darnall L, Hu T, Drescher C, Cotleur AC, et al. CXCR2-positive neutrophils are essential for cuprizone-induced demyelination: relevance to multiple sclerosis. Nat Neurosci. 2010;13(3):319–26. Epub 2010/02/16. doi:10.1038/nn.2491. PubMed PMID: 20154684; PubMed Central PMCID: PMCPMC2827651.

75. Hasty KA, Pourmotabbed TF, Goldberg GI, Thompson JP, Spinella DG, Stevens RM, et al. Human neutrophil collagenase. A distinct gene product with homology to other matrix metalloproteinases. J Biol Chem. 1990;265(20):11421–4. Epub 1990/07/15. PubMed PMID: 2164002.

76. Miranda-Hernandez S, Baxter AG. Role of toll-like receptors in multiple sclerosis. Am J Clin Exp Immunol. 2013;2(1):75–93. Epub 2013/07/26. PubMed PMID: 23885326; PubMed Central PMCID: PMCPMC3714200.

77. Naegele M, Tillack K, Reinhardt S, Schippling S, Martin R, Sospedra M. Neutrophils in multiple sclerosis are characterized by a primed phenotype. J Neuroimmunol. 2012;242(1–2):60–71. Epub 2011/12/16. doi:10.1016/j.jneuroim.2011.11.009. PubMed PMID: 22169406.

78. Wachtel M, Frei K, Ehler E, Fontana A, Winterhalter K, Gloor SM. Occludin proteolysis and increased permeability in endothelial cells through tyrosine phosphatase inhibition. J Cell Sci. 1999;112(Pt 23):4347–56. Epub 1999/11/24. PubMed PMID: 10564652.

79. Alexander JS, Elrod JW. Extracellular matrix, junctional integrity and matrix metalloproteinase interactions in endothelial permeability regulation. J Anat. 2002;200(6):561–74. Epub 2002/08/07. PubMed PMID: 12162724; PubMed Central PMCID: PMCPMC1570742.

80. Konnecke H, Bechmann I. The role of microglia and matrix metalloproteinases involvement in neuroinflammation and gliomas. Clin Dev Immunol. 2013;2013:914104. Epub 2013/09/12. doi:10.1155/2013/914104. PubMed PMID: 24023566; PubMed Central PMCID: PMCPMC3759277.

81. Bauer AT, Burgers HF, Rabie T, Marti HH. Matrix metalloproteinase-9 mediates hypoxia-induced vascular leakage in the brain via tight junction rearrangement. J Cereb Blood Flow Metab Off J Int Soc Cereb Blood Flow Metab. 2010;30(4):837–48. Epub 2009/12/10. doi:10.1038/jcbfm.2009.248. PubMed PMID: 19997118; PubMed Central PMCID: PMCPMC2949161.

82. Nelissen I, Martens E, Van den Steen PE, Proost P, Ronsse I, Opdenakker G. Gelatinase B/ matrix metalloproteinase-9 cleaves interferon-beta and is a target for immunotherapy. Brain. 2003;126(Pt 6):1371–81. Epub 2003/05/24. PubMed PMID: 12764058.

83. Comini-Frota ER, Rodrigues DH, Miranda EC, Brum DG, Kaimen-Maciel DR, Donadi EA, et al. Serum levels of brain-derived neurotrophic factor correlate with the number of T2 MRI lesions in multiple sclerosis. Braz J Med Biol Res = Revista brasileira de pesquisas medicas e biologicas / Sociedade Brasileira de Biofisica [et al.]. 2012;45(1):68–71. Epub 2011/12/21. PubMed PMID: 22183248; PubMed Central PMCID: PMCPMC3854145.

84. Stuve O, Chabot S, Jung SS, Williams G, Yong VW. Chemokine-enhanced migration of human peripheral blood mononuclear cells is antagonized by interferon beta-1b through an effect on matrix metalloproteinase-9. J Neuroimmunol. 1997;80(1–2):38–46. Epub 1997/12/31. PubMed PMID: 9413258.

85. Opdenakker G, Van Damme J. Probing cytokines, chemokines and matrix metalloproteinases towards better immunotherapies of multiple sclerosis. Cytokine Growth Factor Rev. 2011;22(5–6):359–65. Epub 2011/11/29. doi:10.1016/j.cytogfr.2011.11.005. PubMed PMID: 22119009.

86. Agrawal SM, Silva C, Tourtellotte WW, Yong VW. EMMPRIN: a novel regulator of leuko-cyte transmigration into the CNS in multiple sclerosis and experimental autoimmune enceph-alomyelitis. J Neurosci Off J Soc Neurosci. 2011;31(2):669–77. Epub 2011/01/14. doi:10.1523/jneurosci.3659-10.2011. PubMed PMID: 21228176.

87. Festa ED, Hankiewicz K, Kim S, Skurnick J, Wolansky LJ, Cook SD, et al. Serum levels of CXCL13 are elevated in active multiple sclerosis. Mult Scler (Houndmills, Basingstoke, England). 2009;15(11):1271–9. Epub 2009/10/07. doi:10.1177/1352458509107017. PubMed PMID: 19805441.

88. Weiss N, Deboux C, Chaverot N, Miller F, Baron-Van Evercooren A, Couraud PO, et al. IL8 and CXCL13 are potent chemokines for the recruitment of human neural precursor cells across brain endothelial cells. J Neuroimmunol. 2010;223(1–2):131–4. Epub 2010/04/20. doi:10.1016/j.jneuroim.2010.03.009. PubMed PMID: 20400187.

89. Martins TB, Rose JW, Jaskowski TD, Wilson AR, Husebye D, Seraj HS, et al. Analysis of proinflammatory and anti-inflammatory cytokine serum concentrations in patients with mul-tiple sclerosis by using a multiplexed immunoassay. Am J Clin Pathol. 2011;136(5):696–704. Epub 2011/10/28. doi:10.1309/ajcp7ubk8ibvmvnr. PubMed PMID: 22031307.

90. Alatab S, Maghbooli Z, Hossein-Nezhad A, Khosrofar M, Mokhtari F. Cytokine profile, Foxp3 and nuclear factor-kB ligand levels in multiple sclerosis subtypes. Minerva Med. 2011;102(6):461–8. Epub 2011/12/24. PubMed PMID: 22193377.

91. Beard RS, Jr., Haines RJ, Wu KY, Reynolds JJ, Davis SM, Elliott JE, et al. Non-muscle Mlck is required for beta-catenin- and FoxO1-dependent downregulation of Cldn5 in IL-1beta-mediated barrier dysfunction in brain endothelial cells. J Cell Sci. 2014;127(Pt 8):1840–53. Epub 2014/02/14. doi:10.1242/jcs.144550. PubMed PMID: 24522189; PubMed Central PMCID: PMCPMC4074294.

92. Ryan C, Thrash B, Warren RB, Menter A. The use of ustekinumab in autoimmune disease. ExpertOpinBiolTher.2010;10(4):587–604.Epub2010/03/12.doi:10.1517/14712591003724670. PubMed PMID: 20218921.

93. Sorensen EW, Gerber SA, Frelinger JG, Lord EM. IL-12 suppresses vascular endothelial growth factor receptor 3 expression on tumor vessels by two distinct IFN-gamma-dependent mechanisms. J Immunol (Baltimore, Md : 1950). 2010;184(4):1858–66. Epub 2010/01/12. doi:10.4049/jimmunol.0903210. PubMed PMID: 20061409; PubMed Central PMCID: PMCPMC3070472.

94. Mishra M, Kumar H, Bajpai S, Singh RK, Tripathi K. Level of serum IL-12 and its correla-tion with endothelial dysfunction, insulin resistance, proinflammatory cytokines and lipid profile in newly diagnosed type 2 diabetes. Diabetes Res Clin Pract. 2011;94(2):255–61. Epub 2011/08/23. doi:10.1016/j.diabres.2011.07.037. PubMed PMID: 21855158.

95. Jones JL, Coles AJ. New treatment strategies in multiple sclerosis. Exp Neurol. 2010;225(1):34–9. Epub 2010/06/16. doi:10.1016/j.expneurol.2010.06.003. PubMed PMID: 20547155.

96. Neuhaus O, Strasser-Fuchs S, Fazekas F, Kieseier BC, Niederwieser G, Hartung HP, et al. Statins as immunomodulators: comparison with interferon-beta 1b in MS. Neurology. 2002;59(7):990–7. Epub 2002/10/09. PubMed PMID: 12370451.

97. Wang J, Xiao Y, Luo M, Zhang X, Luo H. Statins for multiple sclerosis. Cochrane Database Systematic Reviews. 2010;(12):Cd008386. Epub 2010/12/15. doi:10.1002/14651858. CD008386.pub2. PubMed PMID: 21154395.

98. Pihl-Jensen G, Tsakiri A, Frederiksen JL. Statin treatment in multiple sclerosis: a systematic review and meta-analysis. CNS Drugs. 2015;29(4):277–91. Epub 2015/03/22. doi:10.1007/s40263-015-0239-x. PubMed PMID: 25795002.

99. Weinstock-Guttman B, Zivadinov R, Mahfooz N, Carl E, Drake A, Schneider J, et al. Serum lipid profiles are associated with disability and MRI outcomes in multiple sclerosis. J Neuroinflammation. 2011;8:127. Epub 2011/10/06. doi:10.1186/1742-2094-8-127. PubMed PMID: 21970791; PubMed Central PMCID: PMCPMC3228782.

100. Sasaki M, Bharwani S, Jordan P, Elrod JW, Grisham MB, Jackson TH, et al. Increased disease activity in eNOS-deficient mice in experimental colitis. Free Radic Biol Med. 2003;35(12):1679–87. Epub 2003/12/19. PubMed PMID: 14680690.

101. Sasaki M, Bharwani S, Jordan P, Joh T, Manas K, Warren A, et al. The 3-hydroxy-3-methylglutaryl-CoA reductase inhibitor pravastatin reduces disease activity and inflammation in dextran-sulfate induced colitis. J Pharmacol Exp Ther. 2003;305(1):78–85. Epub 2003/03/22. doi:10.1124/jpet.102.044099. PubMed PMID: 12649355.

102. Izidoro-Toledo TC, Guimaraes DA, Belo VA, Gerlach RF, Tanus-Santos JE. Effects of statins on matrix metalloproteinases and their endogenous inhibitors in human endothelial cells. Naunyn Schmiedebergs Arch Pharmacol. 2011;383(6):547–54. Epub 2011/03/31. doi:10.1007/s00210-011-0623-0. PubMed PMID: 21448567.

103. Desai LP, White SR, Waters CM. Mechanical stretch decreases FAK phosphorylation and reduces cell migration through loss of JIP3-induced JNK phosphorylation in airway epithelial cells. Am J Physiol Lung Cell Mol Physiol. 2009;297(3):L520–9. Epub 2009/07/04. doi:10.1152/ajplung.00076.2009. PubMed PMID: 19574423; PubMed Central PMCID: PMCPMC2739770.

104. Ghosh BC, Shatzkes J, Webb H. Primary epiploic appendagitis: diagnosis, management, and natural course of the disease. Mil Med. 2003;168(4):346–7. Epub 2003/05/08. PubMed PMID: 12733684.

105. Hellwig K, Gold R. Progressive multifocal leukoencephalopathy and natalizumab. J Neurol. 2011;258(11):1920–8. Epub 2011/06/08. doi:10.1007/s00415-011-6116-8. PubMed PMID: 21647730.

106. Streeter PR, Berg EL, Rouse BT, Bargatze RF, Butcher EC. A tissue-specific endothelial cell molecule involved in lymphocyte homing. Nature. 1988;331(6151):41–6. Epub 1988/01/07. doi:10.1038/331041a0. PubMed PMID: 3340147.

107. Yang Y, Cardarelli PM, Lehnert K, Rowland S, Krissansen GW. LPAM-1 (integrin alpha 4 beta 7)-ligand binding: overlapping binding sites recognizing VCAM-1, MAdCAM-1 and CS-1 are blocked by fibrinogen, a fibronectin-like polymer and RGD-like cyclic peptides. Eur J Immunol. 1998;28(3):995–1004. Epub 1998/04/29. PubMed PMID: 9541595.

108. Berger JR, Khalili K. The pathogenesis of progressive multifocal leukoencephalopathy. Discov Med. 2011;12(67):495–503. Epub 2011/12/30. PubMed PMID: 22204766.

109. Seidel P, Merfort I, Hughes JM, Oliver BG, Tamm M, Roth M. Dimethyl fumarate inhibits NF-{kappa}B function at multiple levels to limit airway smooth muscle cell cytokine secretion. Am J Physiol Lung Cell Mol Physiol. 2009;297(2):L326–39. Epub 2009/05/26. doi:10.1152/ajplung.90624.2008. PubMed PMID: 19465513.

110. Wingerchuk DM, Carter JL. Multiple sclerosis: current and emerging disease-modifying therapies and treatment strategies. Mayo Clin Proc. 2014;89(2):225–40. Epub 2014/02/04. doi:10.1016/j.mayocp.2013.11.002. PubMed PMID: 24485135.

111. Kunze R, Urrutia A, Hoffmann A, Liu H, Helluy X, Pham M, et al. Dimethyl fumarate attenuates cerebral edema formation by protecting the blood-brain barrier integrity. Exp Neurol. 2015;266:99–111. Epub 2015/03/01. doi:10.1016/j.expneurol.2015.02.022. PubMed PMID: 25725349.

112. van Kester MS, Bouwes Bavinck JN, Quint KD. PML in patients treated with dimethyl fuma-rate. N Engl J Med. 2015;373(6):583–4. Epub 2015/08/06. doi:10.1056/NEJMc1506151#SA2. PubMed PMID: 26244326.

113. Nishihara H, Shimizu F, Sano Y, Takeshita Y, Maeda T, Abe M, et al. Fingolimod prevents blood-brain barrier disruption induced by the sera from patients with multiple sclerosis. PloS One. 2015;10(3):e0121488. Epub 2015/03/17. doi:10.1371/journal.pone.0121488. PubMed PMID: 25774903; PubMed Central PMCID: PMCPMC4361641.

114. Frohman EM, Havrdova E, Lublin F, Barkhof F, Achiron A, Sharief MK, et al. Most patients with multiple sclerosis or a clinically isolated demyelinating syndrome should be treated at the time of diagnosis. Arch Neurol. 2006;63:614–9. United States.

115. Ubogu EE, Cossoy MB, Ransohoff RM. The expression and function of chemokines involved in CNS inflammation. Trends Pharmacol Sci. 2006;27(1):48–55. Epub 2005/11/29. doi:10.1016/j.tips.2005.11.002. PubMed PMID: 16310865.

116. Rieckmann P, Albrecht M, Kitze B, Weber T, Tumani H, Broocks A, et al. Tumor necrosis factor-alpha messenger RNA expression in patients with relapsing-remitting multiple sclero-sis is associated with disease activity. Ann Neurol. 1995;37(1):82–8. Epub 1995/01/01. doi:10.1002/ana.410370115. PubMed PMID: 7818262.

117. Oshima T, Laroux FS, Coe LL, Morise Z, Kawachi S, Bauer P, et al. Interferon-gamma and interleukin-10 reciprocally regulate endothelial junction integrity and barrier function. Microvasc Res. 2001;61(1):130–43. Epub 2001/02/13. doi:10.1006/mvre.2000.2288. PubMed PMID: 11162203.

118. Swardfager W, Lanctot K, Rothenburg L, Wong A, Cappell J, Herrmann N. A meta-analysis of cytokines in Alzheimer's disease. Biol Psychiatry. 2010;68(10):930–41. Epub 2010/08/10. doi:10.1016/j.biopsych.2010.06.012. PubMed PMID: 20692646.

119. Leitner GC, Vogelsang H. Pharmacological- and non-pharmacological therapeutic approaches in inflammatory bowel disease in adults. World J Gastrointest Pharmacol Ther. 2016;7(1):5–20. Epub 2016/02/09. doi:10.4292/wjgpt.v7.i1.5. PubMed PMID: 26855808; PubMed Central PMCID: PMCPMC4734954.

120. Hegen H, Adrianto I, Lessard CJ, Millonig A, Bertolotto A, Comabella M, et al. Cytokine profiles show heterogeneity of interferon-beta response in multiple sclerosis patients. Neurol Neuroimmunol Neuroinflamm. 2016;3(2):e202. Epub 2016/02/20. doi:10.1212/nxi.0000000000000202. PubMed PMID: 26894205; PubMed Central PMCID: PMCPMC4747480.

121. Matsumoto T, Nakamura I, Miura A, Momoyama G, Ito K. New-onset multiple sclerosis associated with adalimumab treatment in rheumatoid arthritis: a case report and literature review. Clin Rheumatol. 2013;32(2):271–5. Epub 2012/11/15. doi:10.1007/s10067-012-2113-2. PubMed PMID: 23149905.

122. Bitsch A, Kuhlmann T, Da Costa C, Bunkowski S, Polak T, Bruck W. Tumour necrosis factor alpha mRNA expression in early multiple sclerosis lesions: correlation with demyelinating activity and oligodendrocyte pathology. Glia. 2000;29(4):366–75. Epub 2000/02/01. PubMed PMID: 10652446.

123. Plumb J, McQuaid S, Cross AK, Surr J, Haddock G, Bunning RA, et al. Upregulation of ADAM-17 expression in active lesions in multiple sclerosis. Mult Scler (Houndmills, Basingstoke, England). 2006;12(4):375–85. Epub 2006/08/12. PubMed PMID: 16900751.

124. Selmaj KW, Raine CS. Tumor necrosis factor mediates myelin and oligodendrocyte damage in vitro. Ann Neurol. 1988;23(4):339–46. Epub 1988/04/01. doi:10.1002/ana.410230405. PubMed PMID: 3132891.

125. Andreadou E, Kemanetzoglou E, Brokalaki C, Evangelopoulos ME, Kilidireas C, Rombos A, et al. Demyelinating disease following anti-TNFa treatment: a Causal or Coincidental Association? Report of four cases and review of the literature. Case Rep Neurol Med. 2013;2013:671935. Epub 2013/06/14. doi:10.1155/2013/671935. PubMed PMID: 23762678; PubMed Central PMCID: PMCPMC3670521.

126. Enayati PJ, Papadakis KA. Association of anti-tumor necrosis factor therapy with the devel-opment of multiple sclerosis. J Clin Gastroenterol. 2005;39(4):303–6. Epub 2005/03/11. PubMed PMID: 15758624.

127. Naylor SL, Sakaguchi AY, Shows TB, Law ML, Goeddel DV, Gray PW. Human immune interferon gene is located on chromosome 12. J Exp Med. 1983;157(3):1020–7. Epub 1983/03/01. PubMed PMID: 6403645; PubMed Central PMCID: PMCPMC2186972.

128. Schoenborn JR, Wilson CB. Regulation of interferon-gamma during innate and adaptive immune responses. Adv Immunol. 2007;96:41–101. Epub 2007/11/06. doi:10.1016/s0065-2776(07)96002-2. PubMed PMID: 17981204.

129. Ealick SE, Cook WJ, Vijay-Kumar S, Carson M, Nagabhushan TL, Trotta PP, et al. Three-dimensional structure of recombinant human interferon-gamma. Science. 1991;252(5006):698–702. Epub 1991/05/03. PubMed PMID: 1902591.

130. Beck J, Rondot P, Catinot L, Falcoff E, Kirchner H, Wietzerbin J. Increased production of interferon gamma and tumor necrosis factor precedes clinical manifestation in multiple sclerosis: do cytokines trigger off exacerbations? Acta Neurol Scand. 1988;78(4):318–23. Epub 1988/10/01. PubMed PMID: 3146861.

131. Lu CZ, Jensen MA, Arnason BG. Interferon gamma- and interleukin-4-secreting cells in multiple sclerosis. J Neuroimmunol. 1993;46(1–2):123–8. Epub 1993/07/01. PubMed PMID: 7689582.

132. Woodroofe MN, Cuzner ML. Cytokine mRNA expression in inflammatory multiple sclerosis lesions: detection by non-radioactive in situ hybridization. Cytokine. 1993;5(6):583–8. Epub 1993/11/01. PubMed PMID: 8186370.

133. Panitch HS, Hirsch RL, Schindler J, Johnson KP. Treatment of multiple sclerosis with gamma interferon: exacerbations associated with activation of the immune system. Neurology. 1987;37(7):1097–102. Epub 1987/07/01. PubMed PMID: 3110648.

134. Panitch HS, Hirsch RL, Haley AS, Johnson KP. Exacerbations of multiple sclerosis in patients treated with gamma interferon. Lancet (London, England). 1987;1(8538):893–5. Epub 1987/04/18. PubMed PMID: 2882294.

135. Billiau A, Heremans H, Vermeire K, Matthys P. Immunomodulatory properties of interferon-gamma. An update. Ann N Y Acad Sci. 1998;856:22–32. Epub 1999/01/26. PubMed PMID: 9917861.

136. Duong TT, St Louis J, Gilbert JJ, Finkelman FD, Strejan GH. Effect of anti-interferon-gamma and anti-interleukin-2 monoclonal antibody treatment on the development of actively and passively induced experimental allergic encephalomyelitis in the SJL/J mouse. J Neuroimmunol. 1992;36(2–3):105–15. Epub 1992/02/01. PubMed PMID: 1732276.

137. de Lorgeril M, Salen P, Defaye P, Rabaeus M. Recent findings on the health effects of omega-3 fatty acids and statins, and their interactions: do statins inhibit omega-3? BMC Med. 2013;11:13. doi:10.1186/1741-7015-11-5. PubMed PMID: WOS:000318423200002.

138. Wang J, Xiao Y, Luo M, Zhang X, Luo H. Statins for multiple sclerosis. Cochrane Database Syst Rev. 2010 Dec 8;(12):CD008386. doi: 10.1002/14651858.CD008386.pub2.

139. Yun JW, Xiao A, Tsunoda I, Minagar A, Alexander JS. From trash to treasure: The untapped potential of endothelial microparticles in neurovascular diseases. Pathophysiology. 2016 Dec;23(4):265-274. doi: 10.1016/j.pathophys.2016.08.004. Epub 2016 Aug 12.

Multiple Sclerosis: Clinical Features, Immunopathogenesis, and Treatment

2

Alexis A. Lizarraga and William A. Sheremata

List of Abbreviations

ACTH	Corticotrophin
APC	Antigen-presenting cell
CIS	Clinically isolated syndrome
CNS	Central nervous system
CSF	Cerebrospinal fluid
CT	Computerized tomography
DIR	Double inversion recovery
DTI	Diffusion tensor imaging
EAE	Experimental allergic encephalomyelitis
EDSS	Expanded disability status scale
GFAP	Glial fibrillary acidic protein
HIV	Human immunodeficiency virus
IL	Interleukin
MBP	Myelin basic protein
MHC	Major histocompatibility class
MOG	Myelin oligodendrocyte glycoprotein
MRI	Magnetic resonance imaging
MS	Multiple sclerosis
NEDA	No evidence of disease activity
PCR	Polymerase chain reaction
PML	Progressive multifocal leukoencephalopathy
PPMS	Primary progressive multiple sclerosis
RRMS	Relapsing-remitting multiple sclerosis
SLE	Systemic lupus erythematosus

A.A. Lizarraga, MD (✉) • W.A. Sheremata, MD, FRCPC, FACP, FAAN
Miller School of Medicine University of Miami, Miami, FL, USA
e-mail: aalizarraga@med.miami.edu

© Springer International Publishing AG 2017
A. Minagar, J.S. Alexander (eds.), *Inflammatory Disorders of the Nervous System*, Current Clinical Neurology, DOI 10.1007/978-3-319-51220-4_2

Introduction

Great strides in understanding multiple sclerosis (MS) have been made in the areas of immunology, genetics, and most importantly treatment since the first publication of this volume. Advances in drug treatment of MS continue to provide newer, more convenient oral therapies, and potentially more effective options for patients. These areas have been given greater attention for students of this disorder.

History

Charcot first described MS as a unique disorder in the mid nineteenth century in Paris. He attributed the original recognition of this disorder to Cruveillier, the famed professor of anatomy. Others also described the pathological anatomy of the disease in remarkable detail, but it was Charcot who characterized the clinical illness and correlated the illness with its unique neuropathology [1]. From the first descriptions of the illness, it was recognized that MS differed clinically from one patient to another, with the majority of patients experiencing a relapsing-remitting multiple sclerosis (RRMS) [1, 2]. Charcot recognized the illness in a minority of patients was fundamentally different and described them as having an "incomplete" form of illness [1, 2]. From their first symptoms, these patients manifest signs of a progressive spinal cord disease without relapses. They are now designated as having primary progressive (PPMS) [2].

The first person documented to clearly have suffered from MS was a grandson of King George III of England, Sir August D'Este [3]. The course of his illness recorded in his diary was edited and published by Douglas Firth in 1947. While MS is an illness that is more common in the higher socioeconomic strata of society, it is not limited to the well to do by any means [2, 4, 5]. The disease does, however, occur predominantly in persons of European descent [2, 4, 5]. African-Americans have MS diagnosed at approximately half the rate of Caucasians in the United States [4, 5].

Clinical Features of Multiple Sclerosis

Multiple sclerosis is an illness characterized by relapses of neurological deficits followed by remissions with varying degrees of recovery [1–6]. The occurrence and severity of the exacerbations are unpredictable, although several factors are recognized as increasing the risk of attacks. Patients experiencing their initial attacks of MS are more likely to recover "fully," but an experienced neurologist can virtually always find residual evidence of the previous neurological deficit, no matter how complete the recovery seems to have been. For example, retrobulbar neuritis heralds the onset of illness in 10–15% of MS patients. The severity of the visual impairment varies greatly, with a very small percentage of patients suffering complete loss of light perception. Recovery of vision generally occurs, but occasionally, especially if complete loss of vision occurs, there may be little or no recovery. A skilled examiner can find neurological deficits such as an afferent pupillary defect (Marcus Gunn pupil) and color desaturation (impaired color vision) in the vast majority of patients with a history of retrobulbar neuritis who seem to have recovered normal visual acuity.

Multiple sclerosis is typically manifest by recurrent acute onset of neurological difficulties reflecting damage to multiple areas of the brain and spinal cord, defined clinically as "attacks" or "relapses" [1, 2, 4]. Symptoms associated with these events typically remit, but subsequent relapses occur unpredictably and may become more obviously associated with residual disability [1, 3, 4]. It is this *dissemination in time and space* that is so characteristic of multiple sclerosis and its principal diagnostic feature [6–9]. Interval progression between, or in the absence of attacks of illness, signifies the onset of secondary progressive multiple sclerosis (SPMS) [2]. However, approximately 10–15% of the overall patient population will develop a progressive form of illness without relapses, usually appearing in midlife, termed primary progressive multiple sclerosis, PPMS [2, 10]. This form of illness is slightly more common in men. This progressive form of MS is approximately three times more common in Irish and Ashkenazi Jewish populations [2, 10]. Should one or more exacerbations occur after onset of primary progressive illness at outset, patients may be designated as having "relapsing progressive MS" [2]. Although in the past, there has been no agreement that SPMS and relapsing progressive patients differ in any fundamental way; evidence from new studies shows differences in the microscopic neuropathology of RRMS, SPMS, and PPMS. Lesions associated with acute relapse in early disease are cellular with abundant CD3+ T cells and do not show smoldering microglial disease activity. In contrast, in PPMS the central nervous system (CNS) is largely devoid of focal cellular collections and smoldering lesions and markers of microglial activation predominate. Secondary progressive patients have a mixture of four types of microscopic lesions with the presence of CD3+ T cells, antibody in plaques, and microglial activation as well as inactive plaques. The majority of the MS population will experience relapsing-remitting illness, but residual persistent disability may variably follow despite remission [11–13]. The presence of residual disability following exacerbations *does not* signify the onset of secondary progressive illness, however.

Increases in body temperature, or illness, in MS may result in the transient reappearance of neurological symptoms (*Uhthoff phenomenon*). Despite a previous remission of clinical manifestations of MS, those same symptoms may appear with overheating [2]. Although the Uhthoff phenomenon is not an exacerbation, these phenomena in MS patients are commonly misinterpreted as such. Occasionally heat exposure appears to acutely worsen the severity of an exacerbation and, in other circumstances, worsens a minimal or subclinical event making it more clearly apparent clinically [14]. These events probably reflect the ability of heat to impair the blood-brain barrier, allowing activated lymphocytes and immunoglobulins to enter the brain and spinal cord [14].

The most common initial symptoms of MS are sensory disturbances and fatigue but are often ignored by patients and physicians alike. Perceptions of numbness and tingling by the patient may not be accompanied by obvious abnormalities on initial examination, especially if the patient is not examined completely by a neurologist at the onset of their symptoms. Almost half of initially recognized exacerbations principally affect ambulation. Acute paraparesis varies greatly in degree and in symmetry of the weakness. In many MS patients with motor weakness found by examination, they describe their difficulty as a "heaviness" in their "leg(s)." Alternatively, they may seem only to stumble when their foot catches an uneven area on a sidewalk. The difficulty is often initially recognized only by a family member or a friend during ambulation. Gait problems may be due to motor difficulties and/or, ataxia. Ataxia may occur as a result of vestibular, cerebellar, or sensory impairments. Thus, gait difficulty may reflect motor deficits or ataxia due to one or more problems within the brainstem or spinal cord.

About one out of five or six MS patients will have unilateral retrobulbar (optic) neuritis as their initial clinical difficulty [2, 11]. Other common symptoms at onset include diplopia, facial weakness and/or facial myokymia, vertigo, bladder, and bowel symptoms. Seizures will eventually occur in 10% during the clinical illness but rarely (about 1%) are a presenting sign of illness [2]. Some symptoms, such as hearing loss and impaired night vision, can be seen in MS and also acute disseminated encephalomyelitis (ADEM). The speed of recovery is variable and may be slow over several months or may not occur at all. Other less commonly recognized symptoms include extrapyramidal symptoms and a family of paroxysmal manifestations [15].

Recurrent brief (*paroxysmal*) stereotyped manifestations in MS include paroxysmal dystonia or "tonic seizures," paroxysmal dysarthria, paroxysmal akinesis ("paroxysmal falling"), pains (including trigeminal neuralgia and glossopharyngeal neuralgia), and other difficulties [2, 16]. Lhermitte's sign is precipitated by neck flexion and typically consists of transient shocklike sensations radiating down the neck and back, often into the limbs. It is commonly recognized as a sign of MS especially when it occurs in the young, although it may occur with compressive cervical disc disease or spinal tumors. Except for Lhermitte's sign, these paroxysmal symptoms seem to occur in a minority of patients and are often not recognized as part of the spectrum of illness. When recognized, these paroxysmal phenomena are of great diagnostic value since they are rarely associated with other illness. When viewed in a cross section of a patient population, they are evident in only about 3% of patients. We have found, however, that with long-term follow-up that paroxysmal phenomena will eventually occur in up to a quarter of patients. Occasionally paroxysmal dystonia involves all four limbs and the truncal muscles as well and may be accompanied by severe pain. Fortunately there is usually a prompt and complete response to carbamazepine in a 400 mg per day dosage, but a course of parenteral corticotrophin may be needed. Unfortunately, many such patients are incorrectly diagnosed as having an acute psychiatric problem. These paroxysmal symptoms are commonly attributed to ephaptic transmission (cross talk between damaged/demyelinated axons), but we suspect that they may be due to inflammatory mediators such as leukotriene C, and other leukotrienes, produced by macrophages. Leukotrienes are extremely potent depolarizing agents. Often the time course of these paroxysmal events approximates that of an exacerbation and, if so, should be considered to be exacerbations.

Although fatigue and fatigability become more prominent with time, especially during periods of disease activity, they may be prominent presenting signs of MS. Anxiety, depression, and cognitive issues, also, may dominate the presentation of illness and may delay disease recognition. In our experience cognitive problems and accompanying emotional reaction occurring early in the course of illness are more important than physical disability as reasons for social dislocation and patients leaving studies or their workplace. A substantial proportion of patients are dismissed as "functional" early in the course of their illness due to their observed emotional status. A recent oral presentation reported the association of MS with schizophrenia and bipolar disorder, with a rate ratio of 1.42 for schizophrenia and 1.73 for bipolar disorder [17].

A bewildering variety of manifestations may occur in MS, singly or in combination with other difficulties. These include limb weakness, "useless limb" syndrome due to severe proprioceptive loss, memory impairment, word-finding difficulty, acalculia, tremor, unusual nonphysiological patterns of sensory loss, and sexual impotence, among others [2, 11]. Motor impersistence is common in the MS population and accompanies proprioceptive impairment. Geschwind also suggested that frontal lobe involvement was a likely contributing factor (Norman Geschwind – personal communication).

Diagnosis of Multiple Sclerosis

Diagnosis of MS is dependent upon the recognition of symptoms and neurological findings typically accompanying exacerbations of MS *and* affecting different parts of the nervous system over time [7–9]. The importance of an accurate history and physical examination cannot be overemphasized. The senior author's own observation is that a relative's recognition of early manifestations of MS is likely to lead to the diagnosis of MS in a family member, rather than the contrary as is commonly believed.

Diagnostic Criteria The recognition of MS was easy for experienced neurologists in the past. However, long delays in diagnosis were common and many patients were incorrectly diagnosed. The need for standardized criteria for patients entering treatment studies led to the formation of an NIH committee headed by Dr. George Schumacher. Diagnostic criteria have evolved from the 1965 Schumacher criteria [7], that were established primarily for the selection of research subjects for MS studies, to the 1983 Poser criteria [8] which for the first time included laboratory support (magnetic resonance imaging [MRI], evoked response testing, as well as spinal fluid examination). The 2001, 2006, and now 2010 McDonald criteria are based on the original criteria but include validated specific MRI features [9, 10]. These new criteria (Table 2.1) allow the identification of "clinically isolated syndromes" (optic neuritis and brain stem or acute myelitis) with very high (80%)

Table 2.1 2010 RRMS McDonald diagnostic criteria

Clinical attacks	Objective lesions	Additional requirement to make diagnosis
≥2	≥2	*Clinical evidence is enough*
≥2	1	Disseminated in *space* by MRI *or* + CSF and ≥ 2MRI lesions consistent with MS *or* additional clinical attack in different site
1	≥2	Disseminated in *time* by MRI *or* 2nd clinical attack
1 Mono-symptomatic	1	Disseminated in *space* by MRI or await a 2nd attack implicating a different CNS site and disseminated in *time* by MRI or 2nd attack
0 Progressive from start	1 in brain 2 in spinal cord	1 year of disease progression plus two of three of the following: Disseminated in *space* by MRI evidence of 1 or more T2 brain lesions or ≥ 2 cord lesions + CSF

probability of MS. Imaging provides the additional evidence required to establish the presence of dissemination of lesions both in time and space. Early diagnosis of MS with earlier introduction of treatment portends a better outcome in the short-term and prolonged survival, at least for interferon-beta-1a [18, 19]. Consensus definitions of the clinical subtypes of MS were released by the US National Multiple Sclerosis Society Advisory Committee on Clinical Trials in Multiple Sclerosis in 1996 and revised in 2013 [20, 21].

Relapsing MS is characterized by clearly defined relapses with either full recovery or residual deficit, representing about 85% of patients at the outset. *Progressive MS* is characterized clinically by the gradual accrual of disability independent of relapses and can occur with disease onset (primary progressive) or can be preceded by a relapsing disease course (secondary progressive). In most cases, SPMS is diagnosed retrospectively after several years of gradual worsening after a period of clinical relapses. Currently, there are no clear criteria to mark the transition from RRMS to SPMS. The basis of separating the primary versus secondary progressive forms of MS was derived from a meta-analysis of the COP1 trial in progressive MS as an antecedent of the PROMISE trial [22]. The criteria formulated by Thompson et al. grouped suspected PPMS patients into "definite," "probable," and "possible" [21, 23–25]. Multiple sclerosis may be seen as a spectrum with an intense focal inflammatory component in RRMS and more neurodegenerative features with concomitant chronic inflammation and axon loss in progressive forms of MS [26]. Currently, clinical diagnostic criteria exist for both forms. A recent publication provides clear differences in the neuropathological findings separating RRMS, SPMS, and PPMS [27].

Another issue impacting on early diagnosis of MS is the quality of spinal fluid examinations. Importantly, the FDA laboratory standard for oligoclonal banding testing – isoelectric focusing on agarose gel followed by immunoblotting or immunofixation for IgG with paired spinal fluid and serum – avoids technically inadequate studies. The quality of antihuman antibody used in the testing has a major

Table 2.2 Differential diagnosis of MS

Acquired diseases
1. ADEM vs. CIS (MS)
2. Infectious disease
Syphilis
Retroviral infection
HIV
HTLV-I/II
3. CNS vasculitis
Granulomatous vasculitis – sarcoid, HIV, etc.
Primary CNS vasculitis
4. Autoimmune diseases – SLE
5. Tumors of the CNS
6. Trauma to CNS
7. Psychiatric illness
Hereditary diseases
1. Leukodystrophies
2. Spinocerebellar diseases
3. Hereditary spastic paraparesis

impact on the results. Evoked response testing is relied upon less, but can be helpful, especially visual evoked responses [9].

Diagnostic criteria for PPMS were also updated in 2010 and include (1) a minimum of 1 year of disease progression plus two of three of the following: dissemination in space in the brain or spinal cord or positive CSF, defined as the presence of OCBs, and/or elevated IgG index [10].

Differential Diagnosis There is a large differential diagnosis, outlined in Table 2.2. In the past meningovascular syphilis was the "great imitator" and topped the list. Today a variety of granulomatous diseases and other diseases are considered in the differential diagnosis, but sarcoidosis and systemic lupus erythematosus (SLE) are the major differential diagnosis considered. The retroviruses human immunodeficiency virus (HIV) and HTLV-I/II can rarely present as a granulomatous disease or mimic MS.

Central nervous system lymphoma may require brain biopsy to establish a diagnosis, but a positive test for HIV ordinarily rules out the diagnosis of MS. Biopsy is ordinarily required to make a diagnosis of primary central nervous system vasculitis (CNS vasculitis). The disorder "CNS vasculitis" is rare and like progressive multifocal leukoencephalopathy (PML) is associated with MS-like attacks resulting in increasing neurological deficit progressing in a stepwise fashion. Unlike PML there may be at least temporary partial resolution of neurological deficit with high-dose steroids or pulse cyclophosphamide therapy in patients with CNS vasculitis. Despite its rarity, establishing a diagnosis of CNS vasculitis is important because it is regularly fatal if not treated aggressively with chronic systemic immunosuppression.

Multiple sclerosis may occasionally present with prominent sensory complaints and marked, symmetrical weakness of the lower extremities and be mistakenly diagnosed as an acute demyelinating polyneuropathy (Guillain-Barré syndrome). Albumino-cytological dissociation, however, is rarely found in MS.

Symptoms of MS must last 24 hours at a minimum. To be considered a new relapse, a new symptom or a relapse of a prior symptom must occur at least 1 month after the previous exacerbation. The symptoms and findings should be of a type recognized as associated with multiple sclerosis. The diagnosis of multiple sclerosis is accepted only if it is established by a neurologist [7–10].

PPMS is a more difficult diagnosis to establish. This form of MS presents most commonly in midlife (about 40±5 years on average), and distinguishing this form of MS from other potentially treatable illness may be extremely difficult [11, 28]. Manifestations of neurological disease should be observed for at least 6 months before acceptance as evidence supporting a diagnosis of PPMS. Multiple other disorders must be ruled out of the differential diagnosis. Syphilis, vitamin B-12 deficiency (sub-acute combined myelopathy), and retrovirus-associated myelopathy (HIV-associated myelopathy and human T-cell leukemia-associated myelopathy (TSP/HAM)) [2, 11, 29] can be easily ruled out by laboratory testing. Antibody testing by Western blot for HTLV-I/II, if indeterminate, may not be sufficient [30]. Genetic ("PCR," polymerase chain reaction) testing in a reliable laboratory test is the most sensitive and specific test for this purpose. In our experience this test is positive in up to 20% of patients who are Western blot indeterminate but who are infected with either HTLV-I/II virus [31]. Radiation myelopathy continues to be an important differential diagnosis in patients with a history of radiation therapy to the head and neck.

Neuroimaging should be carried out to eliminate spinal cord compression, congenital abnormalities, and intraparenchymal tumors from consideration. At times, imaging will not reveal the presence of one or more intraparenchymal spinal cord lesions that are evidenced by clinical examination, however. The finding of hypothyroidism is common in MS, and myelopathy should not be attributed to thyroid disease alone. Adrenocortical leukodystrophy and hereditary spastic paraplegia are easily distinguished from primary progressive multiple sclerosis by the patient's infantile age of presentation and presence of a family history [2, 32].

It cannot be overemphasized that repeated clinical visits *and* examinations over time, as well as repeated imaging, may clarify the nature of the illness in difficult cases. This is particularly important when cognitive and emotional issues dominate and obscure the presentation [3, 11]. The McDonald criteria, however, greatly assist early diagnosis and justify the institution of treatment. It should be noted that in using the criteria for a clinically isolated syndrome (CIS), the majority will be correctly diagnosed as having MS, but about 20% of patients may never meet criteria for clinically definite MS. On the other hand, we regularly document relapses within weeks to months in many patients with CIS who initially had no evidence of brain lesions in their MRI scans at clinical presentation. Multiple sclerosis remains a clinical diagnosis [9, 10].

Prognosis

Exacerbation rates in MS patients vary greatly but tend to diminish with increasing duration of illness [13, 14, 18, 33]. When a patient has established disability, exacerbations do not appear to correlate with increasing disability [13]. Pregnancy has long been thought to decrease the risk of relapse in the third trimester, as shown in a large prospective study [34]. This is thought, at least in part, to be secondary to high concentrations of estrogen and progesterone, and phase II clinical trials have shown a potential role for estriol in treatment of MS [35]. The risk of relapse in the first trimester, however, is increased. The French study also confirmed a long recognized phenomenon that the risk of exacerbation of MS is markedly increased for 3 months postpartum. This study also showed this risk continued at a somewhat lower level for the 33 months of follow-up in the study. The importance of infection as a precipitating factor for exacerbations has long been recognized [36].

Emotional stress and its impact on MS has been the subject of a number of excellent studies [37–40]. All of these studies have consistently shown a correlation between major life stress and a significantly increased risk of exacerbation of MS. In a remarkable more recent study, Mohr et al. have demonstrated a correlation between stress, including "hassles" and the appearance of new active gadolinium-enhancing brain lesions [40]. The perception of stress, rather than a particular life event, is related to an increased risk of exacerbation [37–40]. While other factors are thought to influence prognosis in MS patients, no similar studies of risk factors has addressed them adequately.

A large number of neurologists at academic centers in the United States and elsewhere have concluded that the majority of MS patients develop secondary progressive disease and then progress rapidly to disability. Confavreux et al. have published their studies of the natural history of a large population of French patients [13]. The French workers have concluded that there is no relationship between relapses and progression, once disability is established. They have further concluded that only 30% of their relapsing-remitting patients had secondary progressive MS. Pittock et al. at the Mayo clinic published important observations of a 10-year follow-up of their MS population from Olmsted County, Minnesota [14]. They too found that disability in the majority of their patients did not progress measurably during the 10-year period of observation. Only 30% of their patients progressed to needing a cane or a wheel chair, but most patients remained stable despite the fact that only 15% had received immunomodulatory therapy. It is obvious that the perception that the vast majority of MS patients develop secondary progressive disease with rapid progression to serious disability is incorrect. The group in Lyon, France, has also found that longer periods of follow-up show that patients thought to have "benign MS" do develop some neurological impairment over 20–30 years of follow-up. Please see Table 2.3 for a list of proposed prognostic indicators.

Neuroimaging in Multiple Sclerosis

Computerized tomography (CT) neuroimaging for the first time revealed areas of decreased radiodensity in the brain as well as occasional enhancing brain and spinal cord lesions in MS. Interestingly, increasing brain atrophy, although reported early, was largely ignored by the MS community [43–45]. Comparative studies of CT and MRI revealed the relative strength of MRI in visualizing plaques as well as brain

Table 2.3 Prognostic indicators in MS [41, 42]

	Favorable	Poor
Race	Caucasian	Black
Age at onset	Young (< 35 years)	Older (>35 years)
Gender	Female	Male
Tobacco abuse	No	Yes
First attack characteristics	Optic neuritis, sensory, unifocal	Motor, cerebellar, sphincter, multifocal incomplete
MRI lesion location	Cerebral	Spinal cord
Brain lesion burden	Low	High
Lesion enhancement on MRI	No	Yes
Recovery after relapse	Complete	Incomplete
Attack rate	Low	High (≥ 2 in 1 year)
MS subtype	Relapsing	Progressive
Disability at 5 years	No	Yes

atrophy in MS [46–48]. In contrast to the limitations encountered with the use of CT, MRI has had an important impact on both the diagnosis and subsequent management of MS because of the relative ease which it can detect white matter lesions in the brain and spinal cord.

Investigators have sought brain MRI correlations with clinical symptoms of MS, prognosis of the illness, other laboratory findings, as well as with central nervous system pathology. Increased T2 signal, reflecting increases in water content of lesions in hemispheric white matter, was emphasized in earlier studies, but their presence correlates poorly with symptoms and neurological findings (Fig. 2.1a). In our initial experience with this imaging modality, we found that very early in the course of clinical disease, only half of patients with clinically definite MS did have cerebral white matter lesions [47, 49]. However, almost half of those that did not have plaques in their brains exhibited spinal cord lesions that were clearly evident [50]. While, not all cerebrospinal fluids (CSF) had "diagnostic" abnormalities, only 5% of patients did not have either brain MRI abnormality or significant CSF abnormality. In part, the difficulty with the MRI findings in these early studies was related to technical issues such as image slice thickness, noncontiguous sections, etc. Use of fluid-attenuated inversion recovery (FLAIR) sequences, which are easier to visualize, has been made practicable by advances in the hardware and software (Fig. 2.1b). Newer acquisition paradigms and the use of gadolinium to identify "active" inflammatory lesions, in particular, as well as continued hardware improvements have remarkably improved the quality and utility of MRI. However, not all patients with MS, particularly those with PPMS, exhibit white matter lesions in their cerebral hemispheres. *The absence of MRI abnormality does not negate the diagnosis of MS* [9]. We found that after 9–12 years, the same proportion of MS patients will have white matter lesions evidence by MRI and by pathology, however [47, 49]. In a recent presentation from the Cleveland Clinic, Dr. Robert Fox revealed that

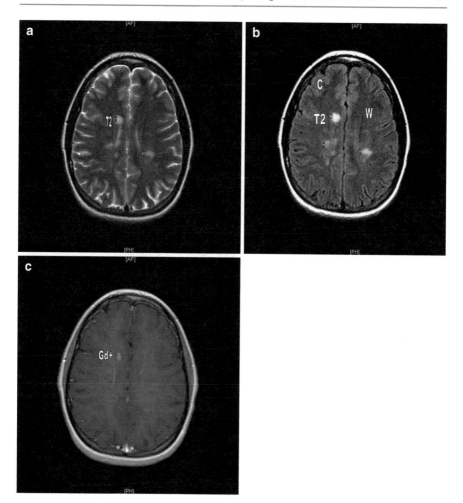

Fig. 2.1 MRI scans of the brain of a 19-year-old woman with relapsing-remitting multiple sclerosis. Axial T2-weighted (**a**) and fluid-attenuated inversion recovery (**b**) views show hyperintense lesions in subcortical white matter. Axial T1-weighted postcontrast (**c**) of the same patient reveals an enhancing lesion, indicating the breakdown of the blood-brain barrier

approximately 20% of their well-documented patients with progressive MS did not have hemispheric white matter lesions at necropsy [50]. They do, however, have cortical as well as spinal cord, i.e., "corticospinal" involvement. Cortical involvement in MS is rarely evident with standard imaging parameters. Double inversion recovery is capable of documenting about 40% of the cortical lesions found in pathological study [51].

A strong correlation between increased volume of cerebral MRI T2 signal and long-term disability in MS has been reported in patients followed for 5 years after the onset of a clinically isolated syndrome. However, further follow-up of this cohort of patients has shown only a moderate correlation at 10 years [52]. A number of short-term correlations between stabilization, or reduction, of T2 volumes and clinical stabilization in patients treated with each of the immunomodulatory drugs are currently approved. After the initial 5 years of illness, with some notable exceptions, changes from 1 year to the next are difficult to see in brain MRI scans. Clearly, there must be some reservation about the use of T2 lesion volumes for assessment of longer-term treatment of any kind.

Gadolinium enhancement of white matter lesions is an accepted indicator of active disease, but enhancing lesions are seen several times more often than acute exacerbations of illness in multiple sclerosis (Fig. 2.1c). This surrogate measure of disease activity has been used effectively in preliminary drug efficacy studies to detect a treatment effect. Despite the earlier negative reports, Leist et al. reported a correlation between gadolinium-enhancing lesions and the subsequent appearance of cerebral atrophy [53]. Unlike the earlier studies reporting on correlation, this NIH study was based on frequent (monthly) gadolinium-enhanced brain MRI studies.

Although T1 hypointensities have been reported to correlate with cerebral atrophy, other studies have shown that this type of MRI lesion does not correlate well with either the amount of demyelination or gliosis in tissue lesions. The lack of correlation with tissue changes makes it difficult to understand and accept these observations at face value [54, 55]. Importantly, De Stefano et al. have reported data supporting a role between early axonal damage and subsequent development of disability in multiple sclerosis [66].

Brain atrophy progresses at a rate of 0.5–1.0% per year in patients with MS, considerably higher than the typical rate seen with normal aging at 0.1–0.3% per year. Once thought to be largely a disease of white matter, MS is now recognized to have significant manifestations in the gray matter [56]. The volumetric changes seen on MRI during the course of MS have been correlated with disability progression and cognitive impairment; however, the quantitative cutoffs to determine physiologic versus pathological brain atrophy in MS remain to be determined.

No evidence of disease activity (NEDA) has been proposed as a potential treatment goal for treatment trials in MS. Elimination of relapses and prevention of disease progression, including cognitive loss and impaired ambulation, are the clinical goals (Fig. 2.2).

NEDA-3 includes (1) no sustained increase in disability lasting 3 months, (2) no relapses, and (3) no MRI activity, defined as no new or enlarging T2 and Gad+ lesions. NEDA-4 includes similar parameters, with the addition of no annual brain volume loss >0.4%. NEDA-3 status appears to correlate with subsequent relapse and focal inflammatory MRI activity. NEDA-4, in utilizing measures for tissue destruction at both the focal inflammatory and diffuse level, may be a more comprehensive predictor for subsequent disability-related outcomes. NEDA-4 data has been collected using post hoc analyses of the FREEDOMS and FREEDOMS-II trials [57, 58].

More advanced imaging methods continue to be explored. Double inversion recovery (DIR) can be used to demonstrate cortical inflammatory lesions, although its use is limited by inadequate resolution and inability to identify purely intracortical, versus juxtacortical or leukocortical, lesions [51]. Diffusion tensor imaging

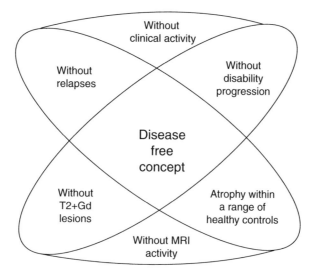

Fig. 2.2 Disease-free concept: NEDA-4

(DTI) is used to evaluate the structural integrity of the white matter tracts. DTI can be used for diffusivity measures including mean diffusivity and fractional anisotropy, which may provide even closer evaluation of tissue integrity and axonal damage [56, 59–61]. The value of proton magnetic resonance spectroscopy continues to be investigated and has resulted in many claims that are not entirely consistent. The advent of higher Tesla field strengths, up to ultrahigh-field 7–8 Tesla, has improved characterization of cortical demyelination, with good pathologic correlation but is restricted to research studies for safety reasons [62].

It is obvious that MRI is especially helpful in the evaluation of patients early in the course of their illness. Unfortunately, the question as to the utility of using MRI or other surrogate measures to evaluate the long-term response to treatment remains essentially unanswered. Cerebral atrophy may very well be the most valuable measure.

Other Laboratory Measures

CSF CSF analysis can be helpful if performed in a specialty laboratory. Increased intrathecal IgG synthesis, measurement of the increase in the proportion of gamma globulin by CSF electrophoresis, and the presence of CSF oligoclonal bands increase the likelihood of a diagnosis of MS [7–9, 11]. *Neurofilament chains* are potential markers for axonal injury as seen in gadolinium-enhancing lesions in RRMS and progressive forms of MS [63, 64].

Glial Fibrillary Acidic Protein (GFAP) Concentration CSF GFAP is raised in SPMS and associated with expanded disability status scale (EDSS) scores [65].

Evoked Response Testing Visual evoked responses carried out in an established laboratory too can be helpful in making a diagnosis [9]. Other evoked responses, brain stem and somatosensory, can be abnormal in other diseases as well as MS, and the studies are technically more difficult. Spinocerebellar degenerations are often associated with markedly abnormal auditory evoked potentials, for example.

Epidemiology

To yield useful data epidemiological studies must be carried out by trained personnel in large populations with good access to good medical care. A number of good studies have been performed, and there is evidence indicating that incidence rates for MS may be increasing.

Age and Sex Distribution Multiple sclerosis of the relapsing-remitting type is more common in women, about 70% of all patients in most recently studied populations, including our large southern population, with onset of illness in both sexes by the age of 30 in two-thirds [11]. Primary progressive MS is slightly more common in men and typically begins in midlife.

Incidence of MS Incidence is the rate of occurrence of newly diagnosed (MS) cases per unit of population (usually described per million) per time period, usually reported on an annual basis. The incidence of MS is relatively low (1–5 per million) but seems to have increased over the last century [11]. In the United States the most useful current data comes from Olmsted County, Minnesota, where the incidence rate increased during the last century from two per million to three times that incidence [11].

A number of confounding factors influence incidence figures. Over the last half century, there has been a dramatic increase in the number of trained neurologists. With the advent of effective therapies, more neurologists are interested in MS and many trained in this subspecialty. Consistent easily interpreted diagnostic criteria, and improved diagnostic testing (especially MRI), have greatly facilitated making the diagnosis. Undoubtedly, these factors partly account for the apparent increased incidence of multiple sclerosis. If we can extrapolate from the experience of neuropathologists, and as reported from Stanford, 1–2% of postmortem examinations reveal tissue evidence of "demyelinating disease" in the absence of a clinical history [66, 67]. It is possible that now, given the availability of neurologists, the increasing awareness of MS, and the diagnostic facilities available, many clinically undiagnosed cases in the past would be labeled as having MS.

Despite the low incidence of MS, this illness is the most common cause of chronic disability in young adults because of the minimal impact on the longevity currently. The observations in Olmsted County, Minnesota, clearly indicate a real increase in the incidence, as well as its prevalence, of MS [9].

It is often stated that there are 250,000–350,000 MS patients in the United States [11]. Figures currently used, however, are not based on any current national epidemiological studies. When prevalence figures were reported to be low for the Southern United States, except for California, there were no neurologists in the South. In Florida, for example, the first neurologist established a practice in Florida in 1953 but then entered the military service, a situation similar to many other areas in the South. The appearance of neurologists in the South since that time, as in virtually all under-serviced communities in the United States, is bound to have had a dramatic impact on the recognition and diagnosis of nervous system disease, especially MS. The impact of MRI on the recognition of neurological disease has been dramatic, especially for MS. Considering the increased availability of neurological consultation, improved diagnostic criteria and the availability to MRI, and improved CSF examination, that larger numbers of MS patients will be recognized in life. The quoted prevalence of MS appears to be unrealistically low.

Environmental Factors   Myriad environmental risk factors for MS have been studied with varying degrees of validation. The most robust data supports the association of *prior Epstein-Barr virus infection and smoking* and development of MS [68]. The significant detrimental effect of smoking has been identified in numerous studies, with a dose-response relationship [69, 70]. Previous infection with EBV and high antibody titers to Epstein-Barr early nuclear antigen are well-established risk factors for MS, especially when contracted as an adolescent or young adult [71, 72].

Other epidemiological factors, which may be associated with an increased risk of MS, include *increased salt intake*. Kleinewietfeld et al. demonstrated that elevated sodium chloride concentrations in human (dietary) and mouse (tissue culture followed by studies of dietary intake) models increase proinflammatory Th17 cells [73, 74]. *Vitamin D* may be an early predictor MS activity and progression, though identification of the optimal Vitamin D supplementation strategies remains undetermined [75]. Unpublished follow-up data beyond 10 years of Aschiero's study group of vitamin D shows maintenance of long-term benefit with vitamin D levels greater than 50 nmol/L. High-dose supplementation with 10,400 IU cholecalciferol daily has been reported as safe [76]. *Adolescent obesity*, defined as a BMI of $> 27 \text{ kg/m}^2$ at age 20, is associated with a twofold increased risk of developing MS. Further study has indicated an interaction between adolescent obesity and HLA risk genes in MS [77, 78].

There is a *geographical pattern distribution* of MS, with higher disease incidence in higher latitudes, though this has become less apparent in recent years in the setting of globalization [79]. In this context, the "hygiene hypothesis" was introduced by Strachan in the 1980s. It proposes that persons with less exposure to microbes early in life are more likely to develop autoimmune disorders, including MS [80]. This hypothesis has fallen out of favor, however, as a result of several studies evaluating MS incidence and helminthic infection, and the role of the *gut microbiome* in MS has become a focus of research. Nonpathogenic intestinal microflora may be mediators of autoimmunity in MS [81–85]. There is no longer evidence for a north-south gradient for MS in the United States.

Pathology of Multiple Sclerosis

Charcot recognized *multiple* areas of discoloration and hardness (*sclerosis*) scattered throughout the brain and spinal cord which he termed *plaques* (plate like) as the cardinal features of MS: hence, the diagnosis of *sclerose en plaque*, or "multiple sclerosis" [1]. By microscopy, Charcot found that plaques exhibited loss of myelin with relative sparing of axons and varying amounts of gliotic scarring. He also described the presence of inflammatory cells, including large numbers of fat-laden cells. The demyelinated plaque remains the pathological hallmark of this disease [85].

Early in the disease small plaques are prominent in subcortical white matter [42], but in the usual necropsy material obtained after many years of disease, large coalesced plaques are predominantly periventricular [85–89]. No regular association between MS plaques and blood vessels was observed by Adams and Kubik [87] and Zimmerman and Netsky [88]. Subsequently, however, Lampert [89], and others, performed whole brain serial sections of a number of cases, including those previously studied and reported that brain *plaques were invariably perivenular* [89]. Although oligodendrocyte loss had earlier been reported as a major feature of MS [87, 88], study of whole brain serial sections did not reveal this to be a consistent feature [89]. Another important finding is that so-called shadow plaques seen at the white matter cortical junction are areas of remyelination, rather than areas of incomplete demyelination, as had previously thought [85].

In recent years, the neuropathology of MS has been revisited [90–92], and a new view of the histopathology of MS has emerged based on a study of 51 biopsies and 37 autopsies. A central role for CD4+ T cells and macrophages in the immuno-pathogenesis of the multiple sclerosis lesions seemed to have been well established (Fig. 2.3) [91]. Lucchinetti et al., however, have suggested four different types of neuropathology in MS, pointing to a predominant role for CD3+ cells and macrophages in type 1, with antibody-mediated demyelination added in type 2, and to loss of oligodendrocytes in others [93].

In type 1, in patients where tissue samples were obtained very early, prominent perivascular infiltrates composed of CD3+ cells and macrophages were present without IgG or complement. In type 2, a similar perivascular picture was seen, except that antibody (IgG) and complement, without cells, were seen at the edge of active demyelination. While prominent loss of myelin basic protein and myelin-associated glycoprotein was found, remyelination was reported to be prominent in types 1 and 2. In type 3 and 4, oligodendrocyte loss was prominent, raising the question of primary oligodendrocyte pathology. Plaques were poorly defined and not related to vessels. However, the authors reported that CD3+ (T) cells and macrophages were present in all four types of multiple sclerosis pathology included in their classification contain, a finding in keeping with other recent analysis of lesions [93]. Their findings that tissue obtained from a small number of patients studied shortly after onset of their illness revealed prominent CD3+ (T) cells and macrophage cellular infiltrates but lacked antibody (type 1) are reminiscent of the findings of patients who died early in the course of their illness, reported by Lumsden [86].

Type 2, where antibody is present in the lesions, is seen at necropsy with some frequency and resembles changes seem in chronic relapsing forms of EAE. In EAE the initial cellular infiltrate is composed primarily of CD4+ cells initially, but this is followed by the appearance of much large numbers of macrophages that induce the damage to myelin and oligodendrocytes [94].

Despite the impressive amount of work their report encompasses [93], the observations that in a proportion of cases the pathology of MS may consist of oligodendrocyte loss, with pathology not associated with blood vessels, raises questions. The numbers of cases are relatively small and many were biopsy specimens, where sampling necessarily was limited and most importantly not based on study of whole brain serial sections. Poser had raised other questions about type 1 pathology [95]. Recently, in 20 patients of a subset of well-documented subset of 150 progressive MS patients without cerebral white matter lesions, pathological evaluation revealed the presence of cortical pathology with an inflammatory component extending from the meninges into the cortex [50]. Spinal cord root entry zone pathology can lead to debilitating pain in MS patients and are rarely identified by neuroimaging [96, 97].

Pathogenesis of Multiple Sclerosis

Genetics

In the past few years, our understanding of the genetic underpinnings of MS has exploded due to the advent of large genome-wide association studies (GWAS). Clustering within families is a well-known phenomenon. Prior to the recent advances, it was found that in a large MS database in Vancouver and our large database in South Florida, a 20% familial incidence was present in both data sets. The Canadian twin study shows a concordance of 31%, similar to other twin studies [98]. Mothers confer a 20–40 times increased risk to their children, greater for girls than boys. Other first-degree relatives also have a much-increased risk of MS [99].

As of press time, more than 159 genetic variants have been associated with an increased risk of developing MS [100, 101]. For several decades, the major histocompatibility (MHC) gene locus located on chromosome 6 has been implicated, and it is clear that the HLA-DRB1 gene in the class II region of the MHC explains up to 10.5% of the genetic variance underlying risk of MS. A monumental linkage study, conducted by the International Multiple Sclerosis Consortium, evaluated 730 families with multiple cases of MS, further emphasized the role of the major histocompatibility (MHC) class II HLA-DRB1*15:01 allele, as the only variant of several genetic loci to achieve statistical significance [102]. Mouse studies also implicate a strong genetic susceptibility for experimental allergic encephalomyelitis (EAE) localized to the region of DQBq*602 [103]. The more complete characterization of MHC contribution to MS and identification of variants outside the MHC region were not appreciated until the advent of the era of GWAS. Using large

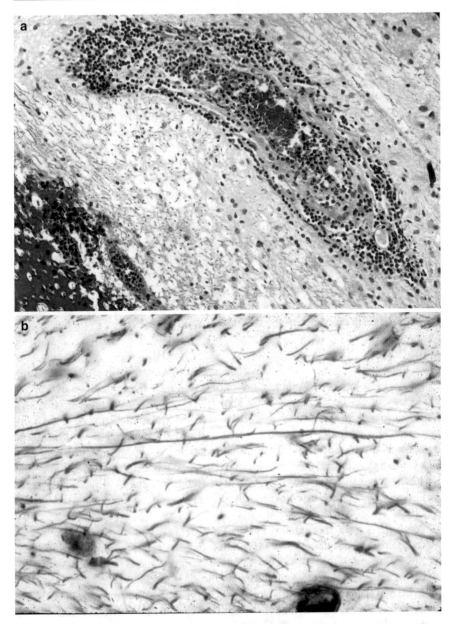

Fig. 2.3 Biopsy of a large left frontal lobe plaque from a 29-year-old woman with new onset multiple sclerosis with recurrent right hemiparesis over 3 months and new mild speech difficulty. (**a**) Specimen is stained with Luxol fast blue counterstained with eosin. A new active plaque is shown which is not sharply demarcated but exhibits prominent perivascular cellularity with varying myelin damage and relative sparing of axons. The inflammatory infiltrate is composed of lymphocytes (predominantly CD4 Th₁ cells) and a large number of macrophages. These cells are predominantly of hematogenous origin and are considered the perpetrators of tissue damage. These features are in contrast to chronic or inactive plaques which exhibit relatively few or no inflammatory cells but contain prominent myelin damage and gliosis. Axonal loss may be prominent. (**b**) *Frontal lobe biopsy*: Luxol fast blue counterstained with eosin. Higher power view showing loss of axons and more prominent myelin loss. Note that axons that are preserved exhibit variable loss of myelin

sample sizes, the largest of which numbered 80,095 subjects, this technique identified 110 non-MHC risk variants in 103 loci. Interestingly, 78% of predicted MS heritability remains undetermined [104]. Improving whole-genome sequencing technologies hold promise to identify rare genetic variants.

A limited number of causative gene variants have been identified. The MS-associated SNP rs6897932, located in the alternatively spliced exon 6 of IL-7Rα, alters the ratio between the soluble and membrane-bound isoforms of the protein by disrupting an exonic splicing enhancer [105]. The risk variant rs1800693 in the tumor necrosis factor (TNF) 1A gene that drives the expression of a novel soluble form of the receptor that can inhibit TNF signaling mimics the effects of TNF-blocking drugs that are known to exacerbate MS pathology [106]. Other variants include rs3453644, acting at the tyrosine kinase 2 protein, and rs12487066 associated with decreased levels of human endogenous retrovirus Casitas B-lineage lymphoma proto-oncogene B in CD4+ T cells [107, 108]. The underlying pathogenic mechanisms for these variants remain unclear. The current collaborative studies arose from early findings by Jersild et al. who found that the alleles A3, B7, and DR2 [109] occurred twice as commonly in MS as compared with the unaffected population. They observed that in patients that possessed both HLA-B7 and DR2, that disease was particularly severe [109]. Many genes important in normal immune function and in immune-mediated tissue damage, such as tumor necrosis factor, are located in the region between HLA-B7 and the DR locus. Several mutations of genes resident in this area are currently being studied. An important study looking for single nucleotide polymorphisms (SNP), modeled on the Crohn's disease study, is currently under way as part of the human genome project. As yet there is no single gene, or combination of genes, implicated in the risk or causation of MS.

Once disease-causing gene variants are identified, the next step is to identify biomarkers that can predict disease progression. Our understanding of the factors leading to neurodegeneration and increased disability in progressive MS remains limited, and genetics may shed significant light on this process.

Several reports have described familial clustering of MS phenotype. The presence of the HLA-B*44 allele is thought to be associated with better neuroimaging outcomes [110]. Variants associated with age of onset and a range of radiologic outlooks include HLA-DRB1*15:01, HLA-DRB1*07:01 and HLA-DRB1*11:04, and HLA-DRB1*01:03 [111–114]. The absence of HLA-B5 independently associates with a marked increase in the severity of MS, as in the Afro-American population [110]. Future directions for pharmacogenetics research in MS include identification of specific genetic variants associated with treatment response, leading to a tailored therapy approach. SNP genotype data led to the discovery of several HLA genes and may be used to identify IFN-β super-responders. An important recent study found an association between the rs9828519 variants, which is intronic to SLC9A9 and implicated as a regulator of proinflammatory lymphocyte activation and MS disease response and nonresponse to IFN-β [115, 116].

Studies of migrant populations have suggested the presence of an environmental factor. Although generally interpreted as evidence that a viral infection is playing a role in multiple sclerosis, no conclusive evidence of a specific virus playing a role in multiple sclerosis has been produced [11, 71, 117, 118].

Myelin Biochemistry

The genetic basis of a number of leukodystrophies has been firmly established. Of these disorders, the most common are adrenocortical leukodystrophy and metachromatic leukodystrophy. At one time both were considered to have some relationship to MS [2, 11]. Of some importance is Marburg's disease, sometimes referred to as "acute multiple sclerosis," which has been attributed to a defect in myelin basic protein (MBP) synthesis and structure [119]. Work on alterations of the 3D structure of MBP and relationship to various demyelinating disease continues. Interestingly, several mutations of the proteolipid of myelin are causative of Pelizaeus-Merzbacher disease, another leukodystrophy, as well as several types of hereditary spastic paraparesis. These disorders ordinarily should not be confused with MS because of early age of presentation of the leukodystrophies, their inexorably progressive course, and their familial setting.

Immunology

Multiple sclerosis is now generally accepted as an immune-mediated illness although its pathogenesis is incompletely understood. The occurrence of MS following about a third of cases of acute disseminated encephalomyelitis complicating infections [120–122] as well as after immunizations, including Semple vaccine (containing spinal cord and killed virus), suggested an autoimmune origin. Although EAE has been studied in animal models for decades, the primary impetus was to elucidate the nature of the immune response [123]. These studies have also provided insight into the pathogenesis of MS as well. Transfer of EAE from immunized to naive animals was first successfully accomplished using lymph node cells but not antibody, thus pointing to a central role for lymphocytes [123]. Nevertheless, antibody from immunized animals, and patients with MS, can induce demyelination in vitro [60, 61].

T cells play a primary role in the pathogenesis of EAE, irrespective of the nervous system antigen used to induce disease [124–127]. A consensus has developed that T cells are the primary effectors both in MS and in EAE [127]. Nevertheless, B cells, plasma cells, and antibody can be found both in EAE pathology and in MS plaques [92, 93]. Despite their emphasis on other findings, these recent studies of pathology in MS show that the predominant cells in active lesions are lymphocytes, in particular CD3+ T cells, and macrophages [93].

Multiple injections of the whole spinal cord were used to induce EAE in early studies, but single immunizations of equivalent amounts of purified myelin or MBP combined with adjuvants were shown to be very effective in disease induction [127]. Myelin proteins other than MBP have also been investigated, notably proteolipid and myelin oligodendrocyte glycoprotein (MOG). Proteolipid protein can induce forms of experimental disease in animal models and, although antibody as well as T cells reactive to this antigen may be present in plaques, no role for sensitization to this antigen has been established [127]. However, an interesting EAE model in marmosets induced using MOG indicates that antibody may mediate demyelination [128, 129]. Passive transfer of the disease by serum from MOG-sensitized animals has been accomplished [129]. However, T cells (CD4+ Th2, rather than CD4+ Th1 cells) may be the primary mediators of myelin damage in MOG-sensitized marmosets [129]. The situation is complicated by the fact that CD4+ cells reactive to MBP, capable of inducing EAE, are present in naive animals as well as in these immunized animals coincidently with anti-MOG antibody [129]. Anti-MOG antibody has been reported at the outset of MS and is common in RRMS [130, 131]. In contrast to anti-MOG antibody being limited to MS relapse, CD4+ cells reactive to MOG are ubiquitous [132].

Antigen presentation by MHC class I or MHC class II by antigen-presenting cells (APC) to T cells results in the initiation of immune responses: antibody production or a cellular immune response. Activated CD4+ T helper (Th) cells fall into three functionally distinct classes, Th1 and Th2, and Th17 with distinctive profiles of lymphokine production. Following antigenic stimulation CD4+ Th1 cells produce interleukin-1 (IL-1), IL-2, IFN-γ, and tumor necrosis factor α (TNF-α) are postulated to mediate inflammatory pathological processes in immune-mediated tissue damage seen in MS and EAE [133]. In contrast, Th2 cells produce IL-4, IL-5, IL-6, and IL-10 and induce upregulation of antibody production and downregulation of Th1 cellular responses (Fig. 2.4) [133]. The observed failure of increased production of the regulatory cytokine IL-10, by myelin-reactive T cells in MS by Ozenci et al. in Sweden, has recently been confirmed by Cao et al. at MIT [134, 135]. More recently a role for Th17 helper cells in a large subpopulation of MS patients has been identified and characterized. Sera from interferon-β-1a treatment failure patients from Denmark were shown to contain IL-17F. Naive patients that had IL-17F and elevated levels of endogenous INF-β failed to respond to IFN-β-1a subsequently also. These IFN-β failure MS patients resemble EAE animals induced by Th17-polarized cells [136, 137].

Macrophages are the principal sources of IL-1, IL-12, and TNF-α, driven by IL-2 production from antigen-activated CD4+ cells. Importantly, IL-12 production is IFN-γ dependent and TNF-α production is IL-12 dependent [138]. Traditionally the macrophage was considered to be the principal APC, but B cells are now recognized as important in this task. However, macrophages are central effector cells in cell-mediated immunity. After antigen presentation, CD4+ cells respond by clonal proliferation and recruitment of other CD4+ cells to participate in the initiation of cellular immune responses. Cytotoxic CD8+ cells, driven by IL-12, may exert their effect directly or target antibody complexed with antigen on target tissue, i.e., *antibody-dependent cytotoxicity* [127, 139]. Macrophages may also target these complexes. The spectrum of CD4+ Th2 responses includes a regulatory role in switching of CD8+ cell cytotoxic function to active suppression of CD4 Th1 responses, *suppressor T cells*. In the CNS microglial cells can function as APC and exhibit certain other macrophage behaviors including an anti-inflammatory response.

The blood-brain barrier (BBB) is a physical barrier that prevents intravascular cellular elements, antibodies, and other proteins free access to the brain and spinal cord [138]. The endothelial cells in the brain and spinal cord possess tight junctions

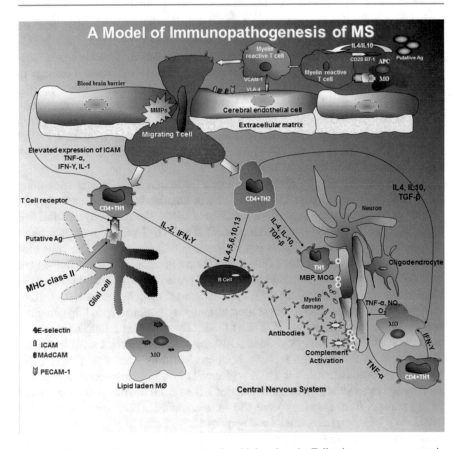

Fig. 2.4 A model of immunopathogenesis of multiple sclerosis. Following exposure to certain environmental antigen(s) in genetically susceptible individuals, myelin-reactive T cells migrate from peripheral circulation to the central nervous system. Interaction between activated T cell and cerebral endothelial cells leads to upregulation of the adhesion molecules (E-selectin, vascular cell adhesion molecule, intercellular adhesion molecule, mucosal addressin cell adhesion molecule, and platelet endothelial cells adhesion molecule). Transendothelial migration of reactive T cells is heralded by the disruption of the blood-brain barrier, which is in part mediated by the activities of the matrix metalloproteinases. Matrix metalloproteinases digest the activated T cells (such as TNF-α and IFN-γ) and upregulate the expression of cell surface molecules on antigen-presenting cells (in this figure, glial cell). Binding of putative multiple sclerosis antigen (e.g., myelin basic protein and myelin oligodendrocyte glycoprotein) by the trimolecular complex T-cell receptor and class II major histocompatibility molecules on the antigen-presenting cells precipitates a massive inflammatory cascade, which leads to production of both pro- and anti-inflammatory cytokines. This inflammatory reaction ultimately results in loss of myelin-oligodendrocyte complexes

that are impervious to intravascular fluids as well as nonactivated cells. These endothelial cells are also surrounded by astrocytic foot processes that further support and maintain the integrity of the BBB. However, activated CD4+ cells do cross the BBB [140–145]. However, the BBB is an actual physical barrier which may be breached only in an organized and well-orchestrated fashion [140, 145, 146]. The mechanisms of cellular transmigration across the blood-brain barrier are now well understood [140–146].

Interleukin-17 and Type 17 Helper T Cells

T cells were found to produce cytokines that could not be classified into either the Th1 or Th2 scheme detailed above. Primary among these cytokines is interleukin-17 (IL-17), and the cells that produce IL-17A have been named Th17 cells. Other cytokines produced include IL-17F, IL-21 and IL-22, IL-26, and TNFα. Their important role in the pathogenesis of MS is increasingly recognized [147, 148]. In vitro studies have suggested that Th17 cells can permeate the blood-brain barrier, and elevated levels of IL-17 have been detected both in serum and CSF in some patients with MS [149]. In addition, an increase in IL-17 mRNA has been detected in MS plaques at autopsy [150, 151]. Th17 cells can induce and regulate tissue inflammation. In the setting of chronic inflammation and autoimmunity, initially studied in rheumatoid arthritis, signaling through Th17 receptors induces production of inflammatory cytokines such as IL-6, IL-1, TNF, IL-8, and matrix metalloproteinases [147]. A recent study has implicated glutamate excitotoxicity as a possible effector mechanism for inflammation in MS [152]. Studies to elucidate the role of Th17 cells in MS are ongoing. Secukinumab, a selective anti-IL-17A monoclonal antibody, is being studied as a potential treatment for MS [153].

Adhesion Molecules

Venules control CD4+ and other cell migration from blood into the nervous system. Attachment requires cellular adhesion molecules and endothelial counter receptors to overcome the considerable shear stresses produced by blood flow. Adhesion molecules on CD4+ cells and macrophages act as functional anchors forming stable bonds with their ligands on the vascular wall. In addition to functioning as mechanical anchors, adhesion molecules function as tissue-specific recognition molecules [140–146].

Entry of CD4+ cells and macrophages into the CNS is accomplished by a series of steps including tethering or rolling, adhesion (binding), and finally transendothelial migration across the BBB [141–146]. Subsequent to their egress, they migrate through the extracellular matrix in the CNS. Selectins mediate the initial step of tethering leading to rolling [146, 154, 155] but selectin-mediated bonds are reversible. To arrest these cells on the endothelium, these low-affinity interactions must be supplemented by high-affinity adhesion molecules, the integrins [153, 154]. The integrins, including α4β1-integrin (VLA-4), are members of the endothelial immunoglobulin superfamily [156, 157]. The predominant function of the β2-integrin leukocyte function antigen-1 (LFA-1) and α4-integrins (integrin-α4β1/VLA-4) is to bind the cells to their ligands intercellular adhesion molecule-1 (ICAM-1) and vascular cell adhesion molecule (VCAM-1) [155–157]. Blocking of attachment of the α4 moiety on lymphocytes by natalizumab is highly effective treatment in MS but is complicated by a risk of progressive multifocal leukoencephalopathy (PML) [158].

Selectins expressed on leukocytes (P-selectin and L-selectin) and endothelium (E-selectin) result in rolling and slowing of the cells. P-selectin and its ligand PECAM-1 appear to play a special role in EAE and MS [159, 160]. As cells roll and are slowed by the interaction of selectins and their ligands, they respond to endothelial cell chemokines. Specific chemokines are fixed on the endothelial surface and are molecular signals that direct cells to tissues and with specific adhesion molecules confer organ specificity [145]. Chemokines are divided into four families that are specific for different T-cell subgroups [145]. Distinctive chemokine receptors on Th1 cells include CCR5 and CXCR3. In MS, all of the infiltrating Th1 cells express these chemokine receptors [161]. They play a central role in the egress of specific lymphocyte subgroups into specific target organs. Selectin binding to ligand is an activating signal that induces rapid activation of α4-integrins and β2-integrins [155–157].

From the first availability of IFN-β, about half of the population placed on this drug did not appear to benefit from it. In a prospective study, Byun and coworkers found that half of MS patients placed on IFN-β were "super-responders" [162]. They found that a number of genes were expressed in this super-responder subpopulation following their first dosage, and this predicted the clinical response. Interestingly, these genes included heparan proteoglycans [160]. Further support for the identification of IFN-β responder/nonresponder populations followed with a report by Axtell et al. in 2010 [136]. They reported that serum from Danish IFN-β-1a nonresponders contained IL-17. Most recently the evidence correlating response or nonresponse to IFN-β to polymorphisms of a specific gene rs9828519, a sodium-hydrogen channel, has been published [115]. Apart from illuminating the mechanisms of the drug response, these observations hopefully will help identify potential "super-responders" and assist in advising them in regard to their therapeutic choices for MS. This should reduce the human and financial cost of treatment failure in managing MS.

T-cell vaccine studies are continuing. The initial approach was to remove immunocompetent cells from patients by immunizing them with antigen analogous to V-beta chains of T-cell receptors that are capable recognizing encephalitogenic fragments of MBP. More recent studies have focused on using CNS antigen-stimulated cells from the patient's own T-cell repertoire and, following irradiation, infusing these *autoreactive* cells back into the donors. There has been a remarkable impact on reducing sustained progression of disability patients with RRMS, and the current study is hoping to replicate these findings in patients with SPMS. A preliminary report in RRMS was encouraging for progressive MS [163].

Treatment of Multiple Sclerosis

Treatment issues in MS generally fall into four categories. These are (1) symptomatic treatment; (2) treatment of acute MS exacerbations; (3) reducing the risk ("prevention") of future exacerbations and, more importantly, reducing the risk of sustained increases in disability; and (4) neurological rehabilitation. In recent years there have been advances in each of these four areas.

In the past, treatment of MS was limited to empirical management of symptoms, i.e., symptomatic treatment. Most treatments were untested and were of questionable value, at best. Interested readers are referred to the Diary of Augustus D'Este where descriptions of treatments employed are recounted [3]. Treatments were really generic, ineffective, and sometimes dangerous remedies such as cathartics, enemas, and bloodletting. Many ineffective empirical treatments continue to be offered by misguided individuals and quacks.

Symptomatic Treatment

Symptomatic treatment covers many areas, but only a few specific issues will be dealt with in this review. Fatigue, spasticity, and bladder symptoms are among the most important areas. Also important is the management of the paroxysmal disorders: paroxysmal dystonia, paroxysmal akinesia, paroxysmal dysarthria, trigeminal neuralgia, facial myokymia, and hemifacial spasm. Treatment can be dramatically effective.

Fatigue is a prominent complaint in the majority of patients. In reality, the fatigue of which patients complain is predominantly fatigability, although the occasional patients with severe exacerbations may awaken with overwhelming fatigue. The first drug for fatigue to be evaluated in double-blind trials (and shown to effective) was amantadine HCl (Symmetrel®) [164]. A dose of 100 mg twice daily is an effective antiviral, initially virtually preventing all influenza type A infections and 90% of type B infections and a lower but important risk reduction for other paramyxovirus infections. The sustained reduction of fatigue observed in the majority of patients is presumably due to its weak dopamine agonist properties, rather than an antiviral effect. In addition, a variety of adrenergic drugs have been used to treat fatigue, but tolerance tends to develop quickly and habituation is also problem [165]. Modafinil (Provigil®), a more selective member of this family of drugs appears safe and tolerated in small (200 mg) daily doses [166]. Unfortunately, in our experience, tolerance seems to develop quickly too. A matter of concern is that in vitro adrenergic drugs appear to promote cellular immune mechanisms, calling into question their use in fatigue management. Fatigue and depression commonly coexist, and fluoxetine (Prozac®) is commonly used to manage these patients. Interestingly, fluoxetine has immunomodulatory properties, with resultant increases in the Th2 lymphokines, IL-4, and TGFβ [167]. Fatigue lessens in patients who stabilize clinically, spontaneously, or in conjunction with immunomodulatory therapy.

Mobility

Dalfampridine (Ampyra®) was approved in 2010 for the improvement of walking ability. It is a nonspecific potassium channel blocker that is thought to improve conduction in focally demyelinated axons by delaying repolarization and prolonging duration of action potentials. Enhanced neuronal conduction is thought to strengthen skeletal muscle fiber twitch activity, resulting in improved motor function [168–170].

Spasticity continues to be a major problem in MS patients [2]. Diazepam (Valium®) was the first drug to be proven to reduce spasticity in MS, and it continues to be a very helpful drug. The use of single oral dose of 5 mg at bedtime is convenient and cost-effective treatment in a large proportion of patients with mild-to-moderate spasticity. Occasionally, a small additional dose can be added in the morning, but the long half-life of the drug usually makes that unnecessary or undesirable. Baclofen (Lioresal®) is an important and useful drug that is less frequently associated with sedation than diazepam, even at high doses. The oral form of the drug, which is a racemic mixture, does not seem to have a predictable dose response in many patients, however. In contrast, those patients with severe refractory spasticity predictably respond to intrathecal baclofen [171]. This, in part, reflects the addition of l-baclofen to the racemic forms of baclofen for intrathecal use. Use of the intrathecal drug requires the implantation of a pump to deliver the drug, however [171]. Tizanidine (Zanaflex®), an alpha-2-adrenergic agonist, has good dose-response characteristics [122]. On the negative side, tizanidine has a short half-life and 40% of patients experience prominent fatigue and dry mouth as side effects. In some patients use of tizanidine avoids the necessity of pump implantation and therefore is a welcome alternative [172]. Hopefully, in the future an oral formulation of l-baclofen will advance to phase III studies and become a clinical option.

Bladder dysfunction occurs in the majority of patients, largely due to hyperreflexia of the detrusor muscle. However, dyssynergia accompanies this in 90% of cases. Managing urinary frequency is usually attempted with the use of low doses of anticholinergic and oral baclofen, but is often unsatisfactory. Often a single dosage of an anticholinergic drug before retiring at night and prior to occasional social outings is more satisfactory than a multiple doses. Incomplete emptying is usually best handed by intermittent catheterization. The management of infections is very important. Avoidance of antibiotics for unproven infections, and obtaining bacterial sensitivities for each infection, is crucial to avoid pseudomonas infections. Often chronic use of oral ascorbic acid 2–4 g daily with hippuric acid 2 g daily to acidify the urine together with six to eight glasses of water successfully prevents recurrent infections. Mirabegron (Myrbetriq®) is a remarkable new adrenergic drug for hyperreflexic bladder with incontinence [173].

More extensively studied in spinal cord injury, botulinum toxin A has recently been approved as an effective alternative for uncontrolled neurogenic detrusor overactivity resulting in incontinence in patients with MS [174, 175]. It is clear that good bladder management significantly contributes to quality of life [176].

Management of the paroxysmal disorders is relatively simple in most patients once they are recognized and identified by physicians [2]. Paroxysmal dystonia (or tonic spasms), paroxysmal akinesia, trigeminal neuralgia, facial myokymia, and hemifacial spasm are often successfully managed with modest doses of anticonvulsant drugs. However, the response in patients with paroxysmal dysarthria tends is less predictable. For patients requiring treatment, carbamazepine in doses of 100 mg orally three times daily controls about 70% of these disorders and 400 mg daily increases the response rate to 80–85%. Higher doses sometimes are helpful but the addition of a second anticonvulsant is often more effective. Some patients require two or more drugs, including gabapentin and topiramate, to control these symptoms, but often carbamazepine can be withdrawn if the second drug is effective [177]. The use of corticotrophin (ACTH) intravenously or intramuscularly, but not steroids, is sometimes necessary to gain control of the situation [178].

Treatment of Acute Exacerbations

In the past management of MS exacerbations consisted principally of continuous enforced rest [2]. At the onset of an exacerbation, rest relieves (or prevents) fatigue. Thankfully, the injudicious use of extended periods of rest has given way to the enthusiastic use of physical rehabilitation.

The senior author's career has spanned the era of validation and FDA approval of corticotrophin (adrenocorticotropic hormone/ACTH) [122] and the subsequent introduction and use of high-dose intravenous steroids for the management of exacerbations of multiple sclerosis. Dr. Leo Alexander, Harvard Medical School, initially used corticotrophin because steroids (that he hypothesized should be helpful) were not available (personal communication). The effectiveness of corticotrophin was established by multiple controlled trials, the first for any MS treatment [178]. The pivotal trial was a multicenter double-blind placebo-controlled trial was published in Neurology 1970 and became the basis of the FDA approval in 1978. No other drug has been validated as an effective treatment for exacerbations of MS. However, 40 years ago neurologists at the Montreal Neurological Institute, including the senior author with other MS physicians, first employed high-dose intravenous steroids in patients diagnosed with MS. The use of high-dose parenteral steroids was limited to patients who had lost vision, in one or both eyes due to optic neuritis, or who were acutely paraplegic due to acute myelitis. In retrospect, these patients probably had neuromyelitis optica rather than MS. On the basis of the analogy with trauma and tumor management, it was hypothesized that that acute severe edematous swelling of the optic nerve or spinal cord resulted in complicating ischemia due to the limited capacity to expand within the dura spaces. Although patients often improved rapidly, frequent complications of high-dose therapy problems were encountered. Gastrointestinal complications are now rare, but psychiatric disturbances, infectious complications, osteoporosis, and aseptic necrosis of the hip and other bones which are side effects are not rare. Despite weak evidence of benefit from the single-blind (intravenous) optic neuritis treatment trial indicating short-term benefit [178, 179], no well-organized appropriate sized, double-blind trials have been carried out to date. The double-blind oral steroid use portion of the optic neuritis trial showed clearly that oral *steroids were deleterious to patients with optic neuritis* (most of whom would develop clinically definite multiple sclerosis). *Patients receiving oral steroids subsequently experienced a doubled relapse rate of optic neuritis, apart from other manifestations of MS compared with oral placebo recipients.* A German trial has confirmed experimental observations of increased damage from the use of steroids equivalent to doses used in human [180]. In patient with optic neuritis treated with steroids, treatment is associated with damage to the affected optic nerve that can be reduced by the concomitant administration of erythropoietin [181]. We interpret these results as evidence that oral steroids, alone, should not be used in the management of MS. It is important to note that a neuroprotective effect for neurons from corticotrophin is well established [182–184]. Methylprednisolone, however, has recently been shown to induce programmed cell death (apoptosis) of neurons [180]. Because of the effectiveness, and the neuroprotective effect, of corticotrophin, we continue to favor its use.

A trial of natalizumab for the management of acute exacerbations failed to influence the outcome of such clinical exacerbations [185]. The drug, however, did reduce the risk of new MRI brain lesions over the subsequent 12 weeks following a single infusion. Despite its failure to induce a more rapid recovery from exacerbations, natalizumab did improve the sense of well-being of the drug recipients, also. Benefit was observed in subsequent studies aimed at reducing the risk of MS exacerbations and/or sustained increase in disability also.

Reduction of Multiple Sclerosis Exacerbations and Disability

For more than a decade and a half, there has been intensive study of several drugs and their potential value in reducing the risk of exacerbations in MS. As a corollary to this outcome, there has been increasing emphasis on their potential impact on reducing the risk of disability due to this disease. At press time, there are ten FDA-approved disease-modifying therapies for relapsing MS (see Table 2.4).

The first drug to be approved (1993) to reduce the frequency of MS exacerbations of (33% reduction) was IFN-β-1b (Betaseron®) [186, 187]. The drug also had a remarkable effect, significantly reducing the burden of disease as measured by brain MRI T2 lesion volumes [187]. Unfortunately, use of IFN-β-1b is consistently associated with flu-like symptoms and local inflammatory reaction at the injection site.

The drug IFN-β-1a is produced using mammalian cell lines and the authentic human genetic sequence, unlike IFN-β-1b that has two genetic alterations and which is made using coliform bacteria. IFN-β-1a is rapidly absorbed from the injection site and local reactions as well as neutralizing antibody formation are less. Avonex® brand of IFN-β-1a was approved in 1996 as a result of a study using 30 micrograms intramuscularly once weekly [188]. Risk of sustained disability for 24 weeks, the primary outcome measure, was reduced for drug recipients to 21.9 vs. 39.7% for placebo recipients in the study. Relapse risk was also reduced, 0.61 vs. 0.90 for those who completed the 104 weeks of the trial. However, data analysis employing "intent-to-treat analysis" showed a reduction in the risk of relapses with active drug treatment of 0.61 vs. 0.82 for placebo. The latter results reflect the fact that 40% of the patients did not complete the study because study drug was not available. Subsequently, the benefits on disability prevention were shown to be sustained [189].

A large three-arm pivotal (PRISMS) trial was reported in 2002, showing results resembling those reported for IFN-β-1b [190]. Subsequently, after additional

Table 2.4 Commonly used disease-modifying therapies in RRMS

Name of medication	Year of approval	Dosing regimen	Proposed mechanism of action	Important side effects
Injectables				
IFN-B-1α Avonex®	1996	Once a week; intramuscular injection; 30 mcg	Modulates T-cell and B-cell function, decreases expression of matrix metalloproteinases, interferes with blood-brain barrier disruption, alters expression of cytokines [121]	Flu-like symptoms, depression, anemia, elevated LFTs, allergic reactions
IFN-B-1α Rebif®	1996	Three times a week; subcutaneous injection; 44 mcg	As above	Flu-like symptoms, injection site reactions, blood dyscrasias, depression, elevated LFTs, allergic reactions
Pegylated IFN-B-1α Plegridy™	2014	Every 14 days; subcutaneous injection; 125 mcg	As above	Flu-like symptoms, injection site reactions, depression, anemia, elevated LFTs, allergic reactions, cardiac abnormalities
IFN-B-1β Betaseron®	1993	Every other day; subcutaneous injection; 250 mcg	As above	Flu-like symptoms, injection site reactions, allergic reactions, depression, elevated LFTs, leukopenia
IFN-B-1β Extavia®	1993	Every other day; subcutaneous injection; 0.25 mg	As above	As above
Glatiramer acetate Copaxone®	1997	Every day; subcutaneous injection; 20 mg OR three times a week; subcutaneous injection; 40 mg	Stimulates regulatory T cells, neuroprotective and repair mechanisms [121]	Injection site reactions; idiosyncratic reaction including anxiety, chest pain, palpitations, SOB, flushing; vasodilation

(continued)

Table 2.4 (continued)

Name of medication	Year of approval	Dosing regimen	Proposed mechanism of action	Important side effects
Oral drugs				
Fingolimod Gilenya®	2010	Every day; capsule taken orally; 0.5 mg	Sphingosine-1-phosphate receptor modulator that inhibits the migration of T cells from lymphoid tissue into the CNS [123]	Headache, flu, diarrhea, back pain, elevated LFTs, cough, prolonged QT interval/bradycardia following first dose, infections, macular edema
Teriflunomide Aubagio®	2012	Every day; pill taken orally; 7 mg or 14 mg	Interferes with de novo synthesis of pyrimidines by inhibition of dihydroorotate dehydrogenase, leads to blocking cell replication in rapidly dividing cells	Hair thinning, diarrhea, flu, nausea, abnormal LFTs, paresthesia, leukopenia, hypertension, hepatic injury
Dimethyl fumarate Tecfidera®	2013	Twice a day; capsule taken orally; 120 mg for 1 week and 240 mg thereafter	Unknown; possibly via action on nuclear factor erythroid2-related factor 2, which upregulates antioxidative pathways; inhibition of the translocation of nuclear factor-κB and therefore inhibits cascade of inflammatory cytokines, chemokines, and adhesion molecules [124]	Flushing, gastrointestinal effects, rash, proteinuria, elevated LFTs, blood dyscrasias
Infusions				
Natalizumab Tysabri®	2003	Every 4 weeks by IV; 300 mg.	Binds α4-integrin and blocks interaction with leukocytes with vascular cell adhesion molecules, resulting in inhibited migrations of leukocytes from the blood into the CNS [122]	PML, allergic, or hypersensitivity reactions within 2 h of infusion, headache, fatigue, urinary tract infections, depression, respiratory tract infections, joint pain, gastrointestinal effects, vaginitis

Table 2.4 (continued)

Name of medication	Year of approval	Dosing regimen	Proposed mechanism of action	Important side effects
Alemtuzumab Lemtrada™	2014	Intravenous infusion on five consecutive days, followed by intravenous infusion on three consecutive days 1 year later; 12 mg	Targets CD52, depletes lymphocytes	Autoimmune disorders including thyroid and ITP, renal failure, rash, headache, fever, nasal congestion, nausea, urinary tract infection, fatigue, insomnia, upper respiratory tract infection, hives, itching, fungal infection, arthralgias, diarrhea, vomiting, flushing, infusion reactions

studies, a head-to-head trial of Rebif® vs. Avonex® was undertaken [191]. The 16-month trial benefit favored Rebif® at each time point in the study. However, the "survival" curve of Avonex® appeared to approach that of Rebif® as the study progressed, however. The PRISM trial extension did show more benefit for patients at the higher dose who initially had received placebo and who were switched to either 22 or 44 micrograms three times weekly [192, 193].

Pegylated IFN-β-1a (Plegridy®) was approved by the FDA in 2014 and is administered subcutaneously at 2-week intervals at a maintenance dose of 125 μcg /0.5 mL, available both as a pen injector and prefilled syringe. It is an IFN-β-1a to which a single, linear 20,000-dalton methoxy poly(ethyleneglycol)-O-2-methylpropionaldehyde molecular is covalently attached to the alpha amino group of the N-terminal amino acid residue. The efficacy of Plegridy® was demonstrated in the ADVANCE study, a randomized, double-blind, placebo-controlled study of RRMS that examined clinical and MRI outcomes at 48 weeks, comparing the treatment group against placebo. The primary outcome of related reduction of annualized relapse rate over 1 year was met, with statistically significant ($p=0.0007$) relative reduction of 36%. MRI outcomes at 48 weeks showed a 67% relative reduction of mean number of new or newly enlarging T2 hyperintense lesions and 86% relative reduction in the mean number of Gd-enhancing lesions ($p \leq 0.0001$) [194]. The side-effect profile is quite similar to that of Rebif®, including flu-like symptoms, injection site reactions, hepatic injury, and depression. The dose-frequency blinded extension study (ATTAIN) is ongoing.

Glatiramer acetate (Copaxone®) was approved in 1997 as a result of a double-blind placebo-controlled trial [195]. The outcome of the trial was a 30% reduction in the risk of relapse for glatiramer, compared with placebo, similar to the IFN-β studies. A follow-up of a subset of patients by the original investigators has shown apparent robust long-term benefits with the majority of the study subjects stabilized [196]. This information has become part of the package insert. More recently in the Glatiramer Acetate Low-Frequency Administration (GALA) study, glatiramer acetate at a dose of 40 mg/mL administered subcutaneously thrice weekly compared to placebo showed a 34.0% reduction in risk of confirmed relapses, and this new dosing regimen is now approved for use [197].

A marked reduction of gadolinium lesion enhancement has been found following initiation of IFN-β-1b [198] and IFN-β-1a [188] and for glatiramer acetate [199]. Similar results for natalizumab have been reported [200]. Interestingly, the serially studied placebo patients showed that while enhancement disappears with steroid administration, enhancement returns, finally disappearing about 2 months after its first appearance [185]. In recent years, increasing emphasis has been placed on techniques of measuring brain atrophy [201–203].

Natalizumab (Tysabri®) is a humanized monoclonal antibody that binds α4-integrin and blocks interaction of α4β1-integrin on leukocytes with vascular cell adhesion molecules (VCAM) and connects segment-1 on fibronectin sites on vascular endothelial cells [204]. Two phase III clinical trials demonstrated the efficacy of natalizumab, administered at a dose of 300 mg intravenously every 4 weeks. The AFFIRM trial showed that natalizumab reduced ARR by 68% over 2 years, disability progression by 42% over 12 weeks and 54% over 24 weeks, an 83% decrease in new or enlarging T2 hyperintense lesions, and decrease in gadolinium-enhancing lesions on MRI by 92% compared to placebo. The SENTINEL trial examined natalizumab in combination with IM IFN-β-1α is more effective than IM IFN-β-1α alone [205–207]. Natalizumab is generally tolerated well. Side effects include infusion-related symptoms, allergic hypersensitivity reactions, anxiety, fatigue, pharyngitis, bladder and respiratory infections, sinus congestion, and peripheral edema. The primary safety concern is the increased risk of PML, the risk of which increases with duration of therapy and serum JCV Ab status and index [208, 209]. Approximately 6% of patients develop persistent anti-natalizumab-neutralizing antibodies [210]. Switching of natalizumab to alternative agents like fingolimod more than 8 weeks after cessation of natalizumab may be associated with lower risk of MRI and clinical disease reactivation [211].

In 2010, Fingolimod (Gilenya®) was the first oral disease-modifying drug to be approved by the Food and Drug Administration for MS. Fingolimod is a sphingosine-1-phosphate receptor (S1P1) modulator, initially acting as an agonist of the S1P1 receptor, and then becomes a potent functional antagonist, leading to internalization of S1P1 receptors on lymph node T cells, resulting in sequestration of lymphocytes in the lymph node. Uniquely, circulating naive T cells and central memory cells are reduced by fingolimod, since both express the chemokine receptor lymph node homing CCR7. Fingolimod does not affect effector memory cells, but some of its mechanisms of action may be explained by the enhancement of function of potent circulating regulatory T cells. Other effects include the modulation of human oligodendrocyte progenitor cells, which potentially could affect myelin repair, astrocyte proliferation, migration and gliosis, and neuroprotection. The clinical efficacy of fingolimod was demonstrated in two large, phase III, double-blind, randomized trials: (1) FTY720 Research Evaluating Effects of Daily Oral Therapy in Multiple Sclerosis (FREEDOMS) and (2) Trial Assessing Injectable Interferon Versus FTY720 Oral in Relapsing-Remitting Multiple Sclerosis (TRANSFORMS). The FREEDOMS trial enrolled 1272 patients who were assigned either oral fingolimod

0.5 mg or 1.25 mg daily versus placebo for 2 years. The primary end point, ARR, was 0.18 in the 0.5 mg dose group, 0.16 in the 1.25 mg dose group, and 0.40 in the placebo group. There was also a statistically significant effect on reduction of sustained disability progression. After 12 weeks progression was seen in 17.7% in the 0.5 mg dose group and 16.6% in the 1.25 mg dose group versus 24.1% in the placebo group. Fingolimod also showed a reduction in the number of new or enlarging lesions on T2-weighted imaged, gadolinium-enhancing lesions at year 2. Importantly, reductions in whole brain volume were less at both 12 and 24 months in the fingolimod group [212, 213]. The TRANSFORMS trial included 1292 patients randomly assigned to the 0.5 mg dose and 1.25 mg dose, but this time a comparator of 30 µg weekly IM interferon-beta-1a. Orally administered fingolimod at a dose of 0.5 mg daily was found to be superior to IFN-β-1a at reducing ARR and MRI activity, although the sustained use of IFN in patients prior to the initiation of the trial is considered a confounder of this data [214]. Fingolimod is generally well tolerated; however, low-frequency specific safety issues including first-dose bradycardia, herpes virus dissemination, macular edema, and elevated blood pressure require screening and regular monitoring. Of note, four cases of PML have now been reported with fingolimod use, without prior exposure to natalizumab.

Teriflunomide (Aubagio®) is an oral medication that interferes with the de novo synthesis of pyrimidines via inhibition of the mitochondrial enzyme dihydroorotate dehydrogenase, resulting in blocking cell replication in rapidly dividing cells. The precise mechanism for its effect in RRMS is unknown. Teriflunomide is a derivative of leflunomide, used for many years in the management of rheumatoid arthritis. Two clinical trials examined the efficacy of teriflunomide: (1) TEMSO and (2) TOWER. The TEMSO study evaluated both 7 mg and 14 mg doses versus placebo in 1088 patients with active relapsing MS. Both doses showed a significant reduction in the primary outcome measure, ARR, compared to placebo by 31.2% (7 mg) and 31.5% (14 mg). Both the 7 mg and 14 mg dose reduced MRI outcomes, slightly more in favor of the14 mg dose. In the TEMSO extension study, adjusted ARR remained low 5 years after initial randomization [215–217]. In the TOWER study, 1169 were randomly assigned to a 7 mg dose, 14 mg dose, and placebo group. The ARR was higher in the placebo group (0.50) compared to the 14 mg (0.32) and 7 mg dose groups (0.39). Teriflunomide at the 14 mg dose reduced the risk of sustained accumulation of disability at 48 weeks; however, the 7 mg dose did not show this effect [218, 219]. A third head-to-head study compared the effectiveness and safety of teriflunomide and subcutaneous interferon-β-1a (44 µg three times per week) in patients with relapsing multiple sclerosis (TENERE) over a 2-year period. The primary end point was time to failure, defined as the first occurrence of confirmed relapse or permanent treatment discontinuation for any reason, and no statistical superiority between IFN-β-1a and the 14 mg dose of teriflunomide was found, although IFN-β-1a was superior to the 7 mg dose of teriflunomide [220]. The ongoing phase III TERACLES trial is examining the clinical usefulness of combination teriflunomide with IFN-β. (ClinicalTrials.gov identifier: NCT01252355)

The most common adverse effects of teriflunomide are mild-moderate, including elevation in transaminases, hair thinning, GI upset, and headache. We have had two apparent allergic reactions to this drug. The greatest concern is the potential for teratogenicity based on animal data, and teriflunomide is contraindicated in women in childbearing potential not using reliable contraception, and men with the potential to father a child are also advised to utilize contraception. As teriflunomide may remain in the serum for up to 2 years, an enhanced drug elimination procedure using cholestyramine or activated charcoal powder is used for patients planning on becoming pregnant or who already are pregnant [221]. Despite these precautions, as of 2013 the AUBAGIO Pregnancy Registry data indicated that 12 newborns have been conceived while on teriflunomide, with no structural or functional deficits reported [222].

Dimethyl fumarate (DMF) (BG-12, Tecfidera®) is the third oral therapeutic option. It is a fumaric acid ester in an enteric-coated microtablet. When it enters the CNS is immediately hydrolyzed by esterases to its metabolite monomethyl fumarate. DMF is associated with decreased GI side effects compared to MMF. It acts on nuclear factor erythroid2-related factor 2 (Nrf-2), which upregulates various antioxidative pathways and inhibits the translocation of nuclear factor-κB into the nucleus, therefore avoiding the expression of a cascade of inflammatory cytokines, chemokines, and adhesion molecules. While the forgoing mechanism is thought to be responsible to it clinical effect, the exact mechanism of action in RRMS, however, is unknown [223].

Two clinical trials have evaluated the efficacy of BG-12 for RRMS: (1) determination of the efficacy and safety of oral fumarate in relapsing-remitting multiple sclerosis (DEFINE) and (2) comparator and an oral fumarate in relapsing-remitting multiple sclerosis (CONFIRM). The DEFINE study evaluated 1234 patients with RRMS and EDSS scores of ≤ 5 who were randomized to a 240 mg twice-a-day dosing regimen, 240 mg three-times-a-day dosing regimen, or placebo. The primary outcome measure was the proportion of patients relapsing at 2 years, whereas unlike other clinical trials, the ARR and risk for disability progression were secondary outcomes. Both doses of BG-12 met the primary outcome measure, with a reduction in the proportion of patients relapsing by almost 50%. Twenty-seven percent of patients on the twice-a-day dosing and 26% of patients on the three-times-a-day regimen had at least one relapse at 2 years, versus 46% of patients on placebo. ARR in both doses of BG-12 was reduced by 53% relative to placebo. EDSS progression was also reduced at 12 weeks in both dosing regimens, with 16% (twice-a-day regimen) and 18% (three-times-a-day regimen) progressing versus 27% of patients on placebo. Other measures, including new or enlarging MRI lesions were significantly lower in the BG-12-treated patients as well. The CONFIRM trial evaluated 1430 patients randomized to one of the two BG-12 dosing regimens or an active comparator glatiramer acetate (GA) 20 mg/d subcutaneously. The primary end point, difference in ARR over a 2-year period, was 44% lower with BG-12 at the twice-a-day regimen, 51% lower with the three-times-a-day regimen, and 29% lower with GA. There was no significant reduction in sustained increase in disability, but a preplanned analysis of the combined outcomes of the DEFINE and CONFIRM studies did reveal a significant reduction in the risk of sustained increase in disability. Of note, the study was powered to evaluate the doses against placebo, but not against GA. The most common adverse effects include abdominal pain, flushing, nausea, and diarrhea. These effects can be ameliorated with the administration of the medication with food and/or regular aspirin at a dose of ≤325 mg 30 minutes prior to administration. Severe lymphopenia may occur, and PML has been reported in four patients. It is recommended that a CBC with differential be obtained at least at 6-month intervals. Reduction of CD8+ T cells is more pronounced than that of CD4+ T cells, and this can be serially monitored with lymphocyte subset panels [224–226].

Despite hopes that oral therapy would lead to increased compliance, it has been shown that oral medications, particularly dimethyl fumarate which is dosed twice daily, is associated with poorer compliance, especially in the young population [227–229]. Alemtuzumab (Lemtrada®) is a humanized anti-CD52 monoclonal antibody. The exact mechanism by which alemtuzumab exerts its therapeutic effects in RRMS is unknown, but is thought to work via depletion and subsequent repopulation of both circulating T and B lymphocytes. These cell populations recover at variable rates, with CD4+ T lymphocytes being the slowest, leading to long-term adaptive immunity. The CARE-MS I trial was a phase III randomized clinical trial of 581 treatment-naive patients comparing alemtuzumab (12 mg/d over a 5-day IV administration with a second 3-day IV administration 1 year later) to subcutaneous IFN-β-1a administered three times a week at a ratio of 2:1. Two primary end points were identified: reduction in relapse rate and 6-month sustained accumulation of disability. Alemtuzumab reduced risk for relapse by 55% compared to IFN-β-1a, with a yearly relapse rate of 0.39 in the IFN-β-1a group compared to 0.18 in the alemtuzumab group, monitored over a period of 2 years. A secondary outcome measure, maintenance of relapse-free status for 2 years, was met in 77.6% of alemtuzumab-treated patients and 58.7% of IFN-β-1a-treated patients. Multiple MRI outcomes also favored alemtuzumab. These included a reduction in the percentage of new and enlarging T2 lesions, new gadolinium-positive lesions, or persistent gadolinium-positive lesions at 24 months and new T1-hypointense lesions. The alemtuzumab group had slower progression of brain atrophy as compared to IFN-β-1a (0.87 versus -1.49 median percent change at year 2) [230]. CARE-MS II evaluated 840 patients who, unlike CARE-MS I, had recently relapsed while taking a standard disease-modifying therapy. Randomization was performed in a 2:2:1 ratio of high-dose (24 mg) alemtuzumab, low-dose (12 mg) alemtuzumab, and IFN-β-1a. Yearly rate of relapse was significantly reduced in the low-dose alemtuzumab group (0.26) compared to the IFN-β-1a group (0.52) over 2 years. A 42% reduction in the risk for sustained accumulation of disability over 6 months was seen in the low-dose alemtuzumab group (12.7%) versus the IFN-β-1a group (21.1%). Of the low-dose alemtuzumab group, 28.8% had sustained improvement in their EDSS score compared to the IFN-β-1a group (12.9%). There was no significant change in total T2 burden, but fewer patients had new or enlarging T2 lesions or new gadolinium-positive lesions over 24 months in the alemtuzumab group. There was less reduction in mean brain parenchymal fraction in the alemtuzumab group (−0.615% versus −0.81%). No advantage of the 24 mg over 12 mg dose of alemtuzumab was seen [231].

Alemtuzumab is associated with several safety issues. Mild-moderate infusion-related reactions are seen in 90%. The incidence of infections is higher, most commonly upper respiratory tract infections, urinary tract infections, and oral herpes. The development of secondary autoimmune disorders is of primary concern, with 16–19% of alemtuzumab-treated patients developing thyroid-related problems and 1% developing immune thrombocytopenia. There is concern for development of antiglomerular basement membrane disease as well. Monthly CBC with differential, serum creatinine levels, and urinalysis with urine cell counts are recommended for 48 months after the last dose of alemtuzumab. Prophylactic medications for pneumocystis pneumonia and herpes viral infections must be administered during treatment and for at least 2 months following the last dose or until CD4+ counts recover to ≥ 200 cells/mm^3 [232].

The management of primary and secondary progressive disease is far from satisfactory but based on prospective studies; two drugs are now approved: mitoxantrone [233, 234] (Novantrone®) and IFN-β-1b [235]. The use of IFN-β-1b varies greatly from one geographic area to another, varying on the impatience and experience of physicians and patients alike. Its use is tempered by the fact that many patients seemingly stabilized initially subsequently begin to progress despite continued use of the drug. In retrospect, this is seen in drug trials that included patients who no longer experienced relapses [235]. This observation is also in keeping with the meta-analysis of the US trial. The use of mitoxantrone resulted in cessation of exacerbations and apparent stabilization in the majority of drug recipients vs. controls in the study. This was accompanied by the realization that the drug is cardiotoxic [233, 234]. The results as published are difficult to under interpret for the non-statistician, and the specter of cardiotoxicity combined with the risk of promyelocytic leukemia has limited its use of this effective drug, despite clear-cut guidelines. It is best used in larger centers with experience with this drug.

High doses of oral biotin (100–300 mg daily) were studied in France for chronic progressive multiple sclerosis [236]. Data in an open-label study of 23 patients showed that 91.3% improved clinically suggested that biotin may have an effect on disability and progression. The results of a randomized, double-blind, multicenter placebo-controlled (2:1) trial of MD1003 (pharmaceutical grade biotin dosed at 300 mg/day) in patients with progressive MS were reported at both the 2015 AAN meeting and 1st Congress of the European Academy of Neurology [237]. A second clinical trial is underway evaluating the effect of biotin in MS patients with permanent visual loss following optic neuritis. A significant reduction in disability progression is preliminarily reported.

Other nonspecific immunosuppressants have been used in the clinical setting. Some were employed in open-label settings, and limited trials of azathioprine, methotrexate, and cyclophosphamide have been carried out. There appears to be a desirable effect from the use of these drugs, but potential infections are real risks, and other problems potentially complicate their use. Hopefully, pivotal trials of one or more of these agents will be organized in the near future. If employed, their use again should be limited or guided by neurologists who are experienced in their use.

Future Directions in Treatment

Though traditionally B cells were not thought to be of central importance in the pathogenesis of MS, and therefore not initially a target for disease-modifying therapy, an anti-B-cell therapy a proof of concept (phase II) study indicated a potential role for rituximab (Rituxan®) in the treatment of RRMS [238]. While a clinical trial evaluating the use of rituximab in primary progressive MS (PPMS) patients did not show a statistically significant difference in time to confirmed disease progression compared to placebo, subgroup analysis revealed a significant difference in patients aged <51 years with gadolinium-enhancing lesions seen on MRI [239].

Data presented at the 2015 ECTRIMS meeting from recently completed pivotal studies of ocrelizumab, a humanized anti-CD20 monoclonal antibody given intravenously, have revealed a highly significant impact on both relapse reduction and reduction in the risk of progression in RRMS. Another anti-CD20 humanized monoclonal antibody under study, ofatumamab, has been successful in *a* proof of concept studies with either intravenous or subcutaneous preparations. The data of three large pivotal (phase III) clinical trials, two evaluating ocrelizumab in the RRMS population (OPERA I and II), and another in the progressive MS population (ORATORIO) were revealed at the 2015 ECTRIMS annual meeting in Barcelona, Spain. Ocrelizumab showed a significant effect for both relapsing-remitting and progressive MS. Ocrelizumab reduced the ARR at 96 weeks by 46% in OPERA I and 47% in OPERA II compared to IFN-β-1a [240]. In the ORATORIO PPMS study, ocrelizumab met the primary end point of a significant 24% reduction in 12-week confirmed disability progression (CDP) [241]. Key secondary end points including a 25% reduction in risk of CDP at 24 weeks, 17.5% reduction in brain volume loss, and 3.4% decrease in T2 lesion volume. The most common adverse events were mild-to-moderate infusion-related reactions [242]. Official publication of the results is newly released [243], [244].

Daclizumab is yet another humanized monoclonal antibody that binds to the α-subunit (CD25) of the high-affinity interleukin-2 (IL-2) receptor expressed on activated T cells and CD4+CD25+FoxP3+ regulatory T cells. Its mechanism of action in MS is thought to be via blockage of the activation and expansion of autoreactive T cells. An important biological effect of daclizumab is the activation and expansion of immunoregulatory CD56 bright natural killer cells. Two phase III trials are recently completed and the drug has been submitted for approval by the Federal Drug Agency. The DECIDE study, which compared subcutaneous daclizumab high-yield process (HYP), administered at a dose of 150 mg every 4 weeks, with intramuscular IFN-β-1a. The annualized relapse rate was significantly lower with daclizumab HYP than with IFN-β-1a (0.22 vs. 0.39, 45% lower rate with daclizumab HYP). The number of new or newly enlarged hyperintense lesions on T_2-weighted magnetic resonance imaging (MRI) over a period of 96 weeks was lower with daclizumab HYP than with IFN-β-1a (4.3 vs. 9.4, 54% lower number of lesions with daclizumab HYP, $P<0.001$). At week 144, the estimated incidence of disability progression confirmed at 12 weeks was 16% with daclizumab HYP and 20% with IFN-β-1a, but this finding was not statistically significant [245]. The results of the

OBSERVE single-arm study, which is evaluating the immunogenicity and pharma-cokinetics of daclizumab HYP, have not been published at press time [246].

There is understandably substantial interest in the development of remyelinating agents in MS to repair damage myelin. The anti-LINGO-1 monoclonal antibody BIIB033 has undergone phase I randomized trials, and phase II results from the SYNERGY trial were reported in Barcelona in 2015 [247, 248]. Another monoclonal antibody under consideration for development is GSK1223249 which targets NOGO-A, an inhibitor of neurite outgrowth [249].

Laquinomod is a derivative of linomide, an agent studied in the 1980s for use in MS whose development was halted due to multiple adverse events including myocardial infarction. As with its parent molecule, serious adverse experience including cardiotoxicity has been recognized, and the pivotal study has been halted.

Other treatments in early clinical studies include secukinumab, an anti-IL-17A monoclonal antibody and firategrast, an oral agent acting against anti-α4-integrin (the target for natalizumab) [250, 251]. Second-generation, more specific sphingosine receptor agents being studied include siponimod and ONO-4641 [252, 253]. Ibudilast is a phosphodiesterase-4 inhibitor that reduces microglial inflammation and hopefully neurodegeneration in MS and is a promising option for treatment of progressive MS. The phase IIb trial Secondary and Primary Progressive Ibudilast NeuroNEXT trial in Multiple Sclerosis (SPRINT-MS) is currently under way.

Rehabilitation

There is renewed interest in exercise in MS both here in the United States and in Europe, and strategies employed in rehabilitation have continued to evolve [254, 255]. The recognition and acceptance of the principal of shorter periods of exercise for MS patients repeated after periods of rest has helped many patients greatly. The use of aquatic exercises, where the patient is cooled during exercise and allowed longer periods of sustained effort, also has resulted in more effective rehabilitation. The impact of daily exercise on experimental models of CNS disease is striking [256–258].

The use of more modern orthotics devices, which are lighter and reduce fatigue in the MS patient, is a major advance in patient management. New neuroprosthetic technology in the form of functional electrical stimulation, such as Bioness® and WalkAide®, can be helpful in selected patients. Fitting these devices and monitoring by experienced physicians and therapists increases their effectiveness and is particularly important. Patients require training and encouragement to adapt to these devices. Similarly, simply giving a patient a prescription for a cane is insufficient. Early introduction of stretching, and judicious use of muscle stretching and use of drugs for control of spasticity prevent contractures and simplify management of most patients. The primary role of the therapist is to instruct the patient and caregivers as to what they must do to decrease the risk of contractures and increase mobility. At the same time they must increase self-confidence of the patient avoid making the patient dependent on the therapist.

Conclusions

The age of rational therapy for MS arrived in the early 2000s with natalizumab and therapeutic options continue to expand. Increased efficacy may be associated with complications such as PML as first evidenced with natalizumab. Its continued use is contingent upon improved risk stratification for PML based on JC virus antibody indices with values less than 1.3 indicative of a low risk (less than 1:10,000). There is continuing concern that other effective drugs may share such risks but the jury is still out. Risks for natalizumab vary with duration of treatment, peaking at the end of the third year of use for high JC virus antibody index subjects and subsequently decreasing to levels resembling those observed after 2 years. Prior use of mitoxantrone or methotrexate raises the risk to especially high levels (1:90) in the presence of high index JVC antibody. L-selectin (CD62L) was thought to be a possible useful biomarker, but a recently published prospective study failed to show any utility [209]. From the available data, fingolimod and dimethyl fumarate appear to be associated with a very low risk for PML, far less than the risk for natalizumab with low JVC antibody indices.

Future trials of compounds discussed in the "emerging therapies" section are exciting prospects. Of particular importance are the anti-B-cell therapies. The focus for disease-modifying therapy has been in relapsing-remitting multiple sclerosis, and there is newfound enthusiasm for treatment of progressive MS stimulated by the recently announced ocrelizumab trial results for PPMS. The FDA has just declared this drug as a "breakthrough" in the treatment of progressive MS.

References

1. Charcot JM. Histologie de la sclerose en plaques. Gaz Hop Paris. 1868;41:554–66.
2. Compston A, Ebers G, Lassman H, McDonald I, Mathews B, Wekerle H. McAlpine's multiple sclerosis. 3rd ed. London: Churchill Livingstone; 1988.
3. Firth D. The case of sir Augustus d'Este. London: Cambridge University Press; 1947.
4. Kurtzke JF. A reassessment of the distribution of multiple sclerosis. Part one. Acta Neurologica Scand. 1975;51:110–36.
5. Kurtzke JF. A reassessment of the distribution of multiple sclerosis. Art two. Acta Neurologica Scand. 1975;51:137–57.
6. Weinshenker BG, Bass B, Rice GPA, et al. The natural history of multiple sclerosis: a geographically based study. 1. Clinical course and disability. Brain. 1989;112:133–46.
7. Schumacher GA, Beebe G, Kibler RF, Kurland LT, Kurtzke JF, McDowell F, Nagler B, Sibley W, Tourtellotte W, Willmon TL. Problems of experimental trials of therapy in multiple sclerosis: report by the panel on the evaluation of experimental trials of therapy in multiple sclerosis. Ann New York Academy of Sciences, NY. 1965;123:552–68.
8. Poser CM, Paty DW, Scheinberg L, et al. New diagnostic criteria for multiple sclerosis: guidelines for research protocols. Ann Neurol. 1983;13:227–31.
9. McDonald WI, Compston A, Edan G, et al. Recommended diagnostic criteria for multiple sclerosis: guidelines from the International Panel on the Diagnosis of Multiple Sclerosis. Ann Neurol. 2001;50:121–7.

10. Polman CH, Reingold SC, Banwell B, Clanet M, Cohen JA, Flippi M, Fujihara K, Havrdova E, Hutchinson M, Kappos L, Lublin FD, Montalban X, O'Connor P, Sandberg-Wollheim M, Thompson AJ, Waubant E, Weinshenker B, Wolinsky JS. Diagnostic criteria for multiple sclerosis: 2010 revisions to the McDonald criteria. Ann Neurol. 2011;69(2):292–302.
11. Noseworthy JH, Luccinetti C, Rodriguez M, Weinschenker BG. Multiple sclerosis. N Engl J Med. 2000;343:938–52.
12. Leibowitz U, Halpern L, Alter M. Clinical studies of multiple sclerosis in Israel. 5. Progressive spinal syndromes and multiple sclerosis. Neurology. 1967;17:988–92.
13. Confavreux C, Vukusic S, Moreau T, Adeline P. Relapses and progression of disability in multiple sclerosis. N Engl J Med. 2000;343:1430–8.
14. Pittock SJ, Mayr WT, McClelland RL, Jorgensen NW, Weigand SD, Noseworthy JH, Weinshenker BG, Rodriguez M. Change in MS-related disability in a population-based cohort: a 10-year follow-up study. Neurology. 2004;62:51–9.
15. Berger J, Sheremata WA. Persistent neurological deficit in multiple sclerosis precipitated by hot bath test. JAMA. 1983;133:1224–6.
16. Berger JR, Sheremata WA, Melmed E. Paroxysmal dystonia as the initial manifestation of multiple sclerosis. Arch Neurol. 1984;41:747–50.
17. Ramagopalan S, Meier U, Goldacre R, Goldacre M. Co-associations of multiple sclerosis with schizophrenia and bipolar disorder: record linkage studies. Presented at: ACTRIMS-ECTRIMS MS, Boston; 2014.
18. Jacobs LD, Beck RW, Simon JH, Kinkel P, Brownscheidle CM, Murray TJ, Simonian NA, Slasor PJ, Sandrock AW, et al. Intramuscular interferon beta-1a therapy initiated during a first demyelinating event in multiple sclerosis. N Engl J Med. 2000;343:898–904.
19. Goodin DS, Reder AT, Ebers GC, et al. Survival in MS: a randomized cohort study 21 years after the start of the pivotal IFNβ-1b trial. Neurology. 2012;78(17):1315–22.
20. Lublin FD, Reingold SC. Defining the clinical course of multiple sclerosis: results of an international survey. National Multiple Sclerosis Society (USA) Advisory Committee on Clinical Trials of New Agents in Multiple Sclerosis. Neurology. 1996;46:907–11.
21. Lublin FD, Reingold SC, Cohen JA, Cutter GR, Sørenson PS, Thompson AJ, Wolinsky JS, Balcer LJ, Banwell R, Barkhof F, Bebo Jr B, Calabresi PA, Clanet M, Comi G, Fox RJ, Freedman MS, Goodman AD, Inglese M, Kappos L, Kieseier BC, Lincoln JA, Lubetzki C, Miller AE, Montalban X, O'Connor PW, Petkau J, Pzzilli C, Rudick RA, Sormani MP, Stüve O, Waubant E, Polman CH. Defining the clinical course of multiple sclerosis: the 2013 revisions. Neurology. 2014;83(3):278–86.
22. Bornstein MB, Miller A, Slagle S, Weitzman M, Drexler E, Keilson M, Spada V, Weiss W, Appel S, Rolak L, et al. A placebo controlled, double-blind, randomized, two-center, pilot trial of Cop 1 in chronic progressive multiple sclerosis. Neurology. 1991;41:533–9.
23. Thompson AJ, Montalban X, Barkhof F, Brochet B, Flippi M, Miller DH, Polman CH, Stevenson VL, McDonald WI. Diagnostic criteria for primary progressive multiple sclerosis: a position paper. Ann Neurol. 2000;47(6):831–5.
24. Ontaneda D, Fox RJ, Chataway J. Clinical trials in progressive multiple sclerosis: lessons learned and future perspectives. Lancet Neurol. 2015;14(2):208–23.
25. Wolinsky JS, Narayana PA, O'Connor P, Coyle PK, Ford C, Johnson K, Miller A, Pardo L, Kadosh S, Ladkani D. PROMiSe Trial Study Group. Glatiramer acetate in primary progressive multiple sclerosis: results of a multinational, multicenter, double-blind, placebo-control trial. Ann Neurol. 2007;61(1):14–24.
26. Lassmann H. Multiple sclerosis: is there neurodegeneration independent from inflammation? J Neurol Sci. 2007;259(1–2):3–6.
27. Frischer JM, Weigand SD, Guo Y, Kale N, Parisi JE, Pirko I, Mandrekar J, Bramow S, Metz I, Brück W, Lassmann H, Lucchinetti CF. Clinical and pathological insights into the dynamic nature of the white matter multiple sclerosis plaque. Ann Neurol. 2015;78:710–21.
28. Cottrell DA, Kremenchutzky M, Rice GPA, et al. The natural history of multiple sclerosis: a geographically based study. The clinical features and natural history of primary progressive multiple sclerosis. Brain. 1999;122:625–89.

29. Sheremata WA, Berger JR, Harrington Jr W, Ayyar R, Stafford JM, Defreitas E. Human lymphotropic (HTLV-I) associated myelopathy: a report of ten cases born in the United States. Arch Neurol. 1992;31:34–8.
30. Biswas HH, Engstrom JW, Kaidarova Z, Garratty G, Gibble JW, Newman BH, Smith JW, Ziman A, Fridey JL, Sacher RA, Murphy EL. Neurologic abnormalities in HTLV-1 and HTLV-II infected individuals without overt myelopathy. Neurology. 2009;73(10):781–9.
31. Lowis GW, Sheremata WA, Minagar A. Epidemiologic features of HTLV-II: serological and molecular evidence. Ann Epidemiol. 2002;12:46–66.
32. Fink JK. Hereditary spastic paraplegia: the pace quickens. Ann Neurol. 2002;51:669–72.
33. Sadovnick AD, Ebers GC. Epidemiology of multiple sclerosis: a critical overview. Can J Neurol Sci. 1993;20:17–9.
34. Confavreux C, Hutchinson M, Hours MM, Cortinovis-Tourniaire P, Moreau T, et al. Rate of pregnancy-related relapse in multiple sclerosis. N Engl J Med. 1998;339:285–91.
35. Voskuhl RR, Wang H, Wu TC, Sicotte NL, Nakamura K, Kurth F, Itoh N, BArdens J, Bernard JT, Corboy JR, Cross AH, Dhib-Jalbut S, Ford CC, Frohman EM, Giesser B, Jacobs D, Kasper LH, Lynch S, Parry G, RAcke MK, REder AT, Rose J, Wingerchuk DM, MacKenzie-Graham AJ, Arnold DL, Tseng CH, Elashoff R. Estriol combined with glatiramer acetate for women with relapsing-remitting multiple sclerosis: a randomized, placebo-controlled, phase 2 trial. Lancet Neurol. 2016;15(1):35–46.
36. Confavreux C. Infections and the risk of relapse in multiple sclerosis. (Editorial). Brain. 2002;125:933–4.
37. Warren S, Greenhill S, Warren KG. Emotional stress and the development of multiple sclerosis: case–control evidence of a relationship. J Chronic Dis. 1982;35:821–31.
38. Grant I, Brown GW, Harris T, McDonald WI, Patterson T, Trimble MR. Severely threatening events and marked life difficulties preceding onset or exacerbation of multiple sclerosis. J Neurol Neurosurg Psychiatry. 1989;52:8–13.
39. Warren S, Warren KG, Cockerill R. Emotional stress and coping in multiple sclerosis and exacerbations. J Psychosom Res. 1991;35:37–47.
40. Mohr DC, Goodkin DE, Bacchetti P, Boudewyn AC, Huang L, Marietta P, Cheuk W, Dee B. Psychological stress and he subsequent appearance of new brain MRI lesions in MS. Neurology. 2000;55:55–61.
41. Scalfari A, Neuhaus A, Degenhardt A, Rice GP, Muraro PA, DAumer M, Ebers GC. The natural history of multiple sclerosis, a geographically based study 10: relapses and long-term disability. Brain. 2010;133:1914–29.
42. Lublin FD, Baier M, Gutter G. Effect of relapses on development of multiple sclerosis. Neurology. 2003;61:1528–32.
43. Cala LA, Mastaglia FL, Black JL. Computerized tomography of brain and optic nerve in multiple sclerosis: observation in 100 patients including serial studies in 16. J Neurol Sci. 1978;36:411–26.
44. Hershey LA, Gado MH, Trotter JL. Computerized tomography in the diagnostic evaluation of multiple sclerosis. Ann Neurol. 1979;5:32–9.
45. Barrett L, Drayer B, Shin C. High-resolution computerized tomography in the diagnostic evaluation of multiple sclerosis. Ann Neurol. 1985;17:33–8.
46. Bradley WG, Walauch Y, Yadley RA, Wycoff RR. Comparison of CT and MR in 400 patients with suspected disease of the brain and cervical spinal cord. Radiology. 1984;152:895–702.
47. Sheldon JJ, Siddharthan R, Tobias J, Sheremata WA, et al. Magnetic resonance imaging of multiple sclerosis: comparison with clinical, paraclinical, laboratory and CT examination. AJNR. 1985;6:683–90.
48. Jacobs L, Kinkel WR, Polachini I, Kinkel RP. Correlations of nuclear magnetic resonance imaging, computerized tomography, and clinical profiles in multiple sclerosis. Neurology. 1986;36:27–34.
49. Honig LS, Siddharthan R, Sheremata WA, Sheldon JJ, Sazant A. Multiple sclerosis: correlation of magnetic resonance imaging with cerebrospinal fluid findings. Neurol Neurosurg Psychiatry. 1988;51:27–280.

50. Fox R et al. Consortium of Multiple Sclerosis Centers annual meeting. Indianapolis; 2015.
51. Seewann A, Kooi EJ, Pouwels PJ, Wattjes MP, van der Valk P, Barkhof F, Polman CH, Geurts JJ. Postmortem verification of MS cortical lesion detection with 3D DIR. Neurology. 2012;78(5):302–8.
52. Honig LS, Sheremata WA. Magnetic resonance imaging of spinal cord lesions in multiple sclerosis. Neurol Neurosurg Psychiatry. 1989;52:459–66.
53. Brex PA, Ciccarelli O, O'Riordan JI, Sailer M, Thompson AJ, Miller DH. A longitudinal study of abnormalities on MRI and disability from multiple sclerosis. N Engl J Med. 2002;348:158–64.
54. Leist TP, Gobbini MI, Frank JA, McFarland HF. Enhancing magnetic resonance imaging lesions and cerebral atrophy in patients with relapsing multiple sclerosis. Arch Neurol. 2000;57:57–60.
55. van Walderveen MA, Kamphorst W, Scheltens P, et al. Histopathologic correlate of hypointense lesions on T1-wighted spin-echo magnetic resonance images in multiple sclerosis. Neurology. 1998;50:1282–8.
56. Bermel RA, Bakshi R. The measurement and clinical relevance of brain atrophy in multiple sclerosis. Lancet Neurol. 2006;5:158–70.
57. Kappos L et al. Predictive value of NEDA for disease outcomes over 6 years in patients with RRMS. Presented at: 31st ECTRIMS Annual Congress; 7–10 Oct 2015; Barcelona; Abstract 570.
58. Cree BAC et al. Long-term effects of fingolimod on NEDA by year of treatment. Poster presented at: 31st ECTRIMS Annual Congress; 7–10 Oct 2015; Barcelona. Poster Session 1; P627.
59. Filippi M, Rocca MA. MR imaging of gray matter involvement in multiple sclerosis: implications for understanding disease pathophysiology and monitoring treatment efficacy. Am J Neuroradiol. 2010;31:1171–7.
60. Moll NM, Rietsch AM, Thomas S, et al. Multiple sclerosis normal-appearing white matter: pathology-imaging correlations. Ann Neurol. 2011;70(5):764–73.
61. Fox RJ, Sakaie K, Lee JC, et al. A validation study of multicenter diffusion tensor imaging: reliability of fractional anisotropy and diffusivity values. ANJR. 2012;33(4):695–700.
62. Pitt D, Boster A, Pei W, et al. Imaging cortical lesions in multiple sclerosis with ultra-high-field magnetic resonance imaging. Arch Neurol. 2010;67(7):812–8.
63. Burman J, Zetterberg H, Fransson M, Loskog AS, Raininko R, Fagius J. Assessing tissue damage in multiple sclerosis: a biomarker approach. Acta Neurol Scand. 2014;130:81–9.
64. Kuhle J, Plattner K, Bestwick JP, et al. A comparative study of CSF neurofilament light and heavy chain protein in MS. Mult Scler. 2013;19:1597–603.
65. Petzold A, Eikelenboom MJ, Gveric D, et al. Markers for different glial cell responses in multiple sclerosis: clinical and pathological correlations. Brain. 2002;125:1462–73.
66. De Stefano N, Narayanan S, Francis GS, et al. Evidence of axonal damage in the early stages of multiple sclerosis and its relevance to disability. Arch Neurol. 2001;5:65–70.
67. Sobel RA. The pathology of multiple sclerosis. In: Multiple sclerosis. Antel J, editor. Neurologic clinics. Philadelphia: Sanders; 1995; 13(1):1–22.
68. Belbasis L, Bellou V, Evangelou E, Ioannidis JP, Tzoulaki I. Environmental risk factors and multiple sclerosis: an umbrella review of systematic reviews and meta-analyses. Lancet Neurol. 2015;14(3):263–73.
69. Wingerchuk DM. Smoking: effects on multiple sclerosis susceptibility and disease progression. Ther Adv Neurol Disord. 2012;5:13–22.
70. Hedström AK, Hiller J, Olsson T, Alfredsson L. Smoking and multiple sclerosis susceptibility. Eur J Epidemiol. 2013;28(11):867–74.
71. Ascherio A, Munger KL. Environmental risk factors for multiple sclerosis. Part I: the role of infection. Ann Neurol. 2007;61:288–99.
72. Thacker EL, Mirzaei F, Ascherio A. Infectious mononucleosis and risk for multiple sclerosis: a meta-analysis. Ann Neurol. 2006;49(3):499–503.

73. Wu C, Yosef N, Thalhamer T, et al. Induction of pathogenic T17 cells by inducible salt-sensing kinase SGK1. Nature. 2013;496:513–51.
74. Kleinewietfeld M, Manzel A, Titze J, et al. Sodium chloride drives autoimmune disease by the induction of pathogenic T17 cells. Nature. 2013;496:518–22.
75. Ascherio A, Munger KL, White R, et al. Vitamin D as an early predictor of multiple sclerosis activity and progression. JAMA Neurol. 2014;71(3):306–14.
76. Sotirchos ES, Bhargava P, Eckstein C, et al. Safety and immunologic effects of high- vs low-dose cholecalciferol in multiple sclerosis. Neurology. 2016;86(4):382–90.
77. Hedström AK, Olsson T, Alfredsson L. High body mass index before age 20 is associated with increased risk for multiple sclerosis in both men and women. Mult Scler J. 2012;18(9):1334–6.
78. Hedström AK, Bomfirm IL, Barcellos L, Gianfrancesco M, Schaefer C, Kockum I, Olsson T, Alfredsson L. Interaction between adolescent obesity and HLA risk genes in the etiology of multiple sclerosis. Neurology. 2014;82(10):867–72.
79. Simpson Jr S, Blizzard L, Otahal P, Van der Mei I, Taylor B. Latitude is significantly associated with the prevalence of multiple sclerosis: a meta-analysis. J Neurol Neurosurg Psychiatry. 2011;82:1132–41.
80. Strachan DP. Family size, infection and atopy: the first decade of the "hygiene hypothesis". Thorax. 2000;55(Suppl 1):S2–10.
81. Correale J. Helminth/parasite treatment of multiple sclerosis. Curr Treat Options Neurol. 2014;16:296.
82. Correale J, Farez MF. The impact of parasite infections on the course of multiple sclerosis. J Neuroimmunol. 2011;233(1–2):6–11.
83. Fleming JO. Helminth therapy and multiple sclerosis. Int J Parasitol. 2013;43(3–4):259–74.
84. Mielcarz DW, Kasper LH. The gut microbiome in multiple sclerosis. Curr Treat Options Neurol. 2015;17:18.
85. Oppenheimer DR. Demyelinating diseases. In: Blackwood W, Corsellis JAN, editors. Greenfield's neuropathology. 3rd ed. London: Edward Arnold; 1976. p. 470–99.
86. Lumsden CE. The neuropathology of multiple sclerosis. In: Vinken PJ, Bruyn GW, editors. Handbook of clinical neurology. New York: Elsevier; 1969. p. 217–309.
87. Adams RD, Kubick CS. The morbid anatomy of the demyelinative disease. Am J Med. 1952;12:510–46.
88. Zimmerman HM, Netsky HG. The pathology of multiple sclerosis. Res Publ Res Nerv Ment Dis. 1950;28:271–312.
89. Lampert PW. Fine structure of the demyelinating process. In: Hallpike JF, Adams CWM, Tourtelotte WW, editors. Multiple sclerosis: pathology, diagnosis and management. Baltimore: Williams and Wilkins; 1983. p. 29–46.
90. Trapp BD, Peterson J, Ransahoff RM, Rudick R, Moerk S, Boe L. Axonal transaction in the lesions of multiple sclerosis. N Engl J Med. 1998;338:278–85.
91. Lassmann H, Vass K. Are current immunological concepts of multiple sclerosis reflected by the Immunopathology of its lesions? Springer Semin Immunopathol. 1995;17:77–87.
92. Lassman H, Raine CS, Antel J, Prineas JW. Immunopathology of multiple sclerosis: report on an international meeting held at the Institute of Neurology of the University of Vienna. J Neuroimmunol. 1998;86:213–7.
93. Lucchinetti C, Brueck W, Paris J, et al. Heterogeneity of multiple sclerosis lesions: implications for the pathogenesis of demyelination. Ann Neurol. 2000;47:707–17.
94. Cannella B, Raine CS. The adhesion molecule and cytokine profile of multiple sclerosis lesions. Ann Neurol. 1995;37:424–35.
95. Poser C. The pathogenesis of multiple sclerosis: a commentary. Clin Neurol Neurosurg. 2000;102:191–204.
96. Khan N, Smith MT. Multiple sclerosis-induced neuropathic pain: pharmacological management and pathophysiological insights from rodent EAE models. Inflammopharmacology. 2014;22(1):1–22.

97. Pender MP, Sears TA. Involvement of the dorsal root ganglion in acute experimental allergic encephalomyelitis in the Lewis rat: a histological and electrophysiological study. J Neurol Sci. 1986;72(2–3):231–42.
98. Sadovnick AD, Armstrong H, Rice GF, et al. A population based study of multiple sclerosis in twins: an update. Ann Neurol. 1993;33:281–5.
99. Sadovnick AD, Baird PA, Ward RH. Multiple sclerosis: update risks for relatives. Am J Med Genet. 1988;29:533–41.
100. Didonna A, Oksenberg JR. Genetic determinants of risk and progression in multiple sclerosis. Clin Chim Acta. 2015;449:16–22.
101. De Jager P et al. ACTRIMS-ECTRIMS. Boston, MA; 2014.
102. Sawcer S, Ban M, Maranian M, et al. A high-density screen for linkage in multiple sclerosis. Am J Hum Genet. 2005;77:454–67.
103. Kaushansky N, Altmann DM, David CS, Lassmann H, Ben-Nun A. DQB1*0602 rather than DRB1*1501 confers susceptibility to multiple sclerosis-like disease induced by proteolipid protein (PLP). J Neuroinflammation. 2012;9:29.
104. International Multiple Sclerosis Genetics Consortium. Analysis of immune-related loci identifies 48 new susceptibility variants for multiple sclerosis. Brain. 2010;133:2603–11.
105. Gregory SG, Schmidt S, Seth P, et al. Interleukin 7 receptor alpha chain shows allelic and functional association with multiple sclerosis. Nat Genet. 2007;39:1083–11.
106. Gregory AP, Dendrou CA, Attfield KE, et al. TNF receptor 1 genetic risks mirrors outcome of ant-TNF therapy in multiple sclerosis. Nature. 2012;488:508–11.
107. Couturier N, Bucciarelli F, Nurtdinov RN, et al. Tyrosine kinase 2 variant influences T lymphocyte polarization and multiple sclerosis susceptibility. Brain. 2011;134:693–703.
108. Sturner KH, Borgmeyer U, Schulze C, Pless O, Martin R. A multiple sclerosis-associated variant of CBLB links genetic risk with type I IFN function. J Immunol. 2014;193:4439–47.
109. Jersild C, Fog T, Hansen GS, Thomsen M, Svejgaard A, Dupont B. Histocompatibility determinants in multiple sclerosis with special reference to clinical course. Lancet. 1973;2:1221–5.
110. Healy BC, Liguori M, Tran D, et al. HLA B*44: protective effects in MS susceptibility and MRI outcome measures. Neurology. 2010;75:634–40.
111. Qju W, Raven S, James I, et al. Spinal cord involvement in multiple sclerosis: a correlative MRI and high-resolution HLA-DRB1 genotyping study. J Neurol Sci. 2011;300:114–9.
112. Okuda DT, Srinivasan R, Oksenberg JR, et al. Genotype-phenotype correlations in multiple sclerosis: HLA genes influence disease severity inferred by 1HMR spectroscopy and MRI measures. Brain. 2009;132:250–9.
113. Masterman T, Ligers A, Olsson T, Andersson M, Olerup O, Hillert J. HLA-DR15 is associated with lower age at onset in multiple sclerosis. Ann Neurol. 2000;48:211–9.
114. Smestad C, Brynedal B, Jonasdottir G, et al. The impact of HLA-A and –DRB1 on age at onset, disease course and severity in Scandinavian multiple sclerosis patients. Eur J Neurol. 2007;14:835–40.
115. Esposito F, Sorosina M, Ottoboni L, et al. A pharmacogenetics study implicates SLC9A9 in multiple sclerosis disease activity. Ann Neurol. 2015;78:115–27.
116. Dhib-Jalbut S, Valenzuela RM, Ito K, Kaufman M, Picone AM, Buyske S. HLA DR and DQ alleles and haplotypes associated with clinical response to glatiramer acetate in multiple sclerosis. Mult Scler Relat Disord. 2013;2(4):340–8.
117. Levin LI, Munger KL, Ruberstone MV, et al. Multiple sclerosis and Epstein-Barr virus. JAMA. 2003;289:1533–6.
118. DeLorenzo GN, Munger KL, Lennette ET, Orentreich N, Vogelman JH, Ascherio A. Epstein-Barr virus and multiple sclerosis: evidence of association from a prospective study with long-term follow-up. Arch Neurol. 2006;63(6):839–44.
119. Woods DD, Bilbao JM, O'Connor P, Moscarello MA. A highly deaminized form of myelin basic protein in Marburg's disease. Ann Neurol. 1996;40:18–24.

120. Schwartz S, Mohr A, Knauth M, Wildemann B, Storch-Hagenlocher B. Acute disseminated encephalomyelitis. A follow-up study of 40 adult patients. Neurology. 2001;56:1312–8.
121. Hartung HP, Grossman RI. ADEM. Distinct disease or part of the MS spectrum? Neurology. 2001;56:1257–60.
122. Murthy JM, Yangala R, Meena AK, Jaganmohan-Reddy J. Acute disseminated encephalomyelitis: clinical and MRI study from South India. J Neurol Sci. 1999;165:133–6.
123. Patterson PY. Transfer of allergic encephalomyelitis in rats by means of lymph node cells. J Exp Med. 1960;111:119–36.
124. Bornstein MB, Appel SH. Application of tissue culture to the study of experimental allergic encephalomyelitis. 1. Patterns of demyelination. J Neuropathol Exp Neurol. 1961;20:141–57.
125. Bornstein MB, Raine CS. Multiple sclerosis and experimental allergic encephalomyelitis: specific demyelination of CNS in culture. Neuropathol Appl Neurobiol. 1977;3:359–67.
126. Ben-Nun A, Cohen IR. Genetic control of experimental autoimmune encephalomyelitis at the level of cytotoxic lymphocytes in guinea pigs. Eur J Immunol. 1982;12:709–13.
127. Owens T, Sriram S. The immunology of multiple sclerosis and its animal model experimental allergic encephalomyelitis. Neurol Clin. 1995;13(1):57–73.
128. Massacesi L, Genain CP, Lee-Parritz D, Letvin NL, Confield D, Hauser SL, et al. Active and passively induced experimental autoimmune encephalomyelitis in common marmosets: as new model for multiple sclerosis. Ann Neurol. 1995;37:519–30.
129. Uccelli A, Giunti D, Capello E, Roccatagliata L, Mancardi GL. EAE in the common marmoset Callithrix jacchus. Int MS J. 2003;10:6–12.
130. Bronstein JM, Lallone RL, Seitz RS, Ellison GW, Myers LW. A humoral response to oligodendrocyte-specific protein in MS. A potential molecular mimic. Neurology. 1999;53:154–61.
131. Berger T, Rubner P, Schautzer F, Egg R, Ulmer H, Mayringer I, Dilitz E, Deisenhammer F, Reindl M. Antimyelin antibodies as a predictor of clinically definite multiple sclerosis after a first demyelinating event. N Engl J Med. 2004;349:139–45.
132. Yu T, Ellison GW, Mendoza F, Bronstein JM. T-cell responses to oligodendrocyte-specific protein in multiple sclerosis. J Neurosci Res. 2001;66:506–9.
133. Adorini L, Singaglia F. Pathogenesis and immunotherapy of autoimmune disease. Immunol Today. 1997;18:209–11.
134. Özenci V, Kouwenhoven M, Huang YM, Xiao BG, Kivisäkk P, Fredrikson S, Link H. Multiple sclerosis: levels of interleukin-10-secreting blood mononuclear cells are low in untreated patients but augmented during interferon-β-1b treatment. Scand J Immunol. 1999;49:554–61.
135. Cao Y, Goods BA, Raddassi K, Nepom GT, Kwok WW, Love JC, Hafler DA. Functional inflammatory profiles distinguished myelin-reactive T cells from patients with multiple sclerosis. Sci Transl Med. 2015;7(287):1–10.
136. Axtell RC, de Jong BA, Boniface K, van der Voort LF, Bhat R, De Sarno P, Naves R, Han M, Zhong F, Castellanos JG, Mair R, Christakos A, Kolkowitz I, Katz L, Killestein J, Polman CH, de Waal MR, Steinman L, Raman C. T helper type 1 and 17 cells determine efficacy of interferon-beta in multiple sclerosis and experimental encephalomyelitis. Nat Med. 2010;16(4):406–12.
137. Wekerle H. Immune pathogenesis of multiple sclerosis. Brain autoimmune reactivity and its control by neuronal function. Mult Scler. 1998;4:136–7.
138. Yang Y, Tomura M, Ono S, Hamaoka T, Fujiwara H. Requirement for IFN-γ in IL-12 production induced by collaboration between Vα14+NKT cells and antigen-presenting cells. Int Immunol. 2000;12:1669–75.
139. Liu C-C, Young LHY, Young JD-E. Lymphocyte-mediated cytolysis and disease. N Engl J Med. 2004;335:1651–9.
140. Minagar A, Alexander JS. Blood-brain barrier disruption in multiple sclerosis. Mult Scler. 2003;9:540–9.

141. Yednock TA, Cannon C, Fritz LC, Sanchez-Madrid F, Steinman L, Karin N. Prevention of experimental autoimmune encephalomyelitis by antibodies against alpha 4 beta 1 integrin. Nature. 1992;356:63–6.
142. Carlos TM, Harlan JM. Leukocyte-endothelial adhesion molecules. Blood. 1994;84:2068–101.
143. Frenette PS, Wagner DD. Adhesion molecules--Part 1. N Engl J Med. 1996;334:1526–9.
144. Frenette PS, Wagner DD. Adhesion molecules--Part II: blood vessels and blood cells. N Engl J Med. 1996;335:43–5.
145. von Andrian UH, MacKay CR. T-cell function and migration. Two sides of the same coin. N Engl J Med. 2000;343:1020–34.
146. von Adrian UH, Engelhardt B. α4 integrins as therapeutic targets in autoimmune disease. N Engl J Med. 2004;348:68–72.
147. Miossec P, Korn T, Kuchroo VK. Interleukin-17 and type 17 helper T cells. N Engl J Med. 2009;361(9):888–98.
148. Bettelli E, Carrier Y, Gao W, Korn T, Strom TB, Oukka M, Weiner HL, Kuchroo VK. Reciprocal developmental pathways for the generation of pathogenic effector Th17 and regulatory T cells. Nature. 2006;441:235–8.
149. Matusevicius D, Kivisäkk P, He B, Kostulas N, Özenci V, Fredikson S, Link H. Interleukin-17 mRNA expression in blood and CSF mononuclear cells is augmented in multiple sclerosis. Mul Scler J. 1999;5(2):101–4.
150. Tzartos JS, Friese MA, Craner MJ, Palace J, Newcombe J, Esiri MM, Fugger L. Interleukin-17 production in central nervous system-infiltrating T cells and glial cells is associated with active disease in multiple sclerosis. Am J Pathol. 2008;172(1):146–55.
151. Lock C, Hermans G, Pedotti R, Brendolan A, Schadt E, Garren H, Langer-Gould A, Strober S, Cannella B, Alalrd J, Klonowski P, Austin A, Lad N, Kaminski N, Galli SJ, Oksenberg JR, Raine CS, Heller R, Steinman L. Gene-microarray analysis of multiple sclerosis lesions yields new targets validated in autoimmune encephalomyelitis. Nat Med. 2002;8:500–8.
152. Kostic M, Dzopalic T, Zivanovic S, Zivkovic N, Cvetanovic A, Stojanovic I, Vojinovic S, Marjanovic G, Savic V, Colic M. IL-17 and glutamate excitotoxicity in the pathogenesis of multiple sclerosis. Scand J Immunol. 2014;79(3):181–6.
153. Elain G, Jeanneau K, Rutkowska A, Mir AK, Dev KK. The selective anti-IL17A monoclonal antibody secukinumab (AIN457) attenuates IL17A-induced levels of IL6 in human astrocytes. Glia. 2014;62(5):725–35.
154. Vestweber D, Blanks JE. Mechanisms that regulate the function of the selectins and their ligands. Physiol Rev. 1999;79:181–213.
155. Takada Y, Elices MJ, Crouse C, Hemler ME. The primary structure of the alpha 4 subunit of VLA-4: homology to other integrins and a possible cell-cell adhesion function. EMBO J. 1989;8:1361–8.
156. Hynes RO. Integrins: a family of cell surface receptors. Cell. 1987;48(4):549–54.
157. Hynes RO. Integrins: versatility, modulation, and signaling in cell adhesion. Cell. 1992;69:11–25.
158. Stüve O, Marra CM, Jerome KR, Cook L, Cravens PD, Cepok S, Frohman EM, Phillips JT, Arendt G, Hemmer B, Monson NL, Racke MK. Immune surveillance in multiple sclerosis patients treated with natalizumab. Ann Neurol. 2006;59(5):745–7.
159. Piccio L, Rossi B, Scarpini E, Laudanna C, et al. Molecular mechanisms involved in lymphocyte recruitment in inflamed brain microvessels: critical roles for P-selectin glycoprotein Ligand-1 and heterotrimeric G$_i$-Linked receptors. J Immunol. 2002;168:1940–849.
160. Minagar A, Jy W, Jimenez JJ, Mauro LM, Horüman L, Sheremata WA, Ahn YS. Elevated plasma endothelial microparticles in multiple sclerosis. Neurology. 2001;56:1319–24.
161. Qin S, Rottman JB, Myers P, et al. The chemokine receptors CSCR3 and CCR5 mark subsets of T cells associated with certain inflammatory reaction. J Clin Invest. 1998;101:746–54.
162. Byun E, Caillier SJ, Montalban X, Villoslada P, Fernandez O, Brassat D, Comabella M, Wang J, Barcellos LF, Baranzini SE, Oksenberg JR. Genome-wide pharmacogenomics

analysis of the response to interferon beta therapy in multiple sclerosis. Arch Neurol. 2008;65(3):337–44.

163. Study of Tecelan (Imilecleucel-T) in secondary progressive multiple sclerosis (Abili-T). ClinicalTrials.gov, Jul 7, 2015. Accessed Feb 27, 2016 from https://clinicaltrials.gov/ct2/show/NCT01684761.

164. Murray TJ. Amantadine therapy for fatigue in MS. Can J Neurol Sci. 1994;21:9–14.

165. Krupp LB, Coyle PK, Doscher C, et al. Fatigue therapy in MS: results of a double-blind, randomized, parallel trial of amantadine, pemoline, and placebo. Neurology. 1995;45:1956–61.

166. Rammohan KW, Rosenberg JH, Lynn DJ, et al. Efficacy and safety of modafinil (Provigil) for the treatment of fatigue in multiple sclerosis: a two centre phase 2 study. J Neurol Neurosurg Psychiatry. 2002;72:150–79.

167. Traugott U. Detailed analysis of immunomodulatory properties of fluoxetine (Prozac) in chronic experimental allergic encephalomyelitis in SJL/J mice. Neurology. 1998;50:1998. (abstract)

168. Goodman AD, Brown TR, Edwards KR, et al. A phase 3 trial of extended release oral dalfampridine in multiple sclerosis. Ann Neurol. 2010;68(4):494–502.

169. Goodman AD, Brown TR, Krupp LB, et al. Sustained-release oral fampridine in multiple sclerosis: a randomised, double-blind, controlled trial. Lancet. 2009;373(9665):732–8.

170. Korenke AR, Rivey MP, Allington DR. Sustained-release fampridine for symptomatic treatment of multiple sclerosis. Ann Pharmacother. 2008;42(10):1458–65.

171. Penn RD, Savoy SM, Corcos D, et al. Intrathecal baclofen for severe spinal spasticity. N Engl J Med. 1989;320:1517–21.

172. Nance P, Sheremata WA, Lynch SG, et al. Relationship of the antispasticity effect of tizanidine to plasma concentration in patients with multiple sclerosis. Arch Neurol. 1997;54:731–06.

173. Rossanese M, Novara G, Challacombe B, Iannetti A, Dasgupta P, Ficarra V. Critical analysis of phase II and III randomized control trials evaluating efficacy and tolerability of a β_3-adrenoreceptor agonist for overactive bladder. BJU Int. 2015;115(1):32–40.

174. Mehnert U, Birzele J, Reueter K, Schurch B. The effect of botulinum toxin type a on overactive bladder symptoms in patients with multiple sclerosis: a pilot study. J Urol. 2010;184(3):1011–116.

175. Goessaert AS, Everaert KC. Onabotulinum toxin A for the treatment of neurogenic detrusor overactivity due to spinal cord injury or multiple sclerosis. Expert Rev Neurother. 2012;12(7):763–75.

176. Browne C, Salmon N, Kehoe M. Bladder dysfunction and quality of life for people with multiple sclerosis. Disabil Rehabil. 2015;37:2350–8.

177. Solaro C, Uccelli MM, Guglieri P, Uccelli A, Mancardi GL. Gabapentin is effective in treating nocturnal painful spasms in multiple sclerosis. Mult Scler. 2000;6(3):192–3.

178. Rose AS, Kuzma JW, Kurtzke JF, et al. Cooperative study in the evaluation of therapy in multiple sclerosis: ACTH vs. placebo. Final Report. Neurology. 1970;20 Part 2:1–19.

179. Beck BW, Cleary PA, Anderson MM, et al. A randomized controlled trial of corticosteroids in the treatment of acute optic neuritis. N Engl J Med. 1992;326:581–8.

180. Diem R, Hobom M, Maier K, Weissert R, Storch MK, Meyer R, Bähr M. Methylprednisolone increases neuronal apoptosis during autoimmune CNS inflammation by inhibition of an endogenous neuroprotective pathway. J Neurosci. 2003;23(18):6993–7000.

181. Diem R, Sättler MB, Merkler D, et al. Combined therapy with methylprednisolone and erythropoietin in a model of multiple sclerosis. Brain. 2005;129(Pt 2):375–85.

182. Botticelli LJ, Wurtman RJ. Septo-hippocampal cholinergic neurons are regulated transynaptically by endorphin and corticotrophin neuropeptides. J Neurosci. 1982;2:1316–21.

183. Spruijt BM, Van Rijzingen I, Masswinkel H. The ACTH 4-9 analog Org2766 modulates the behavioral changes induced by NMDA and the NMDA receptor antagonist AP5. J Neurosci. 1994;14:3225–30.

184. Hol EM, Mandys V, Sodnar P, Gispen WH, Bar PR. Protection by ACTH4-9 analogue against the toxic effects of cisplatin and taxol on sensory neurons and Glial cells in vitro. J Neurosci Res. 1994;39:178–85.
185. O'Connor PW, Goodman A, Willmer-Hulme AJ, et al. Randomized. Multicenter trial of intravenous natalizumab in acute MS relapses: clinical and MRI effects. Neurology. 1994;62:2038–43.
186. The IFNB Multiple Sclerosis Study Group. Interferon beta-1b is effective in relapsing-remitting multiple sclerosis. 1. Clinical results of a multicenter, randomized, double-blind, placebo-controlled trial. Neurology. 1993;43:655–61.
187. Paty DW, Li KDB, the UBC MS/MRI Group and the IFN Multiple Sclerosis Study Group. Interferon beta-1b is effective in relapsing-remitting multiple sclerosis. Neurology. 1993;42:662–7.
188. Jacobs LD, Cookfair DL, Rudick RA, et al. Intramuscular interferon beta-1a for disease progression in relapsing multiple sclerosis. Ann Neurol. 1996;39:285–94.
189. Rudick RA, Goodkin DE, Jacobs LD, et al. Impact of interferon beta-1a on Neurologic disability in relapsing multiple sclerosis. Neurology. 1997;49:358–63.
190. PRISMS (Prevention of Relapses and Disability by Interferon β-1a Subcutaneously in multiple sclerosis) Study Group. Randomised double-blind placebo-controlled study of interferon β-1a in relapsing/remitting multiple sclerosis. Lancet. 2002;352:1498–504.
191. Panitch H, Goodin DS, Francis G, Chang P, Coyle PK, O'Connor P, Monaghan E, Li D, Weinshenker B. Randomized, comparative study of interferon ß-1a treatment regimens in MS: the EVIDENCE Trial. Neurology. 2002;59:1496–506.
192. The PRISMS Study Group and the University of British Columbia MS/MRI Analysis Group. PRISMS-4: longer term efficacy of interferon-beta-1a in relapsing MS. Neurology. 2001;56:1628–36.
193. Cohen BA, Rivera VM. PRISMS: the story of a pivotal clinical trial series in multiple sclerosis. Curr Med Res Opin. 2010;26(4):827–38.
194. Calabresi PA, Kieseier BC, Arnold DL, et al. Pegylated interferon β-1a for relapsing-remitting multiple sclerosis (ADVANCE): a randomized, phase 3, double-blind study. Lancet Neurol. 2014;13(7):657–65.
195. Johnson KP, Brooks BR, Cohen JA, et al. Copolymer 1 reduces relapse rate and improves disability in relapsing-remitting multiple sclerosis: results of a phase III multicenter, double-blind, placebo-controlled trial. Neurology. 1995;45:1268–76.
196. Johnson KP, Brooks BR, Ford CC, et al. Sustained clinical benefits of Glatiramer acetate (Copaxone) in multiple sclerosis patients observed for 6 years. Mult Scler. 2000;6:255–66.
197. Khan O, Rieckmann P, Boyko A, Selmaj K, Zivadinov R, and for the GALA study group. Three times weekly glatiramer acetate in relapsing-remitting multiple sclerosis. Ann Neurol. 2013;73(6):705–13.
198. Stone LA, Frank JA, Albert PS, et al. Characterization of MRI response to treatment with interferon beta-1b: contrast-enhancing MRI lesion frequency as a primary outcome measure. Neurology. 1997;49:862–9.
199. Mancardi GL, Sardanelli F, Parodi RC, et al. Effect of copolymer-1 on serial gadolinium-enhanced RMI in relapsing remitting multiple sclerosis. Neurology. 1998;50:1127–33.
200. Dalton CM, Miszkiel KA, Barker GJ, et al. The effect of natalizumab on conversion of T1 gadolinium enhancing lesions to T1 hypodense lesions. Neurology. 2004;60(Suppl):S484.
201. Rudick RA, Fisher E, Lee J-C, Simon J, Jacobs L, and the Multiple Sclerosis Collaborative Research Group. Us of the brain parenchymal fraction to measure whole brain atrophy in relapsing-remitting MS. Neurology. 1999;53:1698–704.
202. Ge Y, Grossman RI, Udupa JK, et al. Glatiramer acetate (Copaxone) treatment in relapsing-remitting MS. Neurology. 2000;54:813–7.
203. Frank JA, Richert N, Bash C, et al. Interferon-β-1b slows progression of atrophy in RRMS. Neurology. 2004;62:719–25.
204. Ransohoff RM. Natalizumab for multiple sclerosis. N Engl J Med. 2007;356(25):2622–9.

205. Polman CH, O'Connor PW, Hardova E, et al. A randomized, placebo-controlled trial of natalizumab for relapsing multiple sclerosis. N Engl J Med. 2006;354(9):899–910.
206. Miller DH, Soon D, Fernando KT, et al. MRI outcomes in a placebo-controlled trial of natalizumab in relapsing MS. Neurology. 2007;68(17):1390–401.
207. Rudick RA, Stuart WH, Calabresi PA, et al. Natalizumab plus interferon beta-1a for relapsing multiple sclerosis. N Engl J Med. 2006;354(9):911–23.
208. McGuigan C, Craner M, Guadagno J, et al. Stratification and monitoring of natalizumab-associated progressive multifocal leukoencephalopathy risk: recommendations from an expert group. J Neurol Neurosurg Psychiatry. 2016;87(2):117–25.
209. Schwab N, Schneider-Hohendorf T, Pignolet B, et al. PML risk stratification using anti-JCV antibody index and L-selectin. Mult Scler. 2016;22:1048–60. doi:10.1177/135245851607651.
210. Calabresi PA, Giovannoni G, Confavreux C, et al. The incidence and significance of anti-natalizumab antibodies: results from AFFIRM and SENTINEL. Neurology. 2007;69(14):1391–403.
211. Kappos L, Radue EW, Comi G, et al. Switching from natalizumab to fingolimod: a randomized, placebo-controlled study in RRMS. Neurology. 2015;85(1):29–39.
212. Pelletier D, Hafler DA. Fingolimod for multiple sclerosis. N Engl J Med. 2012;366(4):339–47.
213. Kappos L, Radue EW, O'Connor P, et al. A placebo-controlled trial of oral fingolimod in relapsing multiple sclerosis. N Engl J Med. 2010;362(5):387–401.
214. Cohen JA, Barkhof F, Comi G, et al. Oral fingolimod or intramuscular interferon for relapsing multiple sclerosis. N Engl J Med. 2010;362(5):402–15.
215. O'Connor P, Wolinsky JS, Confavreux C, et al. Randomized trial of oral teriflunomide for relapsing multiple sclerosis. N Engl J Med. 2011;365(14):1293–303.
216. Miller AE, O'Connor P, Wolinsky JS, et al. Pre-specified subgroup analyses of a placebo-controlled phase III trial (TEMSO) of oral teriflunomide in relapsing multiple sclerosis. Mult Scler. 2012;18(11):1625–32.
217. O'Connor P, Wolinsky J, Confavreux C, Comi G, Kappos L, Olsson T, et al. Extension of a phase III trial (TEMSO) of oral teriflunomide in multiple sclerosis with relapses: clinical and MRI data 5 years after initial randomisation. Mult Scler. 2011;17(Supp 17):S414. P924
218. Miller A, Kappos L, Comi G, et al. Teriflunomide efficacy and safety in patients with relapsing multiple sclerosis: results from TOWER, a second, pivotal, phase 3 placebo-controlled study (S01.004). Neurology. 2013;80(meeting abstracts 1):S01.004.
219. Confavreux C, O'Connor P, Comi G, et al. Oral teriflunomide for patients with relapsing multiple sclerosis (TOWER): a randomized, double-blind, placebo-controlled, phase 3 trial. Lancet Neurol. 2014;13(3):247–56.
220. Vermersch P, Czlonkowska A, Grimaldi LM, et al. Teriflunomide versus subcutaneous interferon beta-1a in patients with relapsing multiple sclerosis: a randomized, controlled phase 3 trial. Mult Scler. 2014;20(6):705–16.
221. Genzyme Corporation. Aubagio prescribing information. Cambridge, MA; 2012.
222. Jung Henson L, Stüve O, Kieseier B, Benamor M, Benzerdjeb H. Pregnancy outcomes from the teriflunomide clinical development program: retrospective analysis of the teriflunomide clinical trial database. Neurology. 2013;80:1001–11.
223. Gold R, Linker RA, Stangel M. Fumaric acid and its esters: an emerging treatment for multiple sclerosis with antioxidative mechanism of action. Clin Immunol. 2012;142(1):44–8.
224. Gold R, Kappos L, Arnold DL, et al. Placebo-controlled phase 3 study of oral BG-12 for relapsing multiple sclerosis. N Engl J Med. 2012;367(12):1098Y1107.
225. Fox RJ, Miller DH, Phillips JT, et al. Placebo-controlled phase 3 study of oral BG-12 or glatiramer in multiple sclerosis. N Engl J Med. 2012;367(12):1087Y1097.
226. Spencer CM, Crabtree-Hartman EC, Lehmann-Horn K, Cree BAC, Zamvil SS. Reduction of CD8+ T lymphocytes in multiple sclerosis patients treated with dimethyl fumarate. Neurol Neuroimmunol Neuroinflamm. 2015;2(3):e76.

227. Dionne CA, Ganguly R, Camac A, Chaves C. Do oral disease modifying agents improve adherence to MS treatment? A comparison or oral and injectable drugs. CMSC 2015 Indianapolis; Abstract DX19.
228. Munsell M, Locklear JC, Phillips AL, Frean M, Menzin J. An assessment of adherence among MS patients newly initiating treatment with a self-injectable versus oral disease-modifying drug. CMSC 2015 Indianapolis; Abstract DX43.
229. Ko JJ, Nazareth TA, Friedman H, Navaratnam P, Herriott DA, Sasane R. Treatment discontinuation after initiation of oral disease-modifying therapies in patients with MS. CMSC 2015 Indianapolis; Abstract DX44.
230. Cohen JA, Coles AJ, Arnold DL, et al. Alemtuzumab versus interferon beta 1a as first-line treatment for patients with relapsing-remitting multiple sclerosis: a randomized controlled phase 3 trial. Lancet. 2012;380(9856):1819–28.
231. Coles AJ, Twyman CL, Arnold DL, et al. Alemtuzumab for patients with relapsing multiple sclerosis after disease-modifying therapy: a randomized controlled phase 3 trial. Lancet. 2012;380(9856):1829–39.
232. Lemtrada® package insert: http://products.sanofi.us/lemtrada/lemtrada.pdf.
233. Hartung HP, Gonsette R, Koenig N, et al. Mitoxantrone in progressive multiple sclerosis: a placebo controlled, double-blind, randomized, multicentre trial. Lancet. 2002;360:2018–25.
234. Ghalie RG, Edan G, Laurent M, et al. Cardiac adverse effects associated with mitoxantrone (Novantrone) therapy in patients with MS. Neurology. 2002;59:909–13.
235. European Study Group on Interferon β-1b in Secondary Progressive MS. Placebo-controlled multicentre randomised trial of interferon β-1b in treatment of secondary progressive multiple sclerosis. Lancet. 1998;352:1491–7.
236. Sedel F, Papeix C, Bellanger A, et al. High doses of biotin in chronic progressive multiple sclerosis: a pilot study. Mult Scler Relat Disord. 2015;4:159–69.
237. Tourbah A, Frenay CL, Edan G, et al. Effect of MD10003 [high doses of biotin] in progressive multiple sclerosis: results of a pivotal phase III randomized double blind placebo controlled study. Neurology. 2015;84(14):Supplement PL2.002.
238. Hauser SL et al. B-cell depletion in rituximab in relapsing-remitting multiple sclerosis. N Engl J Med. 2008;358(7):676–88.
239. Hawker K, O'Connor P, Freedman MS, et al. Rituximab in patients with primary progressive multiple sclerosis: results of a randomized double-blind placebo-controlled multicenter trial. Ann Neurol. 2009;66(4):460–71.
240. Hauser S. Phase III results in relapsing MS (OPERA I and OPERA II studies). ECTRIMS 2015; Barcelona; Abstract #190.
241. Montalban X. Phase II results of the ORATORIO study. ECTRIMS 2015; Barcelona; Abstract #228.
242. Kappos L et al. Ocrelizumab in relapsing-remitting multiple sclerosis: a phase 2, randomized, placebo-controlled, multicenter trial. Lancet. 2011;378(9805):1779–87.
243. Hauser SL, Bar-Or A, Comi G et al. Ocrelizumab versus interferon beta-1a in relapsing multiple sclerosis. N Engl J Med 2016; doi: 10.1056/NEJMoa1601277.
244. Montalban X, Hauser SL, Kappos L et al. Ocrelizumab versus placebo in primary progressive multiple sclerosis. N Engl J Med 2016; doi: 10.1056/NEJMoa1606468.
245. Kappos L, Wiendl H, Selmaj K, Arnold DL, Havrdova E, Boyko A, Kaufman M, Rose J, Greenberg S, Sweetser M, Riester K, O'Neill G, Elkins J. Daclizumab HYP versus interferon beta-1a in relapsing multiple sclerosis. N Engl J Med. 2015;373(15):1418–28.
246. An immunogenicity and pharmacokinetics study of BIIB019 (daclizumab high yield process) prefilled syringe in relapsing remitting multiple sclerosis (OBSERVE). www.clinicaltrials.gov, last updated Dec 23, 2015. Accessed 27 Feb 2016.
247. Cadavid D, Hupperts R, Dulović et al. Correlation of brain volume and physical measures with cognitive function using baseline data from the anti-LINGO-1 SYNERGY trial in multiple sclerosis. ECTRIMS 2015 Barcelona; Abstract P629.

248. Tran JQ, Rana J, Barkhof F, et al. Randomized phase I trials of the safety/tolerability of anti-LINGO-1 monoclonal antibody BIIB033. Neurol Neuroimmunol Neuroinflamm. 2014;1(2):e18.

249. Wang T, Xiong JQ, Ren XB, Sun W. The role of Nogo-A in neuroregeneration: a review. Brain Res Bull. 2012;87:499–503.

250. Hvardova E. Positive proof of concept of AIN457, an antibody against interleukin-17A, in relapsing-remitting multiple sclerosis, in ECTRIMS. Lyons; 2012.

251. Miller DH et al. Firategrast for relapsing remitting multiple sclerosis: a phase 2, randomised, double-blind, placebo-controlled trial. Lancet Neurol. 2012;11:131–9.

252. Stuve O, Hartung HP, Freedman M, Li D, Hemmer B, Kappos L, Rieckmann P, Montalban X, Ziemssen T, Selmaj K. Phase 2 BOLD extension study efficacy results for siponimod (BAF312) in patients with relapsing–remitting multiple sclerosis. Mul Scler Relat Disord. 2014;3(6):754–5.

253. Komiya T et al. Efficacy and immunomodulatory actions of ONO-4641, a novel selective agonist for sphingosine 1-phosphate receptors 1 and 5, in preclinical models of multiple sclerosis. Clin Exp Immunol. 2013;171:54–62.

254. Aisen ML. Justifying neurorehabilitation. (Editorial). Neurology. 1999;52:8.

255. Thompson A. Symptomatic management and rehabilitation in multiple sclerosis. J Neurol Neurosurg Psychiatry. 2001;71(Suppl 11):112–1127.

256. Heine M, van de Port I, Rietberg MB, van Wegen EE, Kwakkel G. Exercise therapy for fatigue in multiple sclerosis. Cochrane Database Syst Rev. 2015;9:CD009956.

257. Latimer-Cheung AE, Pilutti LA, Hicks AL, et al. The effects of exercise training on fitness, mobility, fatigue, and health related quality of life among adults with multiple sclerosis: a systematic review to inform guideline development. Arch Phys Med Rehabil. 2013;94:1800–28.

258. Motl RW, Pilutti LA. The benefits of exercise training in multiple sclerosis. Nat Rev Neurol. 2012;8:487–97.

HIV Infection of Human Nervous System: Neurologic Manifestations, Diagnosis, and Treatment

Christian Cajavilca, Debra Davis, Oleg Y. Chernyshev, and Alireza Minagar

Introduction

Human immunodeficiency virus (HIV) passes through the blood-brain barrier (BBB) and enters the central nervous system (CNS) at early stages of AIDS in recently seroconverted and yet clinically asymptomatic patients. HIV genetic material can be discovered and extracted from cerebrospinal fluid (CSF), brain, and spinal cord as well as peripheral nerves of AIDS patients. Depending on the severity of the HIV-induced immunosuppression, the clinical manifestations of neuroAIDS vary and entail dementia, myelopathy, opportunistic infections, polyneuropathy, stroke, and HIV-associated neurocognitive disorders (HAND) among other less common complications.

Various pathogenic mechanisms involved in development of neurologic complications of AIDS include direct HIV-induced neurotoxicity, opportunistic infections stemming from immunosuppression, profound abnormalities of the immune system, and impediments and complexities originating from reconstitution of the immune system.

Clinical Manifestations

The extent and spectrum of neurologic complications of HIV infection, to a significant degree, is linked to the depth of AIDS-induced immunosuppression and the underlying mechanism(s) of that particular neurologic complication. Certain opportunistic infections or neoplasms of the nervous system usually develop only when the number of infected T lymphocytes drops below a certain threshold. For

C. Cajavilca, MD • D. Davis, MD • O.Y. Chernyshev, MD, PhD • A. Minagar, MD (✉)
Department of Neurology, LSU Health Sciences Center,
1501 Kings Highway, Shreveport, LA, USA, 71130
e-mail: aming@lsuhsc.edu

© Springer International Publishing AG 2017
A. Minagar, J.S. Alexander (eds.), *Inflammatory Disorders of the Nervous System*, Current Clinical Neurology, DOI 10.1007/978-3-319-51220-4_3

example, significant AIDS-associated neurological manifestations usually begin when the CD4+ T lymphocyte count drops to a number lower than 200 CD4+ T lymphocytes/mm³.

Various mechanisms responsible for the neurologic complications of HIV include neurotoxicity, possible autoimmunity, opportunistic infections, cerebrovascular complications, neoplasms, side effects of antiretroviral therapy (ART), and malnutrition. The early cases of the 1980s were associated with opportunistic infection and neoplasms; however, after the advent of antiretroviral therapies, a myriad of different syndromes such as dementia, myelopathy, and neuropathy have emerged. A list of neurologic complications of HIV and AIDS is presented in Table 3.1.

HIV patients manifest a wide range of neurologic manifestations related to HIV, which demands further diagnostic workup to search for and exclude other possible etiologies. It is important to have a meticulous plan for the state of systemic HIV infection and tendency for opportunistic infections. Diagnostic tests such as serial measurements of peripheral CD4+ lymphocyte count as well as history of exposure to infectious agents should be performed. For example, a demyelinating neuropathy may develop at early stages of infection with a CD4+ count >500/mm³, while a CD4+ lymphocyte count between 200 and 500/mm³ may set the stage for tuberculous meningitis and onset of cognitive impairment. A CD4+ lymphocyte count less than 200/mm³ places the patient at risk for HIV dementia, vacuolar myelopathy, polyneuropathy, toxoplasmosis, encephalitis, progressive multifocal leukoencephalopathy (PML), cryptococcal meningitis, and primary CNS lymphoma. The relative correlation between common neurologic manifestations of AIDS and the serum

Table 3.1 Neurologic manifestations of HIV infection of human nervous system

HIV-associated dementia and encephalopathy
HIV-associated neurocognitive disorders
Demyelinating syndrome (at early stages of infection which imitates multiple sclerosis)
Parkinsonian syndrome and other movement disorders
Sleep abnormalities
Various opportunistic infections of the central nervous system which includes:
Toxoplasmosis, neurosyphilis, progressive multifocal leukoencephalopathy
Cytomegalovirus and varicella zoster encephalitis
Fungal and bacterial infections
Primary nervous system neoplastic processes such as central nervous system lymphoma
Aseptic meningitis and lymphomatous meningitis
Vacuolar myelopathy
Viral and bacterial polyradiculitis
Distal symmetric neuropathy
Mononeuritis multiplex
Acute and chronic inflammatory demyelinating polyneuropathy
Cytomegalovirus mononeuritis multiplex
Neurologic side effect medications used for treatment of AIDS and its complications such as didanosine, zalcitabine, stavudine, dapsone, isoniazid, and pyridoxine
Inflammatory myopathy

CD4+ lymphocyte count is of utmost significance when the neurologist treats AIDS patients. It is significant to bear in mind that the HIV latent period may range from 2 to 10 years. During this time, the CD4+ lymphocyte count declines, while viral load increases, and the patient may remain symptom-free.

Acute Seroconversion: CD4+ Lymphocyte Count >500/mm³

The early signs of retroviral syndrome (also recognized as "acute HIV syndrome") occur within 6 weeks of seroconversion in 50% of the patients. These symptoms, which may remind clinicians of infectious mononucleosis, include fever, headache, myalgia, nuchal rigidity (aseptic meningitis), photophobia, cranial nerve palsies, myelopathy, radiculopathies, acute demyelinating neuropathy, and rarely encephalopathy. As mentioned earlier, HIV can be found in CSF associated with lymphocytic pleocytosis. Rare cases of CNS demyelination and meningoencephalitis have been reported immediately after seroconversion [1]. Peripheral nerve syndromes during the immediate seroconversion stage and latent phase include acute inflammatory demyelinating polyradiculoneuropathy (AIDP), chronic inflammatory demyelinating polyradiculoneuropathy (CIDP), mononeuritis multiplex, and mononeuropathies. Patients at this stage may also develop cranial nerve VII palsy, transverse myelitis, and brachial neuritis [2, 3].

AIDP may manifest at any stage of the illness and clinically presents with distal and proximal weakness, sensory loss, back pain, autonomic dysfunction, cardiac arrhythmias, cranial neuropathies, and urinary retention. CIDP may be monophasic or relapsing. Unlike AIDP, CIDP usually does not include respiratory failure or autonomic dysfunction. The clinical scenario of AIDP and CIDP usually is no different from uninfected patients.

Mononeuritis multiplex is a rare finding in AIDS and usually affects more than two nerves with an asymmetric sensory and motor deficit within the distribution of cranial nerves, peripheral nerves, or nerve roots. Severe dysfunctions are related with cytomegalovirus (CMV) coinfection especially when the CD4+ lymphocyte count is less than 50 cell/mm [3, 4].

Dermatomyositis and polymyositis may also be present during early seroconversion or at the latent phase [5, 6]. They can also be manifestations of drug effect or other infectious entity. Biopsy may help to identify the specific etiology, for example, nemaline rod myopathy is related to HIV. Rhabdomyolysis has been associated with the use of didanosine and statins used for hyperlipidemia related with highly active antiretroviral therapy (HAART) [7]. Other causes of rhabdomyolysis in HIV-infected patients consist of HIV-associated rhabdomyolysis, rhabdomyolysis associated with ART, and rhabdomyolysis at the end stage of AIDS [7].

HIV-Associated Neurologic Manifestations: CD4+ Lymphocyte Count 200–500/mm³

With further drop of CD4+ T lymphocytes, opportunistic infections as well as certain neurologic syndromes present. Patients complain of difficulty with short-term memory and lack of concentration, anxiety, depression, and motor deficits [8].

Disseminated herpes zoster as well as CNS tuberculosis may appear or become activated at this stage of the disease process. In addition, patients with syphilis may proceed to full-blown neurosyphilis at a more rapid rate than HIV-seronegative patients with syphilis. Another interesting and less recognized and understood manifestation in HIV-infected individuals is the diffuse infiltrative lymphocytosis syndrome (DILS), which is defined by persistent circulating CD8+ lymphocytosis, which may be due to oligoclonal expansion of these cells [9]. The expanded CD8+ lymphocytes infiltrate various organs and can imitate Sjogren syndrome. One particular manifestation of DILS is a severe peripheral neuropathy which is accompanied by significant HIV proviral load in peripheral nerves. Other presentations include myositis, hepatitis, and interstitial nephritis.

Patients on therapy with the antiretroviral medication zidovudine (ZDV) may develop myopathy. ZDV is a nucleoside analogue and a nucleoside reverse transcriptase inhibitor with mitochondrial toxicity (inhibiting mitochondrial DNA polymerase) and causes myopathy. Clinically, patients report myalgias, proximal weakness, and muscle atrophy. Muscle biopsy reveals ragged red fibers and cytochrome oxidase negative fibers [10, 11]. The clinical manifestations of ZDV-associated myopathy may correlate with duration of therapy, dosage, and advanced disease stage. Most patients recover with cessation of therapy.

AIDS-Related Neurologic Complications at CD4+ Lymphocyte <200/mm³

As it was previously explained, with more annihilation of the immune system and progressive drop in the number of CD4+ T lymphocytes, more neurologic complications appear. Once the peripheral CD4+ lymphocyte count drops to below 200/mL myelopathy, HIV-associated dementia (HAD) and painful distal sensory polyneuropathy present.

The commonality of HAD among untreated HIV patients may vary between 5 and 20%. Its annual incidence in patients with a CD4+ lymphocyte level 100/mm³ or less is 7.3%. As a significantly subcortical dementia, HAD manifests with cognitive decline, behavioral abnormalities (such as apathy, mania, lack of emotional stability, forgetfulness, mental dullness and slowing, and impaired comprehension), and motor dysfunction such as gait difficulty and loss of fine motor skills. HAD uncommonly presents with psychosis and some of these patients may be at risk for suicidal and homicidal ideation. The progression of dementia may be rapid in untreated patients; however, with the use of HAART, patients with HAD may survive 3–5 years [12].

Vacuolar myelopathy is the most prevalent form of chronic AIDS-associated myelopathy in AIDS patients, with a prevalence of 20–50% in various case series [13, 14]. Clinically, HIV myelopathy presents with progressive spastic paraparesis, hyperreflexia with extensor plantar responses, abnormal gait with tendency to fall, urinary retention or incontinence, ataxia, and sensory loss. Neuropathologically, AIDS myelopathy is recognized by the presence of separate or coalescent intramyelin and peri-axonal vacuolation with loss of spinal cord white matter and presence of lipid-laden macrophages [13]. Vacuolar myelopathy of AIDS should be differentiated from HTLV-1-associated myelopathy.

Peripheral neuropathy is one of the most prominent peripheral neurologic complications of HIV infection, which affects up to 15% of patients. Of the various AIDS-related peripheral nervous system complications of AIDS, distal symmetric polyneuropathy (DSP) is the most common. Patients with DSP complain of numbness, pain, paresthesias, gait instability, and autonomic dysfunction. DSP may occur during latent phases but it affects 30% of people with AIDS. Toxic peripheral neuropathies have increased especially in patients treated with HAART.

Uncommonly, cases of motor neuron disease occur in HIV patients who have CD4$^+$ T lymphocyte count less than 200 cells/mm^3 and may imitate amyotrophic lateral sclerosis (ALS). However, they differ from ALS because of younger age of onset, rapid progression and deterioration, and clinical improvement when treated with ART [15]. In 2001, Moulignier et al. reported six patients with HIV-related motor neuron disease and proposed certain underlying mechanisms such as neuronal infection, reaction to toxic viral products, cytokine effect, and autoimmunity [15].

With a significant drop of the CD4$^+$ T lymphocytes, the risk of opportunistic infections such as toxoplasmosis, cryptococcal meningitis, and mycobacterial infection such as disseminated mycobacterium avium complex and progressive multifocal leukoencephalopathy (PML) rises. In addition, primary CNS lymphoma is a neoplastic process linked to Epstein-Barr virus with poor prognosis in advanced stages of AIDS.

Other AIDS-Related Neurologic Manifestations

Both ischemic and hemorrhagic strokes have been reported in HIV-infected patients and have been attributed to a relatively elevated incidence of vasculitis and hypercoagulability [16]. Other causes of ischemic strokes in these patients include meningitis, cardioembolism, and hypertension.

Neuro-ophthalmologic disorders of AIDS patients occur in up to 60% of patients with case reports on patients with visual field defects, optic neuropathy, papilledema, ocular motor nerve palsies, and one-and-a-half syndrome [17]. Visual evoked potentials may be abnormal in 57% of patients. Movement disorders have also been described in HIV patients. Patients can develop Parkinsonism at seroconversion or advanced stages. Parkinsonism is also related to HAART treatment and antidopaminergic drugs. Another frequent complaint by HIV patients is sleep disorders, particularly those treated with efavirenz.

Immune Reconstitution Inflammatory Syndrome

Immune reconstitution inflammatory syndrome (IRIS) is a fascinating syndrome which is recognized by paradoxical worsening of the patient's clinical and neurological condition once combined antiretroviral therapy (cART) has been initiated.

The pathophysiology of IRIS has been attributed to the recovery of the immune system. IRIS is potentially a dangerous condition. Involvement of the CNS in IRIS is uncommon and may occur in the context of certain opportunistic infections such as tuberculosis, cryptoccocal infection, or PML [18, 19]. It has been hypothesized that IRIS may stem from an aberrant immune response to opportunistic infections. Interestingly, discontinuation of cART is not suggested.

HIV-Associated Neurocognitive Disorders

HIV-associated neurocognitive disorders (HAND) covers a wide range of manifestations from clinically asymptomatic to profound dementia (Table 3.2). Diagnosis of HAND rests on meticulous behavioral neurological examination, detailed neuropsychologic assessment, and evaluation of the patient's functional status and capabilities [20]. HAND is common in the AIDS population and, with further use of cART along with increased survival of AIDS patients, may become more prevalent [21]. In those patients under treatment with cART, the possibility of developing HAND increases with age along with the presence of cardiovascular risk factors [22].

HIV-associated dementia (HAD) constitutes the most severe form of HAND. With the global use of cART, HAD is relatively less common. Present terminology is based on neuropsychological assessment as well as the mental status examination. It categorizes the neurocognitive status of the AIDS patients into three groups: asymptomatic neurocognitive impairment (ANI), mild neurocognitive disorder (MND), and HAD [20].

Patients with MND present with mild to moderate neurocognitive decline (>1 SD below the mean of demographically adjusted normative scores) in at least two

Table 3.2 Classification of HIV-associated neurocognitive disorders

HIV-associated neurocognitive dysfunction (HAND) type[a]	Prevalence in cART-treated HIV+ individuals	Diagnostic criteria [5]
Asymptomatic neurocognitive impairment (ANI)	30%	Impairment in ≥2 neurocognitive domains (≥1 SD) Does not interfere with daily functioning
Mild neurocognitive disorder (MND)	20–30%	Impairment in ≥2 neurocognitive domains (≥1 SD) Mild to moderate interference in daily functioning
HIV-associated dementia (HAD)	2–8%	Marked (≥2 SD) impairment in ≥2 neurocognitive domains Marked interference in daily functioning

Copyright permission obtained Saylor et al. [22]
SD standard deviation
[a]With no evidence of other cause (Adapted from Antinori et al. [20])

cognitive areas. Such impairment generally mildly interferes with the patient's daily function. Patients with HAD experience moderate to severe cognitive decline (≥ 2 SDs below demographically adjusted normative means) with severe cognitive impairment in at least two cognitive areas. There is significant loss and difficulty with activities of daily living. Behaviorally, patients with HAD experience impairment of abstract thinking process, verbal fluency, decision-making, and working memory [8]. Interestingly, other memory domains operated by the posterior neocortical and temporo-limbic systems remain relatively intact [8]. Many of these patients do not develop aphasia or apraxia.

In patients with HAD, HIV especially targets and impairs the fronto-striato-thalamocortical subcortical circuits. In addition, HIV also involves and damages other white matter pathways and neural networks, including but not limited to, the temporal and parietal lobes [23]. Utilizing high-resolution brain MRI scans, Thompson et al. [22] assessed the thickness of the cerebral cortex as well as gray-matter thickness in AIDS patients. They generated three-dimensional maps demonstrating that primary motor, sensory, and language cortices were 15% thinner in AIDS patients compared to healthy controls. The investigators noted that thinner frontopolar and parietal tissue loss revealed correlation with cognitive and motor abnormalities. Based on their view of the findings, HIV specifically injures the cerebral cortex [23].

Headache in HIV Patients

Primary and secondary headache in patients with HIV are very common, seen in 38–61% of HIV-positive individuals [24]. It remains the most common type of pain, even as the natural course of HIV has changed dramatically with widespread use of cART. Early studies conducted prior to about 2005 yielded different headache profiles than recent publications. Before cART was commonly used, secondary headaches were much more prevalent. Since then Kirkland et al. [24] found that whereas 53.5% of a population of 200 HIV patients endorsed problematic headaches, only 2.8% were associated with opportunistic encephalitic infection. The current International Classification of Headache Disorders (ICHD-3-beta) [25] requires certain diagnostic criteria for diagnosis of headache attributed to HIV infection be met (Table 3.3).

Early publications reported that HIV-associated headaches were tension-type in nature [26] or more likely to worsen primary tension-type headache [27]. The headaches were more common with higher viral loads. The clinical features of primary headache in HIV patients in recent years are more similar to migraine, with the exception that nausea is not as prominent [24]. Photophobia and phonophobia (79%) and aggravation by activity (83%) were, in contrast, quite frequently seen. These headaches were frequent (more than 50% of days or 17 days per month), bilateral, and of severe intensity (7.8/10). Half of patients reported the pain as throbbing in nature. Headache severity, frequency, and disability were inversely tightly correlated with lower CD4 counts, but not with duration of HIV. Another

Table 3.3 Headaches attributed to HIV infection: diagnostic criteria

A. Both of the following:
1. Systemic HIV infection has been demonstrated
2. Other ongoing systemic and/or intracranial infection has been excluded
B. Evidence of causation demonstrated by at least two of the following:
1. Headache has developed in temporal relation to the onset of HIV infection
2. Headache has developed or significantly worsened in temporal relation to worsening of HIV infection as indicated by CD4 cell count and/or viral load
3. Headache has significantly improved in parallel with improvement in HIV infection as indicated by CD4 cell count and/or viral load
In most cases, headache is dull and bilateral or has the features of a primary headache disorder (*migraine* or *tension-type headache*)

observation was that the overall CD4 counts in these patients with headache were higher (due to cART treatment) than in the early reports, underscoring that this migraine-like headache more likely represented the direct effect of HIV on the nervous system as opposed to secondary causes [24].

The pathophysiology behind direct HIV-associated headache has been discussed by Joshi and Cho [28]. There is an underlying CNS inflammatory response to the HIV-1 virus resulting in release of cytokines which may be associated with pain. HIV aseptic meningitis (from HIV or an unidentified virus) with an absence of CSF pleocytosis may underlie headaches in those in whom another secondary cause is not found. There is a lack of agreement between those who have found an association of headache with increased CSF viral load and those who point out that some asymptomatic patients also have HIV cultured from their CSF. There are some similarities of the CNS between HIV and migraine patients. For instance, in migraine, alterations of plasma membranes with ionic gradients result in cortical neuronal depolarization. This leads to cortical spreading depression, further resulting in glutamate release. This situation is similar to early HIV infection-related activity of viral proteins *Tat* and gp120 in neurons. Also, N-methyl-d-aspartate (NMDA) receptors are stimulated by *Tat*, sensitizing the nerves to glutamate and causing excitotoxicity. Gp120, implicated in neuronal injury, may have synergism with glutamate, and its effect can be blocked by an NMDA antagonist. NMDA also plays a role in pain. These authors also mention that the metabolism of tryptophan and serotonin are altered in HIV infection, possibly interrupting endogenous pain modifying mechanisms. Viral-mediated cell death in HIV causes mast cell release of histamine. Mast cells also contain high concentrations of CGRP, a key player in the migraine cascade. It has also been suggested that HIV may affect the trigeminovascular system which triggers the neurovascular response leading to the migraine attack [28].

In the HIV-positive population, new headaches can herald the development of secondary disease and should be regarded as a red flag especially if the CD4 count is below 200, as discussed earlier. Other clues to the need for further testing include any focal neurologic findings, changes in cognition or consciousness, "thunderclap" (ultrafast) onset, worst headache of life, increased headache with strain or cough, papilledema, and constitutional symptoms. Of the secondary CNS lesions associated with headache in HIV, the most common include cryptococcus meningitis, CMV encephalitis, toxoplasmosis, primary CNS lymphoma, PML, CNS tuberculosis, and neurosyphilis. HIV aseptic meningitis may cause headache with or without CSF pleocytosis. Primary angiitis of the nervous system early in the course of HIV infection can occur. In addition, headache can be associated with initiation of cART treatment (especially zidovudine) and with IRIS [29].

Sleep Disturbances in HIV-Infected Patients

Sleep disturbances are very common in patients with HIV infection and have been identified as a serious problem ever since the early stage of the HIV epidemic. They have been reported at all stages of HIV infection, including its progression to AIDS [30–32]. Sleep disorders have been recognized as frequent and disabling illnesses for people living with HIV and AIDS both in the pre-combined antiretroviral therapy (cART) and post-cART epoch with a reported prevalence ranging from 30 to 100% [30, 33–36] as compared to 10–35% [37, 38] in the general population.

In one recent study, the prevalence of self-reported sleep disturbances in HIV-infected people was 58.0% (95% CI = 49.6–66.1) based on meta-analysis, taking into account variations in geographic region, gender, age group, CD4 counts, and instrument used to measure sleep disturbances [30].

The mechanisms of sleep disturbances in HIV-infected patients are not very well understood and largely unknown. Previous reports have suggested possible hints, which include the ability of HIV to affect the CNS, opportunistic infections, mental health issues, pharmacological impact of antiretroviral medications, and substance abuse [37–40].

Sleep disturbances have clinically important consequences in this population which include daytime sleepiness, fatigue, depression, cognitive impairment, neurobehavioral dysfunctions, and reduced quality of life in HIV-infected patients [35, 41–44]. Moreover, HIV-infected patients complaining of sleep disturbances are more likely to demonstrate decreased compliance with recommended cART [40, 45], which potentially can cause loss of virologic control, development of drug-resistant strains of HIV, and treatment failure [46, 47]. Daytime fatigue and insomnia are also prevalent symptoms in HIV disease. Between 33 and 88% of adults with HIV experience fatigue [48–50], and 56% have difficulty sleeping. Fatigue in HIV is related to depression, anxiety, sleep problems, comorbidity, and use of cART [48–52].

A recent study showed that self-reported sleep quality, total sleep time (using wrist actigraphy), and fatigue were significantly associated with perception of cognitive problems in adults with HIV, even after controlling for relevant demographic and clinical characteristics. However, disrupted nighttime sleep (WASO) was unrelated to perception of cognitive problems [53]. Moderate-to-severe poor quality of sleep was independently associated with adherence to HAART. Assessing the quality of sleep and complaints about fatigue may be helpful in the comprehensive evaluation of HIV patients which could lead to effective intervention that with greater impact on improving cognition function and quality of life.

The prevalence of insomnia in the HIV-seropositive population is estimated to be 29–97%, far greater than the 10–33% general population prevalence [36, 54–56]. The roles of immune dysregulation, virus progression, and adverse drug effects in contributing to insomnia are unclear. Psychological morbidity is a major determinant of insomnia in HIV infection. It is recommended that sleep quality should be routinely assessed in order to identify the medical treatment needs and the potential impact of sleep problems on antiretroviral therapy outcomes in this population [36].

There are a limited number of studies dedicated to evaluation of sleep architecture in this population. Early reports of sleep-specific electroencephalographic changes were not confirmed.

During the early stages of HIV, before AIDS onset, patients have excess stage 4 non-rapid eye movement (NREM) sleep during the latter half of the night [55]. Alterations in sleep architecture in HIV disease have been associated with increased circulating levels TNF-a and interleukin 1-beta (IL-1b) [56, 57], which have somnogenic effects that may interrupt sleep and daytime function [58–61].

Other sleep disorders including obstructive sleep apnea (OSA) have been reported commonly in HIV-infected patients [62]. Based on recent studies, the prevalence of OSA is ranging from 3.9 to 70% [62, 63]. These patients share the same major risk factors for OSA with the general population, including aging and obesity. The prevalence of OSA among HIV-infected patients has been elevated even among those who are not overweight or obese. Several factors may be responsible in this finding. These factors include:

1. cART-induced adverse events could predispose to OSA. Lipohypertrophy associated with antiretroviral therapy is an increasingly well-recognized problem that may have a range of deleterious effects [63, 64]. Theoretically, HIV-associated lipohypertrophy could be affecting fat deposition around the posterior oropharyngeal airway and adversely affecting pharyngeal mechanics. HIV patients could also experience upper airway neuromuscular dysfunction and neuromuscular instability in ventilator control, although rigorous data remain sparse. Some antiretroviral drugs (i.e., dideoxynucleoside reverse transcription inhibitors) have been associated with neuromyopathy, and thus these drugs should be avoided in patients reliant on upper airway dilator muscle reflexes for the maintenance of pharyngeal airway patency [65–67]. Certain therapeutic agents commonly used in persons living with HIV infection (anxiolytics, antidepressants, analgesics) have sedating properties and as such would be predicted to raise arousal threshold (i.e., difficult to wake up) [67].
2. cART may simply be facilitating restoration of health and concomitant weight gain such that obesity occurs via the natural history of current diet and exercise patterns [67, 68].
3. The prolonged survival of contemporary HIV-infected patients with improved cART may extend the effects of HIV viremia and immune activation/inflammation over time. Systemic inflammation could affect OSA risk via impaired pharyngeal mechanics and/or could affect the risk of OSA cardiometabolic

complications via inflammatory pathways [67–69]. cART may be prolonging survival such that aging effects on the upper airway may have time to manifest. A variety of these factors likely contribute to the observed link between HIV infection and OSA.

Excessive daytime sleepiness is very common in HIV-infected patients (25–30%) [62].

Men with moderate to severe OSA were more likely than men with mild OSA to have sleepiness. One notable finding was that excessive sleepiness was associated with sleep-disordered breathing as defined by the respiratory disturbance index, but not as defined using the apnea-hypopnea index (AHI). Since recurrent arousals are well known to result in sleepiness [70–73], this disparity most likely reflects the fact that the RDI includes respiratory-related arousals in its definition, while the AHI definition does not.

Fatigue is a common symptom in persons living with HIV, and thus OSA may contribute via sleep disruption in these individuals [62]. Recent studies showed that witnessed apnea was the strongest independent predictor of fatigue. Other predictors included opioid use, depression, antidepressant use, and sleep duration<6 h.

These data taken together strongly support the need for increased efforts directed at early screening and treatment of OSA and other sleep disturbances in patients with HIV infection [74].

Etiology of Neurologic Manifestations in HIV

HIV-1 is a lentivirus (a subgroup of retrovirus) retrovirus and contains ribonucleic acid (RNA). Two distinct types are HIV-1 and HIV-2, while HIV-1 is the predominant virus worldwide. HIV strains can be macrophage – or T lymphocyte – tropic and are capable of infecting differentiated cells and macrophages. HIV infection of the brain involves various cells including perivascular macrophages/microglial cells and astrocytes (Table 3.4). HIV invasion and entry to the CNS is associated with neuroinvasion, neurotropism, and neurovirulence. As mentioned before, neuroinvasion most likely occurs early via infected macrophages which cross the BBB and

Table 3.4 Cells in human body which significantly affected by HIV/AIDS

Lymphoreticular system
CD4+ T lymphocyte
Macrophage
Monocyte
B lymphocyte
Endothelial cells
Microglia
Astrocytes
Oligodendrocytes
Neurons

infect adjacent cells. Another mode of entry via the choroid plexus has also been postulated. Infected macrophages/microglia and astrocytes generate and secrete a number of neurotoxic substances, which collectively add to the pathophysiology of HAD. Some of these are inflammatory cytokines such as TNF-α, IFN-Υ, and platelet-activating factor. Levels of cytokines IL-1, IL-6, and TGF-β are elevated in the brain and CSF of patients with HAD. Chemokines are also released by activated and infected macrophages which include MIP-1α/CCL3, MIP-1β/CCL4, RANTES/CCL5, SDF-1/CXCL12, and CX3CCL1. Other released inflammatory mediators include eicosanoids, excitatory amino acids (such as glutamate), reactive oxygen and nitrogen species, TNF-related apoptosis-inducing ligand, and viral proteins (gp120, gp41, Tat, Nef, and Vpr) (Fig. 3.1) [22].

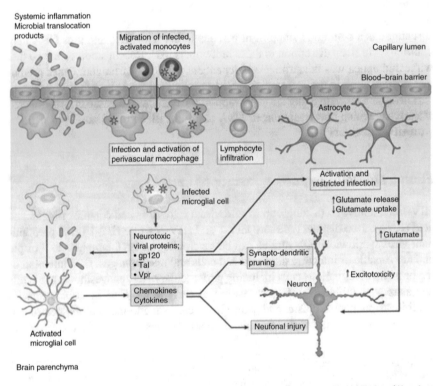

Nature Reviews | Neurology

Fig. 3.1 HIV-infected macrophages and microglial cells release neurotoxic viral proteins that trigger astrocyte activation, which results in increased glutamate release and reduced glutamate uptake. Elevated extracellular glutamate levels cause neuronal bioenergetic disturbances that lead to aberrant synaptodendritic pruning and neuronal injury. Moreover, systemic inflammation and microbial translocation products lead to microglial activation and increased production of chemokines and cytokines that contribute to neuronal injury (From Saylor et al. [22]. Copyright permission obtained; Adapted from Williams et al. [89])

Viral load found in CSF may be related to the severity of HAD. Increased levels of viral protein and RNA detected in CSF have been noted in HAD compared to non-demented AIDS patients.

Neuropathology

Three salient pathological changes observed in HIV encephalitis, both in adults and children, are (1) the presence of multinucleated giant cells or viral antigen, (2) white matter pallor, and (3) microglial nodules [75, 76]. The disruption of the BBB permits egress and deposition of serum proteins into the CNS, which is linked to the white matter pallor. In children, there is also mineralization adjacent to blood vessels. Postmortem examination has demonstrated a number of distinct arrays of neuronal loss [77, 78]. While the larger pyramidal neurons within the cortex are more susceptible to cell death, other neurons expressing somatostatin are resistant to HIV injury.

Vacuolar myelopathy is neuropathologically described as intralaminar edema inside of the myelin sheaths with axonal preservation. Neuropathologically, vacuolar myelopathy of AIDS resembles subacute combined degeneration [13]. Macrophages also play a role as they are found in the posterior columns along with enhanced expression of activation markers. Studies have indicated a relationship of low levels of the protein negative regulatory factor (Nef) in oligodendrocytes with the development of vacuolar myelopathy.

The mechanisms for neuropathy in HIV patients are related to neuronal and axonal injury due to neurotoxicity of HIV and envelope glycoprotein gp120. HIV infection alone in the root ganglia leads to upregulation of IL-1β and TNF-α. As mentioned before, macrophages can play a role in the dorsal root ganglion neurons and Schwann cells. Gp120 is involved in direct toxicity by activation of the mitochondrial caspase pathway which leads to apoptosis and axonal degeneration. HIV patients also exhibit distal sensory polyneuropathy with reduction of epidermal nerve fibers in lower extremities related to macrophage infiltration and activation markers. Other agents like alcohol and illegal drugs in patients with HIV contribute to neuropathy. Nutritional factors like vitamin deficiencies should be addressed in this population. Neuropathy does not seem to be related to viral load or decreased CD4$^+$ T lymphocyte count.

Mitochondrial toxicity has been suggested with the use of nucleoside reverse transcriptase inhibitors. L-carnitine levels are reduced which causes a disruption in the membrane energy balance and fatty acid oxidation. Low levels of L-carnitine are reported in patients with neuropathy likely from the accumulation of fatty acids. L-carnitine is important for peripheral nerve regeneration and its neuroprotective abilities.

HIV patients may develop inclusion body myositis or polymyositis, and histopathologic studies of these cases have revealed the upregulation of Toll-like receptor-3 mRNA [79].

Epidemiology

Mild forms of cognitive impairment happen in about 40% of HIV patients, while the prevalence of HIV-related dementia in advanced stages is 7–27%. The incidence increases by threefold with CD4$^+$ lymphocyte count below 200 cells/mm^3 and by sevenfold if less than 100 cells/mm^3. Coinfection with hepatitis C and coexistence of diabetes mellitus are also other contributing factors in the development of cognitive problems. The introduction of HAART decreased the incidence of dementia in both adults and children.

Neuropathies in HIV patients are on the rise and affect as much as 50% of patients receiving HAART. Risk factors for peripheral neuropathy include male sex, older age, alcohol abuse, and exposure to dideoxynucleosides and protease inhibitors. Sympathetic sensory neuropathy is common with didanosine and stavudine.

Prevention

The incidence of HIV has dropped due to availability of HAART and more widespread use of preventive methods. Public knowledge about AIDS and its devastating consequences has increased, which in turn, may explain lower number of new cases. Primary prevention places emphasis of prevention of occurrence of the infection. Nowadays, society is more aware of the various mechanisms of transmission and modes of prevention such as condom use, substitution of formula for breastfeeding, and avoiding needle sharing in drug abusers. The medical world has witnessed a significant drop in incidence rate since the 1980s due to this approach; however, there still exist areas of concern such as rate of new cases in the minority communities. Early detection and treatment constitute the main target for the secondary prevention. Early treatment maintains patients in the latent period longer and delays symptomatic progression of the disease. Tertiary prevention focuses on limiting disability and rehabilitation. Prophylactic therapy for opportunistic infections is a form of primary prevention but can be successful in secondary and tertiary levels.

Differential Diagnosis

HIV-associated dementia can be mistaken for opportunistic infections, CNS lymphoma, vascular disease, toxic effects, metabolic etiologies, and depression. Each one of these conditions affects the HIV patient's cognition adversely. Meticulous examination is necessary to tease out the correct diagnosis. The patient's age also needs to be considered as a contributing factor in the development of dementia especially as the HIV population is treated with better drugs and living longer. The differential diagnoses of HIV myelopathy include infectious, neoplastic, and metabolic myelopathies. Coinfection with varicella zoster, herpes simplex, and HTLV-I and HTLV-II should be considered and ruled out. Chronic neuropathy may be due to alcoholism, metabolic derangement, paraneoplastic, and paraproteinemic causes. cART-related neurotoxicity-induced neuropathies are dose dependent and improve with cessation.

Diagnostic Workup

Neuroimaging plays a crucial role in diagnosis, differential diagnoses, treatment, and follow-up of patients with neuroAIDS. Obtaining an MRI of the brain and spinal cord with and without contrast is of utmost significance. Patients with HIV encephalitis demonstrate cerebral and basal ganglia atrophy as well as widespread hyperintense white matter lesions on T2-weighted sequences (Fig. 3.2) [80]. 1H MR spectroscopy of patients with HAD has shown an increased myoinositol/creatine (mI/Cr) ratio in the frontal white matter using SV-MRS and an increased choline (Cho)/Cr ratio in the mesial frontal gray matter compared to HIV+ individuals without psychomotor slowing (Fig. 3.3) [12]. It also reveals decreased N-acetyl aspartate peak in the brain – an indicator of neuronal injury or death in the context of HAD [81]. In HIV-seropositive patients without dementia, 1H MRS reveals elevated levels of the glial marker myoinositol/creatinine in the white matter [82, 83]. Other neuroimaging findings of HAD include cerebral atrophy along with atrophy of the basal ganglia and the presence of white matter hyperintensities on FLAIR sequences. Cord atrophy may be seen on spine MR imaging which points to a diagnosis of vacuolar myelopathy.

HIV encephalitis

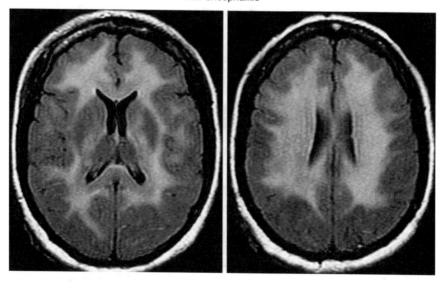

Fig. 3.2 Brain axial view, FLAIR sequence. MRS. Hyperintensity in white matter involving centrum semiovale and internal and external capsule. Widespread demyelination including the corpus callosum

HIV encephalitis

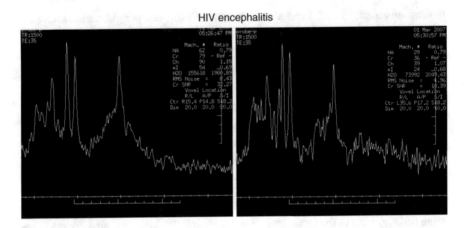

Fig. 3.3 Magnetic resonance spectroscopy in white matter (*left*): parietal region. On the right, frontal region. Decreased NAA indicating neuronal loss, increased myoinositol showing increased membrane metabolism corresponding to an active inflammatory process, increased myoinositol indicating increase in glial component

Examination of CSF reveals pleocytosis along with elevated protein concentration. Other reported CSF abnormalities include the detection of HIV-1 antigen as well as intrathecal generation of anti-HIV-1 antibodies and oligoclonal bands and detection of the inflammatory mediators such as CCL-2 and sCD14. Other markers of active inflammation and potent immune response in the CSF of AIDS patients include elevated levels of beta-2 microglobulin and neopterin. Bossi et al. [84] prospectively measured the level of HIV-1 RNA in the CSF of AIDS patients and reported that the HIV-1 RNA is detectable in CSF of AIDS patients; however, this parameter was not an accurate marker of HIV encephalitis. MRI and CSF examinations, combined, also enable the neurologist to exclude other differential diagnoses.

Electromyography and nerve conductions are routinely performed in AIDS patients with peripheral neuropathy. Diagnosis of AIDP and CIDP in AIDS patients follows the same protocol in HIV-seronegative patients. Certain AIDS patients with HIV-induced myopathy or muscle disease secondary to antiretroviral medications may require muscle biopsy.

Treatment

Presently, AIDS and neuroAIDS remain incurable and existing therapeutic measures only contain the infection and improve patient's clinical symptoms. Available antiretroviral therapies, if successful, can only decelerate the progression of the underlying disease and by altering its natural course, enhance patient's lifespan. There has been a drop in the number of patients with HIV infection and moderate to severe dementia following the use of HAART as of 1996 [85]. Interestingly, the sustained presence of less severe forms of HAND, even in patients with sustained virologic control, fosters the idea that cognitive decline in certain patients may not be responsive to treatment. Multiple antiretroviral agents have been shown to have a better effect than monotherapy or no therapy at all in patient with HIV-related dementia. Another significant finding is that, even in the time of treatment with antiretroviral medications, a significant drop of the number of $CD4^+$ T lymphocytes remains a strong risk factor for development of HAND. This also points to the fact that profound immunosuppression may lead to permanent neuropathology [86].

Improvements in psychomotor activities and speed have been shown in patients treated with HAART. MRI spectroscopy has shown the HAART regimen reverses abnormalities in brain metabolites seen in mild HIV dementia. HAART also has an effect in improving cognitive deficits compared to AZT or dual antiviral therapy. Some patients improve dramatically and may be able to return to employment. Neuropsychological evaluation shows improvement in the areas of attention, verbal fluency, and visuo-construction tasks. Of all FDA-approved antiretroviral medications, most have weak CSF-to-plasma ratios except for AZT, stavudine, abacavir, and nevirapine. Triple therapy is preferred. Viral load elevation following initiation of therapy may indicate resistance. Anti-inflammatory medications, antioxidants, and anti-excitotoxic agents may be utilized to circumvent neurodegeneration.

Psychiatric assessment and treatment of patients with neuroAIDS and HAD are necessary and useful since many of these patients suffer from agitation, anxiety, fatigue, and depression. Antidepressant, antipsychotics, or psychostimulants can help treat mania and psychosis. A multidisciplinary team should be available to these patients. Nutritional therapies can help with cognitive and motor symptoms particularly in those patients with wasting syndrome or toxic nutritional deficiencies. One particular medication, efavirenz, despite having good CNS penetration, may be associated with significant neuropsychiatric side effects (such as depression, anxiety, paranoia, and psychosis) and should be generally avoided in AIDS patients with psychiatric disorders.

Vacuolar myelopathy is incurable with very limited treatment options. The management of these patients significantly relies on physical therapy and symptomatic treatment of spasticity and its related complications. Gait difficulties as well as sphincter dysfunction require symptomatic therapy. There is no treatment for sensory polyneuropathy. However, neuropathy due to nucleoside analogue reverse transcriptase inhibitors may be treated with acetyl-L-carnitine. Supportive therapies such as pain management are also recommended for polyneuropathy.

Syndromes like AIDP and CIDP should be treated as with seronegative HIV patients. Some patient may improve with HAART. Patient with AZT myopathy can be helped with L-carnitine. Movement disorders in HIV patients are treated by treating the underlying opportunistic infection. They are not usually responsive to symptomatic treatment [87, 88]. One exception may be cases of hemiballismus, which may get better with the use of antipsychotics.

Except for eradication of secondary causes, treatment of headache in HIV is geared toward symptom improvement. General preventive and abortive headache treatments can be implemented. However, Sheikh and Cho [29] point out that there are important caveats to drug treatment in HIV patients due to their comorbidities and drug interactions with cART. Because HIV patients are at risk for vascular disease earlier in life, the practitioner must rule this out in each patient prior to using triptans. Triptans and preventives metabolized by the liver may also be contraindicated if the patient has hepatitis C, commonly seen with HIV. Ergots (rarely used for acute migraine anymore) and ergot derivatives such as dihydroergotamine are strictly contraindicated in the presence of protease inhibitors for HIV treatment because of reports of sometimes fatal ergotism. If nonsteroidal anti-inflammatory agents are used for headache, they should not be paired with proton pump inhibitors, which can interact with some cARTs causing decreased efficacy of the latter. Patients treated with corticosteroids to "break" a prolonged headache cycle must be monitored for signs of worsening immunosuppression. Beta-blockers for prevention are okay with the exception of metoprolol, which may act as a substrate for some cART medications. Divalproex sodium and topiramate are relatively safe in this population. Carbamazepine should be avoided due to induction of the CYP450 system leading to lower cART concentrations. Fluoxetine inhibits CYP450 and interferes with cART as well. On the other hand, tricyclic antidepressants and serotonin-norepinephrine reuptake inhibitors are used without problems for pain and headache syndromes in HIV. For chronic migraine, onabotulinum toxin A is the only FDA-approved preventive treatment and should not pose a problem for HIV patients. Injectors should take routine precautions to avoid HIV transmission through blood contact.

Conclusion

Over the past two decades and with widespread utilization of cART, the natural course of HIV infection has altered, and consequently neurologists encounter opportunistic CNS infections, CNS lymphoma, and HIV vacuolar myelopathy uncommonly. More chronic complications of AIDS such as cognitive decline, psychiatric disorders, peripheral neuropathy, and the side effects of antiretroviral therapy constitute most of the present day neurology consults. Proper and timely diagnosis of AIDS and its neurologic complications and early initiation of the therapy do carry a significant effect on the disease process and can potentially improve the quality of life of AIDS patients.

References

1. Hellmuth J, Fletcher JL, Valcour V, Kroon E, Ananworanich J, Intasan J, Lerdlum S, Narvid J, Pothisri M, Allen I, Krebs SJ, Slike B, Prueksakaew P, Jagodzinski LL, Puttamaswin S, Phanuphak N, Spudich S, SEARCH 010/RV254 Study Group. Neurologic signs and symptoms frequently manifest in acute HIV infection. Neurology. 2016;87(2):148–54.
2. Brannagan 3rd TH, Zhou Y. HIV-associated Guillain-Barré syndrome. J Neurol Sci. 2003;208(1–2):39–42.
3. Denning DW, Anderson J, Rudge P, Smith H. Acute myelopathy associated with primary infection with human immunodeficiency virus. Br Med J (Clin Res Ed). 1987;294(6565):143–4.
4. Reus S, Boix V, Priego M, Merino E, Portilla J. Cytomegalovirus polyradiculopathy presenting as bilateral radial nerve palsies in a patient with AIDS. Eur J Clin Microbiol Infect Dis. 1999;18(8):605–6.

5. Carroll MB, Holmes R. Dermatomyositis and HIV infection: case report and review of the literature. Rheumatol Int. 2011;31(5):673–9.
6. Johnson RW, Williams FM, Kazi S, Dimachkie MM, Reveille JD. Human immunodeficiency virus-associated polymyositis: a longitudinal study of outcome. Arthritis Rheum. 2003;49(2):172–8.
7. Chariot P, Ruet E, Authier FJ, Lévy Y, Gherardi R. Acute rhabdomyolysis in patients infected by human immunodeficiency virus. Neurology. 1994;44(9):1692–6.
8. Nath A. Neurologic complications of human immunodeficiency virus infection. Continuum (Minneap Minn). 2015;21(6 Neuroinfectious Disease):1557–76.
9. Couderc LJ, D'Agay MF, Danon F, et al. Sicca complex and infection with human immunodeficiency virus. Arch Intern Med. 1987;147:898–901.
10. Teener JW. Inflammatory and toxic myopathy. Semin Neurol. 2012;32(5):491–9. doi:10.105 5/s-0033-1334467. Epub 2013 May 15.
11. Kiyomoto BH, Tengan CH, Godinho RO. Effects of short-term zidovudine exposure on mitochondrial DNA content and succinate dehydrogenase activity of rat skeletal muscle cells. J Neurol Sci. 2008;268(1–2):33–9.
12. Sacktor N, Skolasky RL, Ernst T, Mao X, Selnes O, Pomper MG, Chang L, Zhong K, Shungu DC, Marder K, Shibata D, Schifitto G, Bobo L, Barker PB. A multicenter study of two magnetic resonance spectroscopy techniques in individuals with HIV dementia. J Magn Reson Imaging. 2005;21(4):325–33.
13. Petito CK, Navia BA, Cho ES, Jordan BD, George DC, Price RW. Vacuolar myelopathy pathologically resembling subacute combined degeneration in patients with the acquired immunodeficiency syndrome. N Engl J Med. 1985;312(14):874–9.
14. Hénin D, Smith TW, De Girolami U, Sughayer M, Hauw JJ. Neuropathology of the spinal cord in the acquired immunodeficiency syndrome. Hum Pathol. 1992;23(10):1106–14.
15. Moulignier A, Moulonguet A, Pialoux G, Rozenbaum W. Reversible ALS-like disorder in HIV infection. Neurology. 2001;57(6):995–1001.
16. Ortiz G, Koch S, Romano JG, Forteza AM, Rabinstein AA. Mechanisms of ischemic stroke in HIV-infected patients. Neurology. 2007;68(16):1257–61.
17. Minagar A, Schatz NJ, Glaser JS. Case report: one-and-a-half-syndrome and tuberculosis of the pons in a patient with AIDS. AIDS Patient Care STDS. 2000;14(9):461–4.
18. Shelburne SA, Visnegarwala F, Darcourt J, Graviss EA, Giordano TP, White Jr AC, Hamill RJ. Incidence and risk factors for immune reconstitution inflammatory syndrome during highly active antiretroviral therapy. AIDS. 2005;19(4):399–406.
19. Zaffiri L, Verma R, Struzzieri K, Monterroso J, Batts DH, Loehrke ME. Immune reconstitution inflammatory syndrome involving the central nervous system in a patient with HIV infection: a case report and review of literature. New Microbiol. 2013;36(1):89–92.
20. Antinori A, Arendt G, Becker JT, Brew BJ, Byrd DA, Cherner M, Clifford DB, Cinque P, Epstein LG, Goodkin K, Gisslen M, Grant I, Heaton RK, Joseph J, Marder K, Marra CM, McArthur JC, Nunn M, Price RW, Pulliam L, Robertson KR, Sacktor N, Valcour V, Wojna VE. Updated research nosology for HIV-associated neurocognitive disorders. Neurology. 2007;69(18):1789–99.
21. Gannon P, Khan MZ, Kolson DL. Current understanding of HIV-associated neurocognitive disorders pathogenesis. Curr Opin Neurol. 2011;24(3):275–83.
22. Saylor D, Dickens AM, Sacktor N, Haughey N, Slusher B, Pletnikov M, Mankowski JL, Brown A, Volsky DJ, McArthur JC. HIV-associated neurocognitive disorder – pathogenesis and prospects for treatment. Nat Rev Neurol. 2016;12(5):309.
23. Thompson PM, Dutton RA, Hayashi KM, Toga AW, Lopez OL, Aizenstein HJ, Becker JT. Thinning of the cerebral cortex visualized in HIV/AIDS reflects CD4+ T lymphocyte decline. Proc Natl Acad Sci U S A. 2005;102(43):15647–52.
24. Kirkland KE, Kirkland K, Many WJ, et al. Headache among patients with HIV disease: prevalence, characteristics, and associations. Headache. 2012;52:455–66.
25. Headache Classification Committee of the International Headache Society (IHS). The International Classification of Headache Disorders, 3rd edition (beta version). Cephalalgia. 2013;33:629–808.

26. Lipton RB, Feraru ER, Weiss G, et al. Headache in HIV-1-related disorders. Headache. 1991;31:518–22.
27. Evers S, Wibbeke B, Tichelt D, et al. The impact of HIV infection on primary headache. Unexpected findings from retrospective, cross-sectional, and prospective analyses. Pain. 2000;85:191–200.
28. Joshi SG, Cho TA. Pathophysiological mechanisms of headache in HIV. Headache. 2014;54:946–50.
29. Sheikh HU, Cho TA. Clinical aspects of headache in HIV. Headache. 2014;54:939–45.
30. Wu J, Wu H, Lu C, Guo L, Li P. Self-reported sleep disturbances in HIV-infected people: a meta-analysis of prevalence and moderators. Sleep Med. 2015;16(8):901–7.
31. Norman SE, Resnick L, Cohn MA, et al. Sleep disturbances in HIV-seropositive patients. JAMA. 1988;260:922.
32. Hand GA, Phillips KD, Dudgeon WD. Perceived stress in HIV-infected individuals: physiological and psychological correlates. AIDS Care. 2006;18:1011–7.
33. Ammassari A, Murri R, Pezzotti P, et al. Self-reported symptoms and medication side effects influence adherence to highly active antiretroviral therapy in persons with HIV infection. J Acquir Immune Defic Syndr. 2001;28:445–9.
34. Robbins JL, Phillips KD, Dudgeon WD, et al. Physiological and psychological correlates of sleep in HIV infection. Clin Nurs Res. 2004;13:33–52.
35. Phillips KD, Mock KS, Bopp CM, et al. Spiritual well-being, sleep disturbance, and mental and physical health status in HIV-infected individuals. Issues Ment Health Nurs. 2006;27:125–39.
36. Reid S, Dwyer J. Insomnia in HIV infection: a systematic review of prevalence, correlates, and management. Psychosom Med. 2005;67:260–9.
37. Ford DE, Kamerow DB. Epidemiologic study of sleep disturbances and psychiatric disorders. An opportunity for prevention? JAMA. 1989;262:1479–84.
38. Ram S, Seirawan H, Kumar SK, et al. Prevalence and impact of sleep disorders and sleep habits in the United States. Sleep Breath. 2010;14:63–70.
39. Vosvick M, Gore-Felton C, Ashton E, et al. Sleep disturbances among HIV-positive adults: the role of pain, stress, and social support. J Psychosom Res. 2004;57:459–63.
40. Omonuwa TS, Goforth HW, Preud'homme X, et al. The pharmacologic management of insomnia in patients with HIV. J Clin Sleep Med. 2009;5:251–62.
41. Wiegand M, Moller AA, Schreiber W, et al. Alterations of nocturnal sleep in patients with HIV infection. Acta Neurol Scand. 1991;83:141–2.
42. Phillips KD, Sowell RL, Rojas M, et al. Physiological and psychological correlates of fatigue in HIV disease. Biol Res Nurs. 2004;6:59–74.
43. Phillips KD, Sowell RL, Boyd M, et al. Sleep quality and health-related quality of life in HIV-infected African-American women of childbearing age. Qual Life Res. 2005;14:959–70.
44. Clifford DB, Evans S, Yang Y, et al. Impact of efavirenz on neuropsychological performance and symptoms in HIV-infected individuals. Ann Intern Med. 2005;143:714–21.
45. Phillips KD, Moneyham L, Murdaugh C, et al. Sleep disturbance and depression as barriers to adherence. Clin Nurs Res. 2005;14:273–93.
46. Gifford AL, Bormann JE, Shively MJ, et al. Predictors of self-reported adherence and plasma HIV concentrations in patients on multidrug antiretroviral regimens. J Acquir Immune Defic Syndr. 2000;23:386–95.
47. Paterson DL, Swindells S, Mohr J, et al. Adherence to protease inhibitor therapy and outcomes in patients with HIV infection. Ann Intern Med. 2000;133:21–30.
48. Jong E, Oudhoff LA, Epskamp C, Wagener MN, van Duijn M, Fischer S, van Gorp EC. Predictors and treatment strategies of HIV-related fatigue in the combined antiretroviral therapy era. AIDS. 2010;24(10):1387–405.
49. Millikin CP, Rourke SB, Halman MH, Power C. Fatigue in HIV/AIDS is associated with depression and subjective neurocognitive complaints but not neuropsychological functioning. J Clin Exp Neuropsychol. 2003;25(2):201–15.
50. Lee KA, Gay C, Portillo CJ, Coggins T, Davis H, Pullinger CR, Aouizerat BE. Symptom experience in HIV-infected adults: a function of demographic and clinical characteristics. J Pain Symptom Manage. 2009;38(6):882–93.

51. Aouizerat BE, Gay CL, Lerdal A, Portillo CJ, Lee KA. Lack of energy: an important and distinct component of HIV-related fatigue and daytime function. J Pain Symptom Manage. 2013;45(2):191–201.
52. Byun E, Gay CL, Lee KA. Sleep, fatigue, and problems with cognitive function in adults living with HIV. J Assoc Nurses AIDS Care. 2016;27(1):5–16.
53. Tello-Velásquez JR, Díaz-Llanes BE, Mezones-Holguín E, Rodríguez-Morales AJ, Huamaní C, Hernández AV, Arévalo-Abanto J. Poor quality of sleep associated with low adherence to highly active antiretroviral therapy in Peruvian patients with HIV/AIDS. Cad Saude Publica. 2015;31(5):989–1002.
54. Low Y, Goforth H, Preud'homme X, Edinger J, Krystal A. Insomnia in HIV-infected patients: pathophysiologic implications. AIDS Rev. 2014;16(1):3–13.
55. Norman SE, Chediak AD, Freeman C, et al. Sleep disturbances in men with asymptomatic human immunodeficiency (HIV) infection. Sleep. 1992;15:150–5.
56. Darko DF, Mitler MM, White JL. Sleep disturbance in early HIV infection. Focus. 1995;10:5–6.
57. Darko DF, Miller JC, Gallen C, White J, Koziol J, et al. Sleep electroencephalogram delta-frequency amplitude, night plasma levels of tumor necrosis factor alpha, and human immunodeficiency virus infection. Proc Natl Acad Sci U S A. 1995;92:12080–4.
58. Chang FC, Opp MR. IL-1 is a mediator of increases in slow-wave sleep induced by CRH receptor blockade. Am J Physiol Regul Integr Comp Physiol. 2000;279:R793–802.
59. Terao A, Matsumura H, Yoneda H, Saito M. Enhancement of slow-wave sleep by tumor necrosis factor-alpha is mediated by cyclooxygenase-2 in rats. Neuroreport. 1998;9:3791–6.
60. Takahashi S, Kapas L, Fang J, Krueger JM. Somnogenic relationships between tumor necrosis factor and interleukin-1. Am J Physiol. 1999;276:R1132–40.
61. Gemma C, Opp MR. Human immunodeficiency virus glycoproteins 160 and 41 alter sleep and brain temperature of rats. J Neuroimmunol. 1999;97:94–101.
62. Patil SP, Brown TT, Jacobson LP, Margolick JB, Laffan A, Johnson-Hill L, Godfrey R, Johnson J, Reynolds S, Schwartz AR, Smith PL. Sleep disordered breathing, fatigue, and sleepiness in HIV-infected and -uninfected men. PLoS One. 2014;9(7):e99258.
63. Kunisaki KM, Akgün KM, Fiellin DA, Gibert CL, Kim JW, Rimland D, Rodriguez-Barradas MC, Yaggi HK, Crothers K. Prevalence and correlates of obstructive sleep apnoea among patients with and without HIV infection. HIV Med. 2015;16(2):105–13.
64. Leung VL, Glesby MJ. Pathogenesis and treatment of HIV lipohypertrophy. Curr Opin Infect Dis. 2011;24:43–9.
65. Saboisky JP, Stashuk DW, Hamilton-Wright A, Carusona AL, Campana LM, Trinder J, Eckert DJ, Jordan AS, McSharry DG, White DP, Nandedkar S, David WS, Malhotra A. Neurogenic changes in the upper airway of patients with obstructive sleep apnea. Am J Respir Crit Care Med. 2012;185:322–9.
66. Nguyen AT, Jobin V, Payne R, Beauregard J, Naor N, Kimoff RJ. Laryngeal and velopharyngeal sensory impairment in obstructive sleep apnea. Sleep. 2005;28:585–93.
67. Darquenne C, Hicks CB, Malhotra A. The ongoing need for good physiological investigation: obstructive sleep apnea in HIV patients as a paradigm. J Appl Physiol (1985). 2015;118(2):244–6.
68. Lakey W, Yang LY, Yancy W, Chow SC, Hicks C. Short communication: from wasting to obesity: initial antiretroviral therapy and weight gain in HIV-infected persons. AIDS Res Hum Retroviruses. 2013;29:435–40.
69. Shapiro SD, Chin CH, Kirkness JP, McGinley BM, Patil SP, Polotsky VY, Biselli PJC, Smith PL, Schneider H, Schwartz AR. Leptin and the control of pharyngeal patency during sleep in severe obesity. J Appl Physiol. 2014;116:1334–41.
70. Guilleminault C, Stoohs R, Clerk A, Cetel M, Maistros P. A cause of excessive daytime sleepiness. The upper airway resistance syndrome. Chest. 1993;104:781–7.
71. Stepanski E, Lamphere J, Badia P, Zorick F, Roth T. Sleep fragmentation and daytime sleepiness. Sleep. 1984;7:18–26.
72. Stepanski EJ. The effect of sleep fragmentation on daytime function. Sleep. 2002;25:268–76.

73. Guilleminault C, Hagen CC, Huynh NT. Comparison of hypopnea definitions in lean patients with known obstructive sleep apnea hypopnea syndrome (OSAHS). Sleep Breath. 2009;13:341–7.

74. Goswami U, Baker JV, Wang Q, Khalil W, Kunisaki KM. Sleep apnea symptoms as a predictor of fatigue in an urban HIV Clinic. AIDS Patient Care STDS. 2015;29(11):591–6.

75. Navia BA, Cho ES, Petito CK, Price RW. The AIDS dementia complex: II. Neuropathology. Ann Neurol. 1986;19(6):525–35.

76. Glass JD, Fedor H, Wesselingh SL, McArthur JC. Immunocytochemical quantitation of human immunodeficiency virus in the brain: correlations with dementia. Ann Neurol. 1995;38(5):755–62.

77. Masliah E, Ge N, Achim CL, Hansen LA, Wiley CA. Selective neuronal vulnerability in HIV encephalitis. J Neuropathol Exp Neurol. 1992;51(6):585–93.

78. Everall IP, Glass JD, McArthur J, Spargo E, Lantos P. Neuronal density in the superior frontal and temporal gyri does not correlate with the degree of human immunodeficiency virus-associated dementia. Acta Neuropathol. 1994;88(6):538–44.

79. Schreiner B, Voss J, Wischhusen J, Dombrowski Y, Steinle A, Lochmüller H, Dalakas M, Melms A, Wiendl H. Expression of toll-like receptors by human muscle cells in vitro and in vivo: TLR3 is highly expressed in inflammatory and HIV myopathies, mediates IL-8 release and up-regulation of NKG2D-ligands. FASEB J. 2006;20(1):118–20.

80. Dousset V, Armand JP, Lacoste D, Mièze S, Letenneur L, Dartigues JF, Caill JM. Magnetization transfer study of HIV encephalitis and progressive multifocal leukoencephalopathy. Groupe d'Epidémiologie Clinique du SIDA en Aquitaine. AJNR Am J Neuroradiol. 1997;18(5):895–901.

81. Yiannoutsos CT, Nakas CT, Navia BA, Proton MRS Consortium. Assessing multiple-group diagnostic problems with multi-dimensional receiver operating characteristic surfaces: application to proton MR Spectroscopy (MRS) in HIV-related neurological injury. Neuroimage. 2008;40(1):248–55.

82. Ernst T, Chang L. Arnold S Increased glial metabolites predict increased working memory network activation in HIV brain injury. Neuroimage. 2003;19(4):1686–93.

83. Chang L, Ernst T, Leonido-Yee M, Walot I, Singer E. Cerebral metabolite abnormalities correlate with clinical severity of HIV-1 cognitive motor complex. Neurology. 1999;52(1):100–8.

84. Bossi P, Dupin N, Coutellier A, Bricaire F, Lubetzki C, Katlama C, Calvez V. The level of human immunodeficiency virus (HIV) type 1 RNA in cerebrospinal fluid as a marker of HIV encephalitis. Clin Infect Dis. 1998;26(5):1072–3.

85. McArthur JC, Brew BJ, Nath A. Neurological complications of HIV infection. Lancet Neurol. 2005;4(9):543–55.

86. Heaton RK, Franklin DR, Ellis RJ, JA MC, Letendre SL, Leblanc S, Corkran SH, Duarte NA, Clifford DB, Woods SP, Collier AC, Marra CM, Morgello S, Mindt MR, Taylor MJ, Marcotte TD, Atkinson JH, Wolfson T, Gelman BB, JC MA, Simpson DM, Abramson I, Gamst A, Fennema-Notestine C, Jernigan TL, Wong J, Grant I, CHARTER Group, HNRC Group. HIV-associated neurocognitive disorders before and during the era of combination antiretroviral therapy: differences in rates, nature, and predictors. J Neurovirol. 2011;17(1):3–16.

87. Estrada-Bellmann I, Camara-Lemarroy CR, Flores-Cantu H, Calderon-Hernandez HJ, Villareal-Velazquez HJ. Hemichorea in a patient with HIV-associated central nervous system histoplasmosis. Int J STD AIDS. 2016;27(1):75–7.

88. Rabhi S, Amrani K, Maaroufi M, Khammar Z, Khibri H, Ouazzani M, Berrady R, Tizniti S, Messouak O, Belahsen F, Bono W. Hemichorea-hemiballismus as an initial manifestation in a Moroccan patient with acquired immunodeficiency syndrome and toxoplasma infection: a case report and review of the literature. Pan Afr Med J. 2011;10:9.

89. Williams DW et al. Monocytes mediate HIV neuropathogenesis: mechanisms that contribute to HIV associated neurocognitive disorders. Curr HIV Res. 2014;12(2):85–96.

Central Nervous System Vasculitis: Immunopathogenesis, Clinical Aspects, and Treatment Options

4

Roger E. Kelley, Ramy El-Khoury, and Brian P. Kelley

Introduction

There continues to be significant challenges in determining the etiology of vascular inflammation of the nervous system. Not only can the clinical presentation be obscure, there is the differentiation of primary central nervous system (CNS) vasculitis from secondary vasculitis related to various systemic illnesses such as connective tissue disorders, sarcoid, infectious etiologies such neuroborreliosis, neoplastic vascular involvement, and an array of other autoimmune processes such as Susac syndrome and demyelinating disorders. Primary CNS vasculitis, also known as angiitis, is often denoted as primary angiitis of the CNS (PACNS). It is considered rare, but enhanced diagnostic measures have led PACNS to be a not uncommonly encountered component of the differential diagnosis in the inflammatory disorders of the CNS. Much has been made of the determination of PACNS by vasculitic changes most sensitively detected by a suggestive pattern on intra-arterial cerebral angiography (Fig. 4.1). However, it is now well recognized that the sensitivity of such imaging is certainly not 100% especially when one is encountering small vessel involvement. On the other hand, the index of suspicion tends to be much higher when there is a so-called smoking gun for inflammatory CNS disorders such as coexistent rheumatological disorders including systemic lupus erythematosus, Sjogren's syndrome, neuro-Behcet's disease, Wegener's granulomatosis, polyarteritis nodosa, Kohlmeier-Degos disease, Cogan's syndrome, sarcoid granulomatosis and angiitis, granulomatous (temporal) arteritis, and scleroderma. The overall differential diagnosis of central nervous system

R.E. Kelley, MD (✉) • R. El-Khoury, MD • B.P. Kelley, BS
Department of Neurology, Tulane University School of Medicine,
1430 Tulane Avenue 8065, New Orleans, LA 70112, USA
e-mail: rkelley2@tulane.edu; relkhour@tulane.edu; bkelley1@tulane.edu

© Springer International Publishing AG 2017
A. Minagar, J.S. Alexander (eds.), *Inflammatory Disorders of the Nervous System*, Current Clinical Neurology, DOI 10.1007/978-3-319-51220-4_4

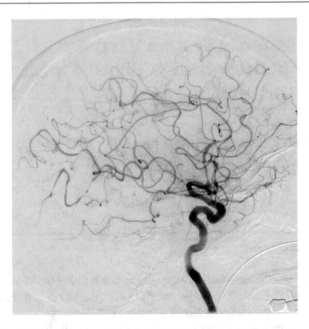

Fig. 4.1 Cerebral arteriogram in patient diagnosed with primary central nervous system angiitis. There is diffuse vessel narrowing in this patient with a stroke-like presentation

Table 4.1 Differential diagnosis of primary central nervous system vasculitis

1. Primary angiitis of the CNS	10. Progressive multifocal leukoencephalopathy
2. Reversible cerebral vasoconstriction syndrome	11. Lymphocytic angioendotheliosis
3. Fibromuscular dysplasia	12. Cerebral autosomal dominant arteriopathy with subcortical infarcts and leukoencephalopathy (CADASIL)
4. Systemic autoimmune disorders (Table 4.2)	
5. CNS lymphoma	13. Chronic lymphocytic inflammation with pontine perivascular enhancement responsive to steroids (CLIPPERS)
6. Multiple sclerosis	
7. Acute disseminated encephalomyelitis	
8. CNS infectious processes (Table 4.3)	14. Mitochondrial encephalopathy with lactic acidosis and stroke-like syndromes (MELAS)
9. Moyamoya disease	

vasculitis is summarized in Table 4.1. Potential autoimmune mechanisms are summarized in Table 4.2.

From a practical standpoint, one must determine if the presentation represents actual PACNS, when confined to the CNS, or the primary mimic of this disorder which is reversible cerebral vasoconstriction syndrome (RCVS). This has major implications, and it will determine whether or not potent immunosuppression, specifically for PACNS, is indicated or not.

Table 4.2 Autoimmune disorders associated with central nervous system vasculitis with subcategories

Large vessel	Medium vessel
1. Giant cell arteritis	1. Polyarteritis nodosa
2. Takayasu arteritis	2. Kawasaki disease
Small vessel rheumatologic	
1. Systemic lupus erythematosus	3. Sjogren's syndrome
2. Rheumatoid arthritis	4. Scleroderma
Antineutrophil cytoplasmic antibody (ANCA) associated	
1. Wegener's granulomatosis	3. Microscopic polyangiitis
2. Churg-Strauss syndrome	
Immune-complex deposition associated	
1. Henoch-Schonlein purpura	2. Cryoglobulinemia
Other inflammatory or undetermined pathogenesis	
1. Neuro-Behcet's syndrome	4. Cogan's syndrome
2. Sarcoidosis disease	5. Churg-Strauss syndrome
3. Susac syndrome	

Primary Angiitis of the Central Nervous System (PACNS)

Overview

PACNS is based upon the determination of unexplained neurological or psychiatric manifestations with demonstration of arteritis of the CNS by either angiography and/or pathological confirmation. Childhood PACNS is similar except for an age range of 1 month of age or older up to 18 years of age [1]. In many patients, the clinical presentation is one of the unexplained stroke-like features along with headache, cerebrospinal fluid (CSF) pleocytosis, and lack of systemic manifestations. In such a clinical setting, routine cerebral angiography remains indicated despite the attractiveness of magnetic resonance angiography (MRA) or computed tomographic angiography (CTA) as less invasive alternative vascular imaging modalities. It has been proposed that the criteria for diagnosis be separated into definite and probable categories [2]. It has also been proposed that subcategorization into granulomatous angiitis of the central nervous system, benign angiopathy of the CNS, and atypical PACNS is also indicated [3].

In certain patients, there can be an insidious course with subtle manifestations predating a more definitive diagnosis by up to several years. This form of granulomatous angiitis is associated with small vessel infarction in different vascular territories along with a meningitic symptoms [4, 5]. There can also be spinal cord involvement [6]. Such small vessel involvement, especially in vessels smaller than 500 μm, limits the sensitivity of even routine angiography with a reported detection rate ranging from 40 to 90% [1]. One study reported a sensitivity of cerebral angiography as low as 27% when compared to documentation by tissue biopsy [7]. In such circumstances, leptomeningeal enhancement on MRI brain scan can be particularly pertinent in helping to raise concern about such a vasculitis process and guiding planned biopsy [8].

Diagnosis

It is expected that MRI brain scan will be of particular value in supporting or refuting CNS vasculitis. MRI brain scan abnormality, along with CSF pleocytosis, is found in greater than 90% of patients [2]. Conversely, a normal MRI brain scan and negative CSF exam are expected to have a high level of confidence in ruling out PACNS as an explanation for the symptoms. The helpful MRI clues to diagnosis are a characteristic vascular pattern in different distributions seen on either T2-weighted or fluid attenuation inversion recovery (FLAIR) images. This along with a leptomeningeal enhancement pattern can be particularly pertinent. However, leptomeningeal enhancement is uncommonly reported to occur in roughly 8% of patients [9]. Enhancement of parenchymal lesions in PACNS is reported to occur in up to one-third of patients [4].

It is reported that the CSF is abnormal in up to 80–90% of patients with PACNS [2], but the findings can be quite subtle and nonspecific such as a modest elevation of the white blood cell count or the total protein. However, CSF analysis also serves to determine if there may be a systemic process such as infection, connective tissue disorder, or malignancy. A pronounced CSF white blood cell elevation, especially with polymorphonuclear leukocytes, rather than a relatively modest lymphocytic pleocytosis, should raise particular concern about alternative explanations. In such circumstances, gram stain and bacterial culture, along with viral culture and appropriate viral polymerase chain reaction (PCR), as well as a fresh, large CSF sample for cytology, will be indicated. White matter signal intensity changes in such a clinical setting should also lead to serious consideration of a multiple sclerosis panel.

PACNS remains a diagnostic challenge, and this is probably compounded by the fairly routine substitution of routine intra-arterial cerebral arteriography with less invasive modalities specifically MRA and CTA which have lower diagnostic yield. This mandates higher levels of suspicion for PACNS when features in Table 4.3 are present. The sensitivity of brain/leptomeningeal biopsy varies from 36 to 83% [2]. The supportive histologic findings include lymphocytic cellular infiltrates, granulomatous inflammation, and vessel wall fibrinoid necrosis [6]. In the Mayo Clinic cohort [10], of 163 patients diagnosed with PACNS, 105 were diagnosed on the basis of cerebral angiographic findings, while 58 were diagnosed by biopsy. The authors were able to identify some differentiations in their cohort with biopsy-proven subjects more likely to present with cognitive impairment as well as had higher CSF protein, less frequent cerebral infarction pattern, more frequent enhancing lesions on

Table 4.3 Features which can raise concern about primary angiitis of the central nervous system in a patient with stroke-like presentation

1. Unexplained ischemic stroke	4. Leptomeningeal enhancement
2. Multiple vascular territories involved	5. Cerebrospinal fluid pleocytosis
3. Accompanying headache	6. Suspicion of cerebral arterial narrowing, especially beading pattern, on angiography

MRI, as well as lesser mortality and morbidity. On the other hand, those identified by cerebral angiography had more frequent stroke-like presentations both clinically and by imaging along with greater mortality. It was theorized that this was attributable to larger vessel involvement in the angiogram-positive group.

Treatment

The importance of accurate diagnosis is underscored by the dilemma of an unrecognized and untreated serious disease process, with potentially devastating consequences, versus empiric therapy with potent immunosuppressive agents which can have serious long-term side effects. The treatment for PACNS remains empiric with no randomized clinical trials available to provide convincing guidance. Because of the inflammatory nature of the disease process, immunosuppression is considered the underpinning of effective management. This must factor in the risks versus potential benefits of such therapy especially with the absence of specific biomarkers for disease activity. This is in distinction to giant cell arteritis where both the erythrocyte sedimentation rate (ESR) and C-reactive protein (CRP) can be of value in monitoring the course of the disease and response to therapy [11].

Birnbaum and Hellman [2] outlined a therapeutic approach for PACNS in 2008 based upon presently available information. They combined cyclophosphamide at 2 mg/kg/day with prednisone at 1 mg/kg/day. In severe acute presentations, they initiated methylprednisolone intravenously with 1000 mg daily for 3 days. This reflected some alteration of the recommendation of Salavarani et al. [4] in which corticosteroid therapy alone was felt to be adequate. In a recent review from 2013 [12], the combination of a corticosteroid and cyclophosphamide is felt to be the "gold standard." However, in light of concerns about the longer-term side effects of daily oral cyclophosphamide, intravenous pulse therapy is reported to be less toxic and of equivalent efficacy [13].There is also increasing acceptance of limiting the course of oral cyclophosphamide therapy to no more than 3–6 months in light of these concerns over longer-term toxicity [14]. Over the longer term, it has been recommended that prednisone be tapered and discontinued over a 12-month period [2], and cyclophosphamide be replaced with lower-risk immunosuppressants such as azathioprine at 1–2 mg/kg/day, methotrexate at 20–25 mg/week, or mycophenolate mofetil at 1–2 gram/day [15]. Most patients are felt to go into remission after a 12–18-month course of immunosuppression [16], but treatment for up to 2–3 years may be necessary [2].

Reversible Cerebral Vasoconstriction Syndrome (RCVS)

Overview

This is an increasingly recognized entity that has been invoked with various terminologies such as Call-Fleming syndrome [17] as well as a migraine-related vasospasm [18]. RCVS is characterized by severe headache in association with diffuse segmental vasoconstriction of the cerebral arteries that are generally reversible within a 3-month time frame [19]. This "string of beads" pattern is most definitively detected by intra-arterial digital subtraction angiography (DSA). However, the yield of detection is reported to be as high as 80% by less invasive cranial tomographic angiography (CTA) or magnetic resonance angiography (MRA) [20]. RCVS, despite being viewed as a reversible process, is not only associated with what can be incapacitating severe headache, which has been termed thunderclap to underscore its severity [21, 22], it can also be associated with seizures, ischemic and hemorrhagic stroke, as well as subarachnoid hemorrhage not in association with cerebral aneurysm [23].

The incidence of RCVS is unknown as its detection is predicated on pursuit of cerebrovascular imaging in the clinical setting which is often arbitrary for a particular institution. There can also be a difference of opinion as to what constitutes RCVS depending upon the criteria used by the reporting physicians [23]. This is often dependent on the duration of the headache and any possible associated focal neurological deficit. Most patients have headache as the sole manifestation [24], and, unlike the headache associated with aneurysmal subarachnoid hemorrhage, the duration is usually no more than several hours [23].

Associated Conditions

Table 4.4 summarizes conditions that can be associated with reversible cerebral vasoconstriction syndrome. There are particularly pertinent associations including migraine; postpartum period vascular complications, including that associated with preeclampsia and eclampsia; posterior reversible encephalopathy syndrome (PRES); and convexity subarachnoid hemorrhage. It has been reported that two-thirds of patients with postpartum RCVS have onset of symptoms within 1 week of delivery and typically after an uncomplicated delivery [25]. RCVS can overlap with PRES in between 8 and 39% of those affected [21, 26]. PRES is an encephalopathic condition associated with seizures, headache, and visual loss [27]. Like RSCV, the onset is usually sudden and is associated with reversible vasogenic edema seen either on CT or more readily defined on MRI brain scan, particularly T2-weighted and FLAIR images [28]. The DWI/ADC image pattern of hyperintensity on DWI and ADC has been reported to be most common with some subjects showing hyperintensity on DWI with hypointensity of ADC or normointensity on DWI and hyperintensity on ADC [29].

Table 4.4 Conditions associated with reversible cerebral vasoconstriction syndrome

1. Migraine angiopathy	5. Post-carotid endarterectomy
2. Postpartum angiopathy	6. Cerebral venous thrombosis
3. Posterior reversible encephalopathy syndrome	7. Convexity subarachnoid hemorrhage
4. Vasoactive drugs including triptans, ergotamines, sympathomimetic agents, immunosuppressants	8. Head trauma
	9. Autonomic dysreflexia

PRES tends to be self-limited with resolution of the vasogenic edema within several days. However, despite the "reversible" connotation, one can see resultant cerebral infarction, associated with cytotoxic edema, as well as intracerebral hemorrhage [30]. PRES is associated with numerous conditions, including infection, markedly elevated blood pressure, autoimmune disease, immunosuppressants, cytotoxic agents, as well as eclampsia and preeclampsia. Naturally, the manifestations of PRES, as well as the outcome, might well reflect the underlying associated condition.

Migraine was previously thought to represent a vasoconstriction in the aura phase followed by vasodilatation in the headache phase, at least in regard to migraine with aura. However, this simplified approach has been abandoned to a considerable degree. Despite this, concerns about vessel narrowing in migraine, especially when there is focal neurological deficit, such as in hemiplegic migraine, have raised concerns about the potential for infarction (Fig. 4.2). This is of particular concern with vasoconstrictive agents such as triptans and ergot alkaloids. Of note, migraine is often seen in association with RCVS and terminologies previously used, such as migraine angiitis [31], or migrainous vasospasms [32] may have been reflective of this association. Also of interest, in terms of potential overlap mechanism, triptans and ergots have been reported to precipitate RCVS in certain patients [33] with potentially serious consequences [34]. In addition, migraine in association with RCVS is reported to increase the risk of cerebral hemorrhage [35].

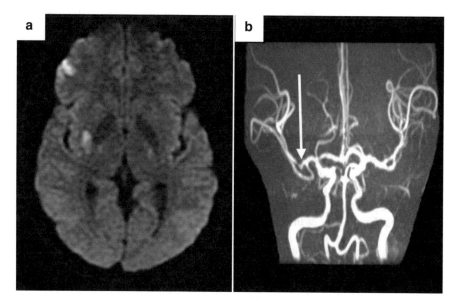

Fig. 4.2 (**a**) Diffusion-weighted image (DWI) on magnetic resonance imaging (MRI) brain scan of a 36-year-old woman with severe migraine-type headache in association with acute left side weakness. There are multiple areas of increased signal intensity in the distribution of the right middle cerebral artery (MCA). (**b**) Magnetic resonance angiography (MRA) revealed focal right MCA narrowing (*arrow*) believed reflective of migrainous arteriopathy

Treatment

Any potential factor possibly contributing to RCVS should be as effectively removed as feasible. This would include discontinuation of vasoactive medications. Management of associated hypertension is imperative as are symptomatic management approaches to headache, avoidance of physical exertion, and relaxation measures for anxiety. There have been reports of response to vasodilating agents, such as verapamil or nimodipine, as well as to magnesium [23], but no systematic randomized control trials are presently available to support this in an evidence-based approach.

Giant Cell (Temporal) Arteritis

Overview

This is a larger- and medium-size vessel inflammatory disorder typically seen in older subjects, beyond age 50, with the peak incidence at 70–80 years of age [36]. It is most commonly seen in Caucasians of European descent [37]. An association has been reported between HLA-DR4 and HLA-DRB1 suggestive of a genetic susceptibility [38]. The female to male ratio is reported to be 3:1 [39]. There is considerable overlap with a diffuse inflammatory disorder of the muscles, polymyalgia rheumatica (PMR). Roughly 50% of patients with giant cell arteritis (GCA) develop PMR either before, during, or after the time of presentation of GCA [40]. GCA is a T-cell-mediated disorder with recruitment of both T cells and macrophages to form a granulomatous infiltrate within the affected vessels [41]. On temporal artery biopsy, one sees inflamed vascular tissue with various cytokine and other inflammatory mediators [41]. Of interest, in terms of pathogenesis, Gilden and Nagel [42] have reported a relationship between varicella zoster virus (VZV) antigen and positive GCA pathology on temporal artery biopsy. In an extension of this study [43], they found VZV antigen in 74% of 82 GCA-positive biopsies. They theorize that GCA has a viral-mediated trigger.

It is expected that the incidence of GCA will increase as the population has greater longevity, and there is a present reported incidence of 27 cases per 100,000 for those 50 years of age and older [37]. The recognition is extremely important in a timely fashion in light of the potential for ischemic optic neuritis with irreversible blindness. This is reported to affect 10–15% of patients with GCA [44]. The protection of such an occurrence with early administration of steroid therapy is utmost urgency in the clinical setting.

Manifestations

A patient presenting with new onset headache at 50 years or beyond should always raise concern about GCA. Localization to the superficial temporal artery region

Table 4.5 Features of giant cell (temporal) arteritis

1. Moderate to severe head pain in region of the superficial temporal artery	6. Elevation of the erythrocyte sedimentation rate (ESR)
2. Age ≥ 50 years	7. Elevation of the C-reactive protein (CRP)
3. Predilection for female Caucasians	8. Systemic complaints which can include fever, malaise, and weight loss
4. Jaw claudication	
5. Neck pain	9. Temporal biopsy with characteristic granulomatous inflammation

along with tenderness to palpation of this region should heighten the degree of concern. These are the most common manifestations. There can be accompanying jaw claudication and neck pain. It is also important to recognize that there can be systemic manifestations including fever of unknown origin, lassitude, and malaise, as well as loss of appetite with weight loss. The vasculitic process can involve not only the temporal arteries but also the carotid distribution, the aortic arch, as well as the axillary, iliac, and femoral arteries [45]. There can be both arterial and venous occlusive events associated with such inflammation including both myocardial infarct and stroke [46]. Features of GCA are summarized in Table 4.5.

Diagnosis and Treatment

The American College of Rheumatology criteria [38] factors in such features as head pain in the region of the superficial temporal artery, age ≥ 50, and elevation of the erythrocyte sedimentation rate (ESR) to > 40 mm/h to formulate their criteria for diagnosis with a reported sensitivity of 93.5% and specificity of 91.2% [45]. However, Murchison et al. [47] reported that the use of these criteria alone, without confirmatory temporal artery biopsy findings, could miss up to 25% of cases. The ESR is often quite high at 80 mm/h or above, and the C-reactive protein (CRP) is often quite elevated. These are not 100% in terms of degree of detection, however. One study of 764 subjects [48] reported a sensitivity of the ESR of 84% and the CRP of 86% but with a specificity of 30%. Overall, the yield is quite high with only 4% of patients having normal ESR and CRP values at the time of diagnosis.

Because of the low specificity for the ESR and CRP, and the need to support ongoing steroid therapy if indeed the patient has GCA, then a temporal artery biopsy is mandatory. The granulomatous inflammatory findings expected on biopsy are detected in 85–95% of GCA cases [49]. The urgency to protect against potential blindness, with steroid therapy, can lead to misdiagnosis. Saedon et al. [50] reported that clinical criteria for diagnosis, without confirmatory biopsy findings, led to immunosuppressive treatment in 61% of 112 patients which raises some concern about possible unnecessary treatment in some subjects.

A generally accepted approach is the initiation of prednisone at 1 mg per kg of body weight per day. For those patients with worrisome visual symptoms, a 3-day course of daily 1000 mg intravenous methylprednisolone would be indicated. Assuming response, various tapering courses have been implemented. It has been suggested that a reasonable approach is reduction of the dose of prednisone by 10–20% every 2 weeks down to less than 10 mg a day, and then a slower taper follows by 1 mg per month [40]. The course of tapering is obviously influenced by the ESR, and CRP results with such studies recommended monthly the first year, bimonthly the second year, and every 3–6 months for longer-term follow-up. Alternative agents for those patients either not responsive or intolerant of glucocorticoids include cyclophosphamide, methotrexate, azathioprine, and infliximab [51]. Antiviral therapy will certainly be investigated in light of the recent identification of an association with VZV [42, 43].

Polyarteritis Nodosa (PAN)

Overview

PAN usually presents in the fourth or fifth decade but can present in childhood. Men are affected twice as commonly as women. There can be an association with hepatitis B or C infection [12]. There is typically multi-organ involvement. The systemic inflammatory process can be reflected in systemic signs such as fever, malaise, and weight loss. This can be supported by an elevated ESR, and renal involvement is usually accompanied by proteinuria as well as hypertension. Dermatological manifestations and peripheral neuropathy tend to be particularly common.

Despite potentially devastating effects, PAN is not uncommonly associated with CNS vascular involvement. In one report, 12% of 26 patients had only CNS involvement, while 34% had combined CNS and peripheral nervous system (PNS) involvement [52]. This systemic vasculitis is associated with necrotizing inflammatory vascular lesions of primarily small- and medium-size muscular arteries. There tends to be preferential involvement of vessel bifurcations. There is microaneurysm formation with the potential for hemorrhage as well as thrombosis with infarction [53]. Cumulative involvement of the brain can result in a multifocal encephalopathy in up to 40% of affected patients [54], but isolated cerebral infarction or hemorrhage can be the presenting manifestation. One can see a lacunar-type infarction pattern related to thrombotic microangiopathy [55]. Generally speaking, in light of the potential for smaller vessel involvement, cerebral arteriography is recommended for evaluation of patients suspected of having the disease.

Diagnosis and Treatment

The spectrum of manifestation of a systemic vascular inflammatory process should raise suspicion for PAN in the differential diagnosis. Pathological confirmation is most readily determined when there is associated dermatological or PNS involvement available for biopsy. The diagnostic challenge of CNS involvement is lessened by the tendency for cerebral, or spinal, vasculitis to develop 2–3 years later than other manifestations.

The treatment is immunosuppression. In uncomplicated disease, corticosteroids can have a very positive impact on prognosis including survival [56]. In more aggressive disease, cyclophosphamide combined with steroid can have a positive impact [57]. Anecdotally, rituximab may provide benefit in refractory cases of PAN [12]. Antiviral therapy combined with immunosuppression is reported to be of particular benefit in hepatitis B- and C-related PAN [58] especially in severe disease [59].

Antineutrophil Cytoplasmic Antibody (ANCA)-Associated CNS Vasculitis

Overview

Antibodies reflective of ANCA are directed against certain cytoplasmic proteins within neutrophils and appear to be part of the pathogenesis in certain vasculitides. This is an evolving process both in terms of insight into mechanism and terminology. For example, "Wegener's granulomatosis" has been suggested to be replaced with "granulomatosis polyangiitis" (GPA). Churg-Strauss syndrome has been proposed to be replaced with eosinophilic granulomatosis with polyangiitis (EGPA). The other commonly cited ANCA-related vasculitic process is microscopic polyangiitis (MPA) [60].

CNS involvement by Wegener's granulomatosis is quite uncommon [61]. It can be associated with either small to medium-sized cerebral vasculitis, meningitis, or orbital granuloma [62]. There can be extension of the granulomatous process to the cavernous sinus with resultant cavernous sinus syndrome [63]. Cerebral vasculitis is seen in up to 4% of patients and is reported to be the most frequent CNS manifestation [64].

MPA affects small vessels such as arterioles, capillaries, and venules and can be associated with cerebral infarction [65] although reports tend to be few and far between reflective of the rarity of such a disorder. There is the potential for lacunar-type infarct as well as hemorrhagic stroke, and support for the diagnosis can come from elevated ESR and CRP, positive ANCA, and pathological confirmation such as sural nerve biopsy [66].

EGPA affects small- and medium-size vessels. This is a systemic process typically affecting the lungs with asthma and eosinophilia and often with gastrointestinal involvement as well. The necrotizing small vessel vasculitis can also affect the CNS with resultant stroke, ischemic or hemorrhagic [54]. Although rare, it has been proposed that this diagnostic possibility be raised in patients with stroke and hypereosinophilia [12].

Diagnosis and Treatment

Recognition of the clinical manifestations is key with such a systemic granulomatosis processes as Wegener's, aka GPA, and Churg-Strauss, aka EGPA. Pathological confirmation of available tissue for biopsy is of utmost importance as aggressive immunosuppressive therapy can be of clear benefit in most patients. In EGPA, for

Table 4.6 Antineutrophil cytoplasmic antibody (ANCA)-associated vasculitis types and patterns

Designation	Alternative name	Areas of involvement	CNS manifestations
Wegener's granulomatosis	Granulomatosis with polyangiitis	Small and medium blood vessels of multiple organs	Ischemic and hemorrhagic stroke small- and medium-size vessel pattern
Churg-Strauss syndrome	Eosinophilic granulomatosis with polyangiitis	Pulmonary with eosinophilic asthma, gastrointestinal, and other organs	Ischemic and hemorrhagic stroke with nodular small vessel polyangiitis, seizures, cranial nerve palsies
Microscopic polyangiitis		Micro-arteriolar necrotizing systemic pattern	Ischemic small vessel infarcts, sino-venous occlusion, hemorrhagic stroke, basilar meningitis

example, the small epineural arteriolar inflammatory process is often identified on peripheral nerve biopsy as neuropathy is a common manifestation of this illness [67] with CNS involvement much less common [68]. Characteristically, one sees necrotizing vasculitis with eosinophilic infiltration along with extravascular granulomas. In this disorder, corticosteroid therapy can be highly effective with one study demonstrating remission in 94% of patients during the first year of therapy [69].

More aggressive ANCA-associated inflammatory disease, especially when associated with cerebral vasculitis, often calls for more potent immunosuppression such as a combination of cyclophosphamide and high-dose glucocorticoids. Gaining acceptance as a replacement for cyclophosphamide is rituximab shown to be non-inferior in two ANCA-associated vasculitis studies [70, 71]. Both azathioprine and methotrexate can be alternatives for chronic immunosuppression [72].

It is important to point out that the role of ANCA autoantibodies in the pathogenesis is not clearly defined. For example, Wegener's granulomatosis can be associated with polyangiitis in ANCA-negative patients [73]. In addition, the presence of ANCA antibodies can overlap with other autoimmune disorders, such as Sjogren's syndrome, and possibly contribute to the spectrum of manifestations [74]. ANCA-associated vasculitic disorders are outlined in Table 4.6.

Takayasu Disease

Overview

This is a larger-vessel granulomatous vasculitis with particular involvement of the aorta and its major branches. It is typically seen in patients less than 40 years of age [54]. It is much more commonly seen in women than men. Aortic imaging in patients suffering from large artery occlusive disease, with loss of pulses (pulseless disease), is vital in diagnostic evaluation. Systemic manifestations can precede occlusive events and include fever, malaise, and loss of appetite. Elevated ESR and CRP call attention to the inflammatory nature of this rare disorder. The natural history can range from mild to severe [75]. Involvement of the carotid arteries can result in ischemic optic neuropathy and stroke. Corticosteroid therapy is traditionally the first line of immunosuppression. Unfortunately, the ongoing need for such therapy often leads to side effects. Agents used for steroid sparing include azathioprine, methotrexate, antitumor necrosis factor receptor agents, rituximab, and cyclophosphamide with some degree of response reported in open-label trials [76].

Neuro-Behcet's Disease

Overview

Unlike Takayasu disease, Behcet's syndrome is more common in men. There is a triad of oral and genital ulcers with uveitis. There can be CNS involvement in up to 30% of cases which can include small vessel vasculitis and meningovascular inflammatory cell deposition. Neuro-Behcet's disease can be either acute or chronic progressive [77]. The acute form can be set off by cyclosporine A. The acute form is associated with a meningoencephalitis with focal lesions seen on T2-weighted and FLAIR MRI [78]. This form tends to be very steroid responsive and self-limited.

The chronic form is characterized by a slowly progressive neurological impairment with dementia, ataxia, and dysarthria [79]. There is an elevation of cerebrospinal fluid interleukin-6 activity [54]. High-dose methylprednisolone tends to be the first line of therapy with well-recognized resistance to such therapy along with cyclophosphamide and azathioprine. However, low-dose methotrexate may be of particular benefit for disease suppression in the chronic progressive form [80].

Cogan's Syndrome

Overview

This rare autoimmune syndrome is characterized by bilateral interstitial keratitis with profound sensorineural hearing loss. There can be systemic vasculitic manifestations, and there are both typical and atypical presentations described [81]. There can be an association with both ANCA antibodies and rheumatoid factor suggestive of a potential overlap in terms of pathogenesis and potential contribution to vasculitis. There can be associated larger artery aneurysm formation which can include the carotid artery [82]. This is reflective of the larger vessel involvement seen in both Cogan's syndrome and Behcet's disease [83]. Of note, there is considerable overlap in the manifestations of these two disorders with both diagnosed on the basis of clinical manifestations with lack of confirmatory diagnostic testing. Despite its recognition as a cause of CNS vasculitis, it is felt that Cogan's syndrome is not only quite rare but uncommonly results in neurological manifestations [84].

Susac Syndrome

Overview

The clinical trial of this rare, apparent autoimmune process consists of CNS involvement, branch retinal artery occlusions, and sensorineural hearing loss. As of a review published in 2012, 304 cases of this syndrome had been reported worldwide at that time [85]. There is an inflammatory process affecting microvessels of the brain, retina, and inner ear. It has most commonly been reported in young women and is felt to be underdiagnosed [86]. Retinal artery branch occlusions can be documented by fluorescein angiography, and compatible changes on MRI brain scan have been reported in patients presenting with the triad. Antiendothelial cell antibodies are found in some patients [86]. Response to immunosuppression has been reported with corticosteroid therapy as the usual initial first choice.

Cryoglobulinemia-Associated CNS Vasculitis

Overview

Vasculitic involvement in cryoglobulinemia is characterized by the triad of purpura, weakness, and arthralgia [12]. The presentation can be quite insidious, but aggressive multi-organ involvement can be life threatening. This smaller vessel arteritis is related to the deposition of cryoglobulins within the vessel wall with activation of the complement cascade. Type I represents single monoclonal immunoglobulin formation related to B-cell lymphoproliferative disorders, while types II and III are often referred to mixed cryoglobulinemias. These are reflective of polyclonal IgG immunoglobulin formation with or without monoclonal IgM associated with rheumatoid factor activity [87]. Hepatitis C virus infection is observed to be the most common cause of mixed cryoglobulinemic vasculitis [88].

There can be associated cerebral infarction, and there is also the potential for the associated hyperviscosity to promote cerebral ischemia. The treatment consists of various forms of immunosuppression with the potential for rituximab to be particularly effective [89, 90]. Hyperviscosity in cryoglobulinemia is best managed with early plasma exchanges.

CNS Vasculitis in Association with Connective Tissue Disorders

Overview

The following disorders fall into this category: systemic lupus erythematosus (SLE), rheumatoid arthritis (RA), systemic sclerosis (scleroderma), and Sjogren's syndrome. SLE is the best recognized for association with CNS vasculitis although alternative mechanisms can be related to coexistent antiphospholipid antibody syndrome, resulting in a hypercoagulable state, as well as potential cardio-embolic events from Libman-Sacks endocarditis. The most common CNS presentation is a multifactorial encephalopathy which can include cognitive impairment with psychosis, seizures, headache, and chorea. The autoimmune-mediated pathology tends to be non-thrombotic in such a presentation but instead is a combination of deposition of immune complexes and vasculitis. SLE is prominently listed in the differential diagnosis of stroke in the young [91]. There can be vascular occlusion with ischemic stroke as well as hemorrhagic insults which can be related to vasculitic mediated aneurysm formation [92]. Involvement of the CNS is relatively common in SLE, but the exact frequency of involvement varies considerably among reported studies [54, 93].

Systemic sclerosis is not commonly associated with CNS vasculitis but is recognized for potential PNS effects. Amaral et al. [94] reported on 180 studies of systemic sclerosis and identified the following pattern of potential CNS involvement: headache in 23.73%, seizures in 13.56%, and cognitive impairment in 8.47% with anxiety/depression also commonly seen.

Rheumatoid arthritis (RA), like lupus, is now a much more indolent disease with advances in immunosuppression. Furthermore, the incidence of RA is reported to be declining [54]. Cerebral infarction can be seen related to vasculitis. Of note, there is the potential for atlantoaxial subluxation with resultant ischemia or compression to the brainstem. It is reported that this is a not uncommon cause of death attributable to RA [95].

Sjogren's syndrome, also known as keratoconjunctivitis sicca, can be associated with vasculitis of the CNS. It is reported that the vascular insult may be related to the presence of anti-Ro and antineuronal antibodies [54]. There have been reports of both ischemic and hemorrhagic strokes with this disorder. However, the risk appears to be quite small and, as mentioned previously, may be part of an autoimmune overlap such as with coexistent ANCA antibodies [74].

Infection-Related CNS Vasculitis

Overview

The classic infectious CNS vasculopathy, from years past, was meningovascular syphilis. After effective eradication of this former common cause of stroke, there has been somewhat of a reemergence related to coinfection with human immunodeficiency virus (HIV) resulting in less resistance to CNS penetration by the spirochete. It is still fairly standard to obtain syphilis serology for any unexplained stroke, either ischemic or hemorrhagic, especially in a younger patient. A biologically false-positive test, such as the VDRL (Venereal Disease Research Laboratory) test or RPR (rapid plasma reagin) test, could be an indicator of the presence of antiphospholipid antibodies, while a true positive, such as that seen with a positive fluorescent treponemal antibody absorption (FTA-ABS) study, would point toward CSF evaluation for possible meningovascular syphilis. According to recent reports, the yield of such a pursuit is now greater with coexistent HIV disease.

Table 4.7 Vasculopathy of the CNS associated with infection

1. Varicella zoster	7. Meningovascular from bacterial, fungal, and tuberculosis infection
2. HIV	
3. Neurosyphilis	8. Septic emboli from subacute bacterial endocarditis
4. Hepatitis C	9. Septic aortitis
5. Rickettsial	10. Q fever
6. Viral encephalitis	11. Mycoplasma
7. Ehrlichial vasculitis	12. Toxoplasma vasculitis

HIV can be associated with CNS vasculopathy with resultant infarction. There is often a heterogeneous pattern to the vascular involvement, related to coexistent disease, but there is the potential for either a primary granulomatous angiitis, eosinophilic vasculitis, or a necrotizing vasculitis [97, 98]. The pathogenesis of the vasculitis may involve overlap with autoimmune antibodies such as antinuclear antibodies and ANCA antibodies [98].

VZV can be associated with a combined meningoencephalitis and vasculitis [99]. There can be either small or larger vessel involvement. As mentioned previously, there is recently reported evidence of the potential for VZV to promote GCA [42, 43]. Despite the recognition that VZV can affect the CNS in a number of ways [100], a recent review of this topic [101] concluded that VZV-associated cerebral infarction is uncommon. When cerebral infarction does occur, the reported cerebral angiographic findings can include segmental constriction and occlusion often with post-stenotic vessel dilatation [102]. However, this would be reflective of larger vessel involvement with negative cerebral arteriography not necessarily excluding small vessel disease. Such VZV-associated infarcts are often treated with a combination of corticosteroids and acyclovir after support for such a process with a positive VZV polymerase chain reaction (PCR) result.

Other infection-related vasculitides include endovascular microbial disease related to bacterial endocarditis and septic aortitis, rickettsial, Q fever, ehrlichial, mycoplasma, toxoplasmosis, tuberculosis, fungal, parvovirus, cytomegalovirus, herpes simplex virus, human T-cell lymphotropic virus-1, Epstein-Barr virus, and West Nile virus [103] outlined in Table 4.7.

Neoplastic-Related CNS Vasculitis

Overview

Vascular invasion with an inflammatory response can be seen in certain neoplastic disorders. Both Hodgkin's and non-Hodgkin's lymphoma have been implicated along with angioimmunolymphoproliferative disorder [3]. The clinical picture can mimic PACNS with the potential for both ischemic and hemorrhagic strokes. The presentation can be quite insidious for intravascular lymphomatosis also known as neoplastic angioendotheliosis [104]. The presentation can mimic disseminated encephalomyelitis and encephalomyelopathy [105]. A clue to the variable presentations [106] is an unexplained elevation of the serum lactate dehydrogenase level [104, 107]. Naturally, the treatment is directed toward the neoplastic process, and outcome is reflective of response to therapy.

References

1. Hajj-Ali RA, Singhal AB, Benseler S, Molloy E, Calabrese LH. Primary angiitis of the CNS. Lancet Neurol. 2011;10:561–72.
2. Birnbaum J, Hellman DB. Primary angiitis of the central nervous system. Arch Neurol. 2009;66:704–9.
3. Calabrese LH, Duna GF, Lie JT. Vasculitis in the central nervous system. Arthritis Rheum. 1997;40:1189–201.
4. Salvarani C, Brown Jr RD, Calamia KT, et al. Primary central nervous system vasculitis: analysis of 101 patients. Ann Neurol. 2007;62:442–51.
5. Lie JT. Angiitis of the central nervous system. Curr Opin Rheumatol. 1991;3:36–45.
6. Salvarani C, Brown Jr RD, Calamia KT, et al. Primary CNS vasculitis with spinal cord involvement. Neurology. 2008;70:2394–400.
7. Vollmer TL, Guarnaccia J, Harrington W, Pacia SV, Petroff OA. Idiopathic granulomatous angiitis of the central nervous system. Diagnostic challenges. Arch Neurol. 1993;50:925–30.
8. Parisi JE, Moore PM. The role of biopsy in vasculitis of the central nervous system. Semin Neurol. 1994;14:341–8.
9. Salvarani C, Brown Jr RD, Calamia KT, et al. Primary central nervous system vasculitis with prominent leptomeningeal enhancement: a subset with a benign outcome. Arthritis Rheum. 2008;58:595–603.
10. Salvarani C, Brown Jr RD, Christianson T, et al. An update of the Mayo Clinic cohort of patients with adult primary central nervous system vasculitis. Description of 163 patients. Medicine. 2015;21:1–15.
11. Weyand CM, Goronzy JJ. Giant-cell arteritis and polymyalgia rheumatica. N Engl J Med. 2014;4(371):50–7.
12. Broussalis E, Trinka E, Draus J, McCoy M, Killer M. Treatment strategies for vasculitis that affects the nervous system. Drug Discov Today. 2013;18:818–35.
13. Berlit P. Diagnosis and treatment of cerebral vasculitis. Ther Adv Neurol Disord. 2010;3(3):29–42.
14. Hoffman GS, Kerr GS, Leavitt RY, et al. Wegener granulomatosis: an analysis of 158 patients. Ann Intern Med. 1992;116:488–98.
15. Mukhtyar C, Guillevin L, Cid MC, et al. EULAR recommendations for the management of primary small and medium vessel vasculitis. Ann Rheum Dis. 2009;68:310–7.
16. Salvarani C, Brown Jr RD, Hunder GG. Adult primary central nervous system vasculitis. Lancet. 2012;380:767–77.
17. Call GK, Fleming MC, Sealfon S, Levine H, Kistler JP, Fisher CM. Reversible cerebral segmental vasoconstriction. Stroke. 1988;19:1159–70.
18. Sendara M, Chiras J, Cujas M, Lhermitte F. Isolated benign cerebral vasculitis or migrainous vasospasm? J Neurol Neurosurg Psychiatry. 1984;47:73–6.
19. Calabrese LH, Dodick DW, Schwedt TJ, Singhal AB. Narrative review: reversible vasoconstriction syndromes. Ann Intern Med. 2007;146:34–44.
20. Ducros A, Bousser MG. Reversible cerebral vasoconstriction syndrome. Pract Neurol. 2009;9:256–67.
21. Wang SJ, Fuh JL, Wu JA, Chen SP, Lai TH. Bath-related thunderclap headache: a study of 21 consecutive patients. Cephalalgia. 2008;28:524–30.

22. Hu CM, Lin YJ, Fan YK, Chen SP, Lai TH. Isolated thunderclap headache during sex: orgasmic headache or reversible cerebral vasoconstriction syndrome? J Clin Neurosci. 2010;17:1349–51.
23. Ducros A. Reversible cerebral vasoconstriction syndrome. Lancet Neurol. 2012;11:906–17.
24. Ducros A, Boukobaza M, Porcher R, Sarow M, Valade D, Bousser MG. Brain. 2007;130:3091–101.
25. Edlow JA, Caplan LR, O'Brien K, Tibbles CD. Diagnosis of acute neurlological emergencies in pregnant and post-partum women. Lancet Neurol. 2013;12:175–85.
26. Fugate JE, Ameriso SF, Ortiz G, et al. Variable presentations of postpartum angiopathy. Stroke. 2012;43:67–676.
27. Bartynski WS. Posterior reversible encephalopathic syndrome. Part 1: fundamental neuroimaging and clinical features. AJNR Am J Neuroradiol. 2008;29:1036–42.
28. Fugate JE, Claassen DO, Cloft HJ, Kallmes DF, Kozak OS, Rabinstein AA. Posterior reversible encephalopathy syndrome: associated clinical and radiologic findings. Mayo Clin Proc. 2010;85:427–32.
29. Ibrahim NMA, Badawy ME. MR imaging of posterior reversible encephalopathy syndrome associated with pregnancy. Egypt J Radiol Nucl Med. 2014;45:505–10.
30. Staykov D, Schwab S. Posterior reversible encephalopathy syndrome. J Intensive Care. 2012;27:11–24.
31. Jackson M, Lennox G, Jaspan T, Jefferson D. Migrainous angiitis precipitated by sex Headache and leading to watershed infarction. Cephalalgia. 1993;13:427–30.
32. Serdaru M, Chiras J, Cujas M, Lhermitte F. Isolated benign cerebral vasculitis or migrainous vasospasm? J Neurol Neurosurg Psychiatry. 1984;47:73–6.
33. Singhal AB, Caviness VS, Begleiter AF, Mark EJ, Rordorf G, Korosshetz WJ. Cerebral vasoconstriction and stroke after use of serotonergic drugs. Neurology. 2002;58:130–3.
34. Meschia JF, Malkoff MD, Biller J. Reversible segmental cerebral arterial vasospasm and cerebral infarction: possible association with excessive use of sumatriptan and Midrin. Arch Neurol. 1998;55:712–4.
35. Ducros A, Fiedler U, Porcher R, Boukobza M, Stapf C, Bousser MG. Hemorrhagic manifestations of reversible cerebral vasoconstriction syndrome: frequency, features and risk factors. Stroke. 2010;41:2505–11.
36. Gonzalez-Gay MA, Vazquez-Rodriquez TR, Lopez-Diaz MJ, et al. Epidemiology of giant cell arteritis and polymyalgia rheumatica. Arthritis Rheum. 2009;61:1454–61.
37. Chacko JG, Chacko JA, Salter MW. Review of giant cell arteritis. Saudi J Ophthalmol. 2015;29:48–52.
38. Hunder GG, Da B, Michel BA, et al. The American College of Rheumatology 1990 criteria for classification of giant cell arteritis. Arthritis Rheum. 1990;33:1122–8.
39. Ly K-H, Regent MC, Mouthon L. Pathogenesis of giant cell arteritis: more than just an inflammatory condition? Autoimmun Rev. 2010;9:635–45.
40. Weyand CM, Goronzy JJ. Giant-cell arteritis and polymyalgia rheumatica. N Engl J Med. 2014;371:50–7.
41. Weyand CM, Goronzy JJ. Immune mechanisms in medium and large-vessel vasculitis. Nat Rev Rheumatol. 2013;9:731–40.
42. Gilden D, Nagel M. Varicella zoster virus in temporal arteries of patients with giant cell arteritis. J Infect Dis. 2015;212(Supple 1):S37–9.
43. Gilden D, White T, Khmeleva N, et al. Prevalence and distribution of VZV in temporal arteries of patients with giant cell arteritis. Neurology. 2015;84:1948–55.
44. Aiello PD, Trautmann JC, McPhee TJ, Kunselman AR, Hunder GG. Visual prognosis in giant cell arteritis. Ophthalmology. 1993;100:550–5.
45. Azhar SS, Tang RA, Dorotheo EU. Giant cell arteritis: diagnosing and treating inflammatory disorders in older adults. Geriatrics. 2005;60:26–30.
46. Guida A, Tufano A, Perna P, et al. The thromboembolic risk in Giant Cell Arteritis: a critical review of the literature. Int J Rheumatol. 2014;1:1–7.

47. Murchison AP, Gilbert ME, Bikyk JR, et al. Validity of the American College of Rheumatology Criteria for the diagnosis of giant cell arteritis. Am J Ophthalmol. 2012;154:617–9.
48. Kermani TA, Schmidt J, Crowson CS, et al. Utility of erythrocyte sedimentation rate and C-reactive protein for the diagnosis of temporal arteritis. Semin Arthritis Rheum. 2012;41:866–71.
49. Kermani TA, Warrington KJ, Crowson CS, et al. Large-vessel involvement in giant cell arteritis: a population-based cohort study of the incidence and prognosis. Ann Rheum Dis. 2013;72:1989–94.
50. Saedon H, Saedon M, Goodyear S, Papettas T, Marshall C. Temporal artery biopsy for giant cell arteritis. Retrospective audit. JRSM Short Rep. 2012;3:73.
51. Kotter I, Henes JC, Wagner AD, Loock J, Gross WL. Does glucocorticosteroid-resistant Large-vessel vasculitis (giant cell arteritis and Takayasu arteritis) exist and how can remission be achieved? A critical review of the literature. Clin Exp Rheumatol. 2012;30(Suppl 70):S114–29.
52. Samson M, Puechal X, Devilliers H, et al. Long-term follow-up of a randomized trial on 118 patients with polyarteritis nodosa or microscopic polyangiitis without poor-prognosis factors. Autoimmun Rev. 2014;13:197–205.
53. Younger DS. Vasculitis of the nervous system. Curr Opin Neurol. 2004;17:317–36.
54. Bougea A, Anagnostou E, Spandideas N, Triantafyllou N, Kararizou E. An Update of neurological manifestations of vasculitides and connective tissue diseases: a literature review. Einstein (Open Access). 2015;13:627–35.
55. Reichart MD, Bogousslavsky J, Janzer RC. Early lacunar strokes complicating polyarteritis nodosa: thrombotic microangiopathy. Neurology. 2000;54:883–9.
56. Vishwanath S, Relan M, Shen L, Ambrus Jr JL. Update on the use of biologics in vasculitides. Curr Pharm Biotechnol. 2014;15:558–62.
57. Ribi C, Cohen P, Pagnous C, et al. French Vasculitis Study Group. Treatment of polyarteritis nodosa and microscopic polyangiitis without poor prognosis factors. A prospective randomized study of one hundred twenty-four patients. Arthritis Rheum. 2010;62: 1186–1197.
58. Pagnoux C, Seror R, Henegar C, et al. for the French Vasculitis Study Group. Clinical features and outcomes in 348 patients with polyarteritis nodosa: a systematic retrospective study of patients diagnosed between 1963 and 2005 and entered into the French Vasculitis Study Group database. Arthritis Rheum. 2010;62:616–626.
59. Semmo AN, Baumert TF, Kreisel W. Severe cerebral vasculitis as primary manifestation of hepatitis-B-associated polyarteritis nodosa. J Hepatol. 2002;37:414–6.
60. Salvarani C, Pipitone N, Hunder GG. Management of primary and secondary central nervous system vasculitis. Curr Opin Rheumatol. 2016;28:21–28.
61. Seror R, Mahr A, Ramanoelina J, et al. Central nervous system involvement in Wegener's granulomatosis. Medicine. 2006;85:54–65.
62. Holle JU, Gross WL. Neurological involvement in Wegener's granulomatosis. Curr Opin Rheumatol. 2011;23:7–11.
63. Fadil H, Gonzalez-Toledo E, Kelley RE, Henley J. Wegener's granulomatosis with extension to the cavernous sinus. J La State Med Soc. 2007;159:212–4.
64. Nishino H, Rubino FA, DeRemee RA, et al. Neurological involvement Wegener's granulomatosis: an analysis of 324 consecutive patients at the Mayo Clinic. Ann Neurol. 1993;33:4–9.
65. Ku BD, Shin HY. Multiple bilateral non-hemorrhagic cerebral infarctions associated with microscopic polyangiitis. Clin Neurol Neurosurg. 2009;111:904–6.
66. Ozkul A, Tataroglu C, Kiylioglu N, Akoyi A, Tataroglu C. Microscopic polyangiitis presenting with medullary infarct. J Neurol Sci. 2011;300:173–5.
67. Masi AT, Hunder GG, Lie JT, et al. The American College of Rheumatology 1990 criteria for classification of Churg-Strauss syndrome (allergic granulomatosis and angiitis). Arthritis Rheum. 1990;33:1094–100.

68. Wolf J, Bergner R, Mutallib S, Buggle F, Grau AJ. Neurological complications of Churg-Strauss syndrome-a prospective monocentric study. Eur J Neurol. 2010;17:582–8.
69. Ribi C, Cohen P, Pagnoux C, et al. Treatment of Churg-Strauss syndrome without poor- prognosis factors: a multicenter, prospective, randomized open-label study of seventy-two patients. Arthritis Rheum. 2008;58:586–94.
70. Stone JH, Merkel PA, Spiera R, et al. Rituximab versus cyclophosphamide for ANCA- associated vasculitis. N Engl J Med. 2010;363:221–32.
71. Jones RB, Tervaert JW, Hauser T, et al. Rituximab versus cyclophosphamide in ANCA- associated renal vasculitis. N Engl J Med. 2010;363:211–20.
72. Pagnoux C, Mahr A, Hamidou MA, et al. Azothrioprine or methotrexate maintenance for ANCA-associated vasculitis. N Engl J Med. 2008;359:2790–803.
73. Kashiwagi T, Hayama N, Fujita E, et al. A case of (double) negative granulomatosis with polyangiitis (Wegener's). CEN Case Rep. 2012;1:104–11.
74. Guellec D, Cornec-Le Gall E, Groh M, et al. ANCA-associated vasculitis in patients with primary Sjogren's syndrome: detailed analysis of 7 new cases and systemic review of the literature. Autoimmun Rev. 2015;14:742–50.
75. Subramanyan R, Joy J, Balakrishman KG. Natural history of aortoarteritis (Takayasu's disease). Circulation. 1989;80:429–37.
76. Wen D, Du X, Ma CS. Takayasu arteritis: diagnosis, treatment and prognosis. Int Rev Immunol. 2012;31:462–73.
77. Hirohata S. Central nervous system involvement in Behcet's disease. Rinsho Shinkeigaku. 2001;41:1147–9.
78. Kidd D. Neurological complications of Behcet's syndrome. Curr Neurol Neurosci Rep. 2012;12:675–9.
79. Saip S, Akman-Demir G, Siva A. Neuro-Behcet syndrome. Handb Clin Neurol. 2014;121:1703–23.
80. Kikuchi H, Aramaki K, Hirohata S. Low dose MTX for progressive neuro-Behcet's disease. A follow-up for 4 years. Adv Exp Med Biol. 2003;528:575–8.
81. Espinoza GM, Prost A. Cogan's syndrome and other ocular vasculitides. Curr Rheumatol Rep. 2015;17:24–7.
82. Angiletta D, Wiesel P, Marinazzo D, Bortone AS, Regina G. Endovascular treatment of multiple aneurysms complicating Cogan syndrome. Ann Vasc Surg. 2015;29:361–0.
83. Singer O. Cogan and Behcet syndromes. Rheum Dis Clin North Am. 2015;41:75–9.
84. Antonios N, Silliman S. Cogan syndrome: an analysis of reported neurological manifestations. Neurologist. 2012;18:55–63.
85. Dorr J, Krautwald S, Wildeman B, et al. Characteristics of Susac syndrome: a review of all reported cases. Nat Rev Neurol. 2013;9:307–16.
86. Kleffner I, Duning T, Lohmann H, et al. A brief review of Susac syndrome. J Neurol Sci. 2012;322:35–40.
87. Cacoub P, Comarmond C, Domont F, Savey L, Saadoun D. Cryoglobulinemic vasculitis. Am J Med. 2015;128:950–5.
88. Ferr C, Sebastiani M, Colaci M, Poupak F, Piluso A, Antonelli A, Zignego AL. Hepatitis C virus syndrome: a constellation of organ- and non-organ specific disorders, B-cell non-Hodgkins lymphoma, and cancer. World J Hepatol. 2015;7:327–43.
89. De Vita S, Quartuccio L, Isola M, et al. A randomized controlled trial of rituximab for the treatment of severe cryoglobulinemic vasculitis. Arthritis Rheum. 2012;64:843–53.
90. Lally L, Spiera R. B-cell-targeted therapy in systemic vasculitis. Curr Opin Rheumatol. 2016;28:15–20.
91. Greenberg BM. The neurological manifestations of systemic lupus erythematosus. Neurologist. 2009;15:115–21.
92. Kelley RE, Stokes N, Reyes P, Harik S. Cerebral transmural angiitis and ruptured aneurysm. Arch Neurol. 1980;37:526–7.
93. Streifler JY, Molad Y. Connective tissue disorders: systemic lupus erythematosus, Sjogren's syndrome and scleroderma. Handb Clin Neurol. 2014;119:463–73.

94. Amaral TN, Peres FA, Lapa AT, Marques-Neto JF, Appenzeller S. Neurologic involvement in Scleroderma: a systematic review. Semin Arthritis Rheum. 2013;43:335–47.
95. de Corte FC, Neves N. Cervical spine instability in rheumatoid arthritis. Eur J Orthop Surg Traumatol. 2014;24(Suppl 1):S83–91.
96. Nogueras C, Sala M, Sasal M, et al. Recurrent stroke as a manifestation of primary angiitis of the central nervous system in a patient infected with human immunodeficiency virus. Arch Neurol. 2002;59:468–73.
97. Garcia-Garcia JA, Macias J, Castellanos V, et al. Necrotizing granulomatous vasculitis in advanced HIV infection. J Infect. 2003;47:333–5.
98. Savige JA, Chang L, Horn S, Crowe SM. Antinuclear, anti-neutrophil cytoplasmic and anti-glomerular basement membrane antibodies in HIV-infected individuals. Autoimmunity. 1994;18:205–11.
99. McKelvie PA, Collins S, Thyagarajan D, Trost N, Sheorey H, Byrne E. Meningoencephalo-myelitis with vasculitis due to varicella zoster virus: a case report and review of the literature. Pathology. 2002;34:88–93.
100. Gilden DH, Kleinschmidt-DeMasters BK, LaGuardia JJ, Mahalingam R, Cohrs RJ. Neurologic complications of reactivation of varicella-zoster virus. N Engl J Med. 2000;342:635–45.
101. Grahn A, Studahl M. Varicella-zoster virus infections of the central nervous system-Prognosis, diagnostics and treatment. J Infect. 2015;71:281–93.
102. Russman AN, Lederman RJ, Calabrese LH, Embi PJ, Forghani B, Gilden DH. Multifocal Varicella-zoster virus vasculopathy without rash. Arch Neurol. 2003;60:1607–9.
103. Teng GG, Chatham WW. Vasculitis related to viral and other microbial agents. Best Pract Res Clin Rheumatol. 2015;29:226–43.
104. Smadja D, Mas JL, Fallet-Bianco C, Sicard D, de Recondo J, Rondot P. Intravascular lym-phomatosis (neoplastic angioendotheliosis) of the central nervous system: case report and literature review. J Neurooncol. 1991;11:171–80.
105. Gaul C, Hannisch F, Neureiter D, Behrmann C, Neundorfer B, Winterhoffer M. Intravascular lymphomatosis mimicking disseminated encephalomyelitis and Encephalomyelopathy. Clin Neurol Neurosurg. 2006;108:486–9.
106. Berger JR, Jone R, Wilson D. Intravascular lymphomatosis presenting with sudden hearing loss. J Neurol Sci. 2005;232:105–9.
107. Vieren M, Sciot R, Robberecht W. Intravascular lymphomatosis of the brain: a diagnostic problem. Clin Neurol Neurosurg. 1999;101:33–6.

Neurosarcoidosis: Clinical Features, Pathogenesis, and Management

5

Ragav Aachi, Marjorie Fowler, Eduardo Gonzalez-Toledo, Jeanie McGee, and Alireza Minagar

Introduction

Sarcoidosis is an idiopathic, multi-organ, immune-mediated, inflammatory disorder of unrecognized cure characterized by the development of non-caseating epithelioid granulomas. As a systemic disorder, it heavily involves the respiratory and lymphatic systems (particularly intrathoracic lymph nodes) as well as the skin. Nervous system involvement in the course of sarcoidosis (neurosarcoidosis) is uncommon and occurs only in 5–10 % of cases. Interestingly, neurologic symptoms can be the only presentation of sarcoidosis in 10–17 % of individuals [1]. Despite these figures, the exact prevalence of nervous system involvement in the course of sarcoidosis is believed to be higher since subclinical involvement of the nervous system has been reported in up to 27 % of patients with sarcoidosis on autopsy [2]. Neurosarcoidosis comprises a wide gamut of clinical presentations which stem from involvement of both central and peripheral components of the human nervous system; therefore, it can imitate many other neuropathologies. Clinically, neurosarcoidosis presents with cranial nerve(s) involvement (facial nerve palsy is particularly common), aseptic meningitis, diencephalic syndromes (particularly hypopituitarism), epilepsy, cognitive decline, myelopathy, and peripheral neuropathy.

R. Aachi, MD • J. McGee, DHEd, MSHS • A. Minagar, MD (✉)
Department of Neurology, LSU Health Sciences Center,
1501 Kings Highway, Shreveport, LA 71130, USA
e-mail: aminag@lsuhsc.edu

M. Fowler, MD
Departments of Pathology, LSU Health Sciences Center, Shreveport, LA 71130, USA

E. Gonzalez-Toledo, MD, PhD
Department of Neurology, LSU Health Sciences Center,
1501 Kings Highway, Shreveport, LA 71130, USA

Departments of Radiology, LSU Health Sciences Center, Shreveport, LA 71130, USA

© Springer International Publishing AG 2017
A. Minagar, J.S. Alexander (eds.), *Inflammatory Disorders of the Nervous System*, Current Clinical Neurology, DOI 10.1007/978-3-319-51220-4_5

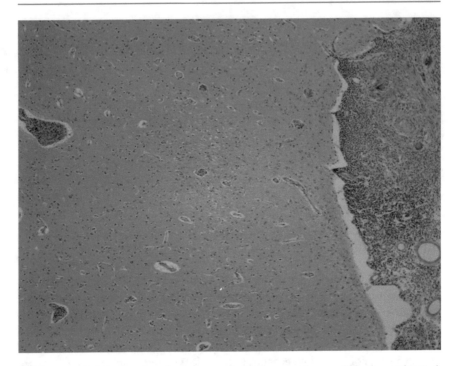

Fig. 5.1 10×4XX: Low-power photomicrograph showing granulomas within the meninges. A small granuloma is seen in the parenchyma of the brain (H&E, original magnification × 40)

Neuropathologically, sarcoidosis is characterized by the presence of epithelioid, non-caseating granulomas, including clusters of activated and highly differentiated macrophages and other epithelioid cells surrounded by T lymphocytes (Figs. 5.1 and 5.2). Langerhans-type multinucleated giant cells are commonly present, and further examination of the granulomas reveal that the center consists mainly of CD4+ lymphocytes, while the CD8+ lymphocytes exist in the periphery (Figs. 5.1, 5.2, and 5.3). Also, tumor necrosis factor-α (TNFα) is implicated in the pathogenesis of nervous system inflammation [3].

Epidemiology

Sarcoidosis, more frequently, affects African-Americans as well as individuals of Scandinavian origin. The estimated incidence of neurosarcoidosis in these ethnic groups is 15–20 and 35–80 cases per 100,000, correspondingly. However, a review of a number of retrospective case series reports indicates that 5–10 % of patients with sarcoidosis suffer from neurological complications and in 50–70 % of these individuals neurologic abnormalities are the initial clinical presentations. These neurologic abnormalities commonly develop during the first 2 years of systemic involvement. Isolated neurosarcoidosis, which means exclusive involvement of the

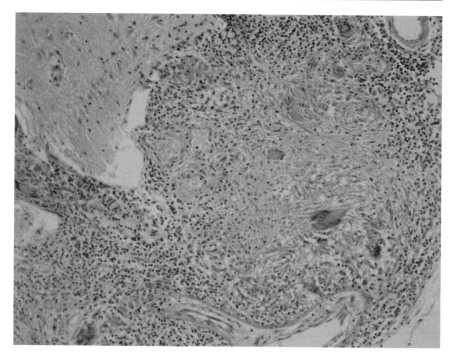

Fig. 5.2 0×10XX: Medium-power photomicrograph showing meningeal granulomas containing a few giant cells and a surrounding lymphocytic infiltrate (H&E, original magnification × 100)

nervous system without systemic involvement, is uncommon and its prevalence differs among various studies between 1–3 % and 10–17 % [4, 5]. Usually, sarcoidosis peaks in the third to fifth decades for most individuals, and neurologic symptoms commonly manifest during the first 2 years of disease. Women often have been reported to have a later age of onset and are more frequently affected compared to men. Various genetic, infectious, and environmental causes have been associated with sarcoidosis but without any proven cause and effect relationship.

Clinical Manifestations

Sarcoidosis is a great masquerader of other systemic diseases (particularly tuberculosis) and in a large number of patients with neurosarcoidosis presents with non-neurologic issues. Neurologists should always be aware of certain clues such as pulmonary involvement, eye disease (especially uveitis), dermatologic manifestations such as erythema nodosum, lymphadenopathy, joint pain, and other systemic symptoms (such as unexplained fever), which can eventually guide them to a correct diagnosis.

As a complicated multisystemic disease, sarcoidosis affects various parts of human nervous system and such widespread process leads to a wide range of

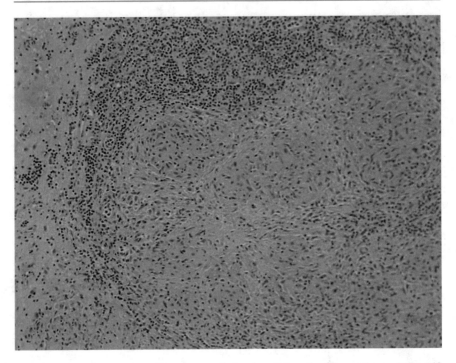

Fig. 5.3 ×10: Medium-power photomicrograph showing a parenchymal granuloma with central epithelioid cells and surrounding lymphocytic infiltrate (H&E, original magnification × 100)

neurological manifestations. Cranial nerve palsy and neuropathy, either due to granuloma, elevated intracranial pressure, or granulomatous basal meningitis, is the most common neurological presentation of neurosarcoidosis. Among the cranial nerves, the facial and the optic nerves are the most commonly affected. Bilateral facial nerve palsy due to neurosarcoidosis may occur, or the seventh cranial nerve may be affected sequentially.

While patients with neurosarcoidosis may present with rapidly progressing papilledema, other cranial nerves including olfactory, optic, oculomotor, vestibulocochlear, and uncommonly trigeminal, may be affected either alone or in combination. The pathologic process of the sarcoidosis can affect the cranial nerve nucleus or at any point within their anatomic pathway. Patients with Heerfordt's syndrome present with cranial neuropathy (most commonly facial nerve palsy), uveitis, fever, and enlargement of parotid gland. Such a unique combination is highly suggestive of neurosarcoidosis. Also, Horner's syndrome which develops from the disruption of cervical sympathetic fibers could be a manifestation of neurosarcoidosis. Pupillary abnormalities including Argyll-Robertson pupil and Adie's pupil have also been described in sarcoidosis.

Leptomeningeal involvement due to widespread meningeal infiltration of brain occurs in the presence or absence of parenchymal brain lesions and clinically may be symptomatic or may manifest as subacute or chronic aseptic meningitis, basilar polycranial neuropathy, and neuroendocrine abnormalities. Clinicians who manage these patients should bear in mind that headache and seizures may stem from meningitis, hydrocephalus, space-occupying lesions, or opportunistic infections (particularly in immunocompromised patients). Headache in these patients less often originates from trigeminal neuropathy or worsening of coexisting migraines [6]. In patients with neurosarcoidosis, seizures may be the initial presentation of the underlying disease process, and they may experience any type of seizures. Manifestation of the seizure in these patients may designate chronicity and an unfavorable prognosis [7].

Rarely, neurosarcoidosis may result in stroke due to penetration of the endothelial layers of small or large blood vessels, with disruption of the media and internal elastic lamina, resulting in obstruction of the vessel and ischemic cerebral infarct [8]. Other possible stroke pathology suggested includes sarcoidosis-associated mass lesion compression of an intracranial artery, necrotizing arteritis with fibrinoid necrosis of the media and massive leukocyte invasion [9], and cardiac granulomatous inflammation resulting in cardiogenic emboli. Cerebral and dural venous sinus thrombosis is also a potential, however, rare complication of this inflammatory process [5, 10].

With more diffuse leptomeningeal disease, headache may be accompanied by gait dysfunction, cognitive changes, and/or seizures, suggesting involvement of the brain parenchyma. Patients presenting acutely with this complex of symptoms should be evaluated urgently for hydrocephalus, which can often complicate severe cases of leptomeningeal inflammation and is considered a neurologic emergency. Hydrocephalus is another interesting clinical feature of neurosarcoidosis, which may be due to meningeal infiltration of the arachnoid granulations or cerebral aqueduct. Patients with neurosarcoidosis may develop cauda equina syndrome due to meningeal infiltration of the lumbosacral nerve roots.

Myelopathy in the context of neurosarcoidosis occurs as a result of spinal leptomeningeal infiltration, extensive myelitis, or both. Cases of neurosarcoidosis with longitudinally extensive myelitis which span an average of 3.9 segments (a significant differentiating feature from multiple sclerosis with smaller and patch cord lesions) have been reported. The most significant differential diagnoses of neurosarcoidosis patients with such extensive myelitis include multiple sclerosis, neuromyelitis optica, lupus myelitis, Sjogren's syndrome, and infectious diseases.

Neuroendocrine abnormalities of neurosarcoidosis, which stem from hypothalamic and pituitary involvement by the subependymal granulomatous invasion of the third ventricle region, includes hypothalamic hypothyroidism, hypogonadotropism, SIADH, diabetes insipidus, growth hormone deficiency, and hyperprolactinemia [11].

Neurosarcoidosis may be associated with various nonspecific neuropsychiatric symptoms such as memory loss, fatigue, mood disturbances, and other behavioral issues, without evidence of a CNS lesion. These are attributed primarily to underlying systemic disease, medication side effects, depression, and sleep disorders such as sleep apnea syndrome and primary hypersomnia.

Peripheral nervous system involvement in the process of neurosarcoidosis includes asymmetric polyradiculoneuropathy, mononeuritis multiplex, small fiber sensory neuropathy with autonomic dysfunction, AIDP, CIDP, and subacute length-dependent axonal polyneuropathy. Mononeuropathy is another manifestation of neurosarcoidosis and the ulnar and peroneal nerves are the most frequently affected. Autonomic dysfunction symptoms include orthostatic hypotension, gastrointestinal dysmotility, and disorders of sweating. Small fiber neuropathy of neurosarcoidosis can involve autonomic nerve fibers and cause cardiac sympathetic denervation with cardiac arrhythmias and may cause restless leg syndrome [12]. Patients with neuro-sarcoidosis may develop myopathy with granulomatous muscle involvement, and this may be clinically symptomatic or remain asymptomatic. In symptomatic cases, patients complain of myalgia, weakness, and muscle tenderness and suffer from cramps and muscle atrophy. Acute myositis in the context of neurosarcoidosis is uncommon and the myopathy more often takes a chronic course.

Sleep Disorders in Neurosarcoidosis Patients

The exact incidence of sleep disorders in patients with neurosarcoidosis remains unrecognized, and the only diagnostic polysomnographic studies in these patients include cases of narcolepsy with cataplexy [13–15]. Recently, May et al. had reported the HLA DQB1*0602-negative case of hypocretin deficiency and respiratory dys-function (hypoventilation and hypercapnia) from extensive destruction of hypocretin neurons and key diencephalic structures secondary to the underlying sarcoidosis [13–15]. In another HLA DR2/DQ1-positive case of neurosarcoidosis, patients pre-sented with hypothalamic lesion, excessive daytime sleepiness, sleep attacks, and cataplexy, and multiple sleep latency tests (MSLT) were characteristic of narcolepsy [14]. Anecdotally, low-dose, whole-brain irradiation, but not high dose of corticoste-roids, led to complete resolution of the narcoleptic features in patients with struc-tural neurosarcoidosis lesion in the hypothalamus [15]. Even though sleep-disordered breathing (SDB) is very prevalent in sarcoidosis patients ranging from 17 to 67 % [16–18], overall prevalence of SDB and obstructive sleep apnea in neurosarcoidosis population is unknown. Epidemiologic distribution of other primary and secondary sleep disorders in neurosarcoidosis remains largely unknown.

Neuropathology

On growth appearance, neurosarcoidosis most frequently involves the meninges at the base of the brain, particularly in the area of the infundibulum and optic chiasm, although it may involve other meningeal areas including the brain stem, convexities, cerebellum, and spinal cord. It may involve both cranial and spinal nerves where they traverse the meningeal space. The involved meninges are thickened, gray yel-low, and frequently gelatinous (Fig. 5.1). Long-standing sarcoidosis results in pro-gressively more fibrosis resulting in a tough fibrous-thickened membrane.

Occasional cases also exhibit involvement of the choroid plexus and/or ependymal lining of the ventricular system. Dural involvement is unusual but would have similar gross features.

Although less common, the granulomas of sarcoidosis may be seen within the parenchyma of the brain where they are usually small, discrete, gray, firm nodular lesions that may be solitary or multifocal. The infundibulum and hypothalamus are the favored parenchymal areas of involvement followed by the brain stem.

Microscopic Appearance

The granulomas are composed of numerous central epithelioid macrophages with abundant eosinophilic cytoplasm and vesicular nuclei. Multinucleated giant cells representing a fusion of these macrophages may be seen, but are not always present (Figs. 5.2 and 5.3). Although not common, giant cells may contain asteroid bodies or calcified nodular Schaumann bodies. The central cluster of epithelioid macrophages is surrounded by a cuff of benign lymphocytes and plasma cells. Necrosis is uncommon but rarely may be seen. Although blood vessels may be seen within rare granulomas, this is not common. With age progressively more fibrosis is seen in the meninges.

The tissue surrounding parenchymal granulomas contains gemistocytic astrocytes and may exhibit edema or loss of neuropil. Small perivascular cuffs of benign lymphocytes are frequently seen in the tissue surrounding the parenchymal granulomas. Microglial nodules are usually absent. Special stains for mycobacteria, fungi, and amyloid are negative.

Differential Diagnosis

The histologic differential diagnosis includes fungal and mycobacterial infections. These can usually be excluded using special stains. Special stains are also useful in excluding amyloid angiopathy with a granulomatous response. The presence of granulomas within the parenchyma and the rarity of blood vessels within the granulomas help distinguish sarcoidosis from primary angiitis of the CNS. As in all cases, the clinical history and presence of disease elsewhere are essential for making the correct diagnosis. Clinically, the most significant differential diagnoses of neurosarcoidosis include multiple sclerosis, CNS tuberculosis, neuromyelitis optica, transverse myelitis, HIV infection, and neuro-Behcet's disease.

Diagnosis

Neuroimaging plays a crucial role in diagnosing of neurosarcoidosis, and all suspected patients should undergo magnetic resonance imaging of the brain and spinal cord with and without gadolinium contrast. Interestingly, many of neuroimaging abnormalities of neurosarcoidosis mimic other inflammatory, neoplastic, demyelinating, and

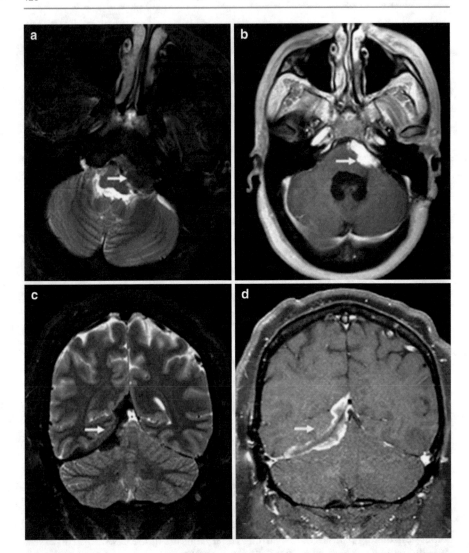

Fig. 5.4 Extra-axial masses in sarcoidosis. (**a**, **b**) Axial T2- and enhanced axial T1-weighted images demonstrate an enhancing T2-hypointense extra-axial mass in the left cerebellopontine angle cistern (*arrow*). (**c**, **d**) Coronal T2 and enhanced coronal T1 images from a different patient show a T2-hypointense enhancing right tentorial mass (*arrow*). Noncontrast CT (not shown) did not demonstrate any calcification. Biopsy (not shown) revealed granulomatous inflammation (From Shah et al. [19]. Copyright permission obtained from American Society of Neuroradiology)

infectious neurological diseases. Also, the disease may manifest as meningeal involvement either as a focal thickening concerning for meningioma or diffuse pachymeningeal involvement as seen in intracranial hypotension or leptomeningeal disease. Hydrocephalus, either communicating or noncommunicating, may develop as a result of severe meningeal inflammation. Various neuroimaging abnormalities of the neurosarcoidosis are presented in Figs. 5.4, 5.5, 5.6, 5.7, 5.8, and 5.9 [19].

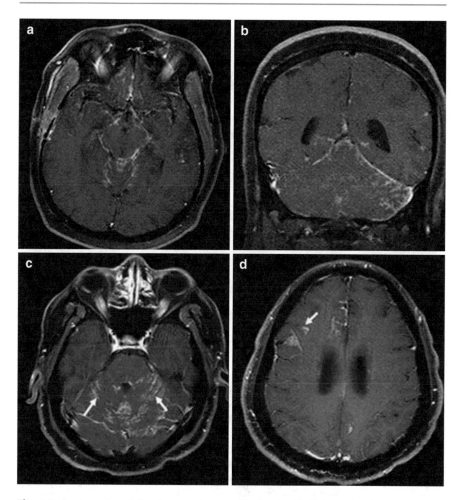

Fig. 5.5 Leptomeningeal involvement in sarcoidosis. (**a, b**) Enhanced axial and coronal T1-weighted images demonstrate nodular leptomeningeal enhancement in the basilar cisterns and posterior fossa. (**c, d**) Enhanced axial T1-weighted images in a different patient demonstrate nodular leptomeningeal enhancement along the cerebellar folia (*arrows*). Involvement of perivascular spaces is seen at a higher level in **d** (*arrow*) (From Shah et al. [19]. Copyright permission obtained from American Society of Neuroradiology)

The classification by Zajicek and colleagues [20] is by far the most acceptable and utilized diagnostic criteria for neurosarcoidosis (Table 5.1). As per them the disease process can be categorized as definite (direct neural tissue confirmation), probable (neurologic inflammation along with evidence of systemic sarcoidosis), and possible (typical clinical presentation but no other criteria met except for the exclusion of other potential etiologies).

In almost half of patients with neurosarcoidosis, intramedullary spinal cord lesions are present with involvement of ≥3 segments with a patchy and noncontiguous dissemination which may or may not enhance and is usually accompanied by

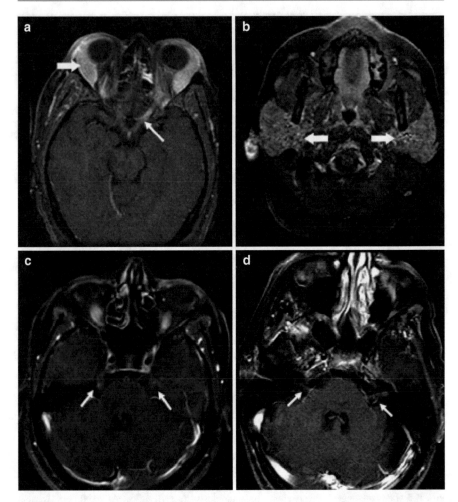

Fig. 5.6 Cranial nerve enhancement in sarcoidosis. (**a, b**) Axial fat-suppressed T1 images show enhancement of the left optic nerve (*thin arrow*). Lacrimal and parotid glands are enlarged (*thick arrows* in **a** and **b**, respectively). (**c**) Bilateral trigeminal nerve enhancement is seen in a different patient (*arrows*). (**d**) Enhancement of bilateral seventh to eighth nerve complexes is seen in another patient (*arrows*) (From Shah et al. [19]. Copyright permission obtained from American Society of Neuroradiology)

meningeal enhancement. In acute phase the affected spinal cord appears swollen and expanded, while chronic cases manifest with spinal cord atrophy. However, acute lesions may at times be nonenhancing as well.

Examination and analysis of cerebrospinal fluid (CSF) also assists clinicians to establish the correct diagnosis and exclude other differential diagnoses. The authors of this chapter routinely perform spinal tap on all patients suspected of having neurosarcoidosis. CSF examination of these patients reveals inflammatory features such as increased protein concentration (≥ 200 mg/dL) and elevated white blood

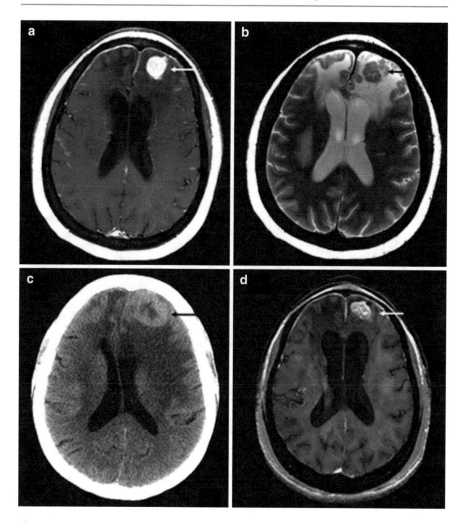

Fig. 5.7 Parenchymal lesion in sarcoidosis. (**a, b**) Enhanced axial T1- and T2-weighted images at presentation demonstrate an enhancing T2-hypointense left frontal mass (*arrow*). There is surrounding nonenhancing T2-hyperintensity due to vasogenic edema. Also note thin dural enhancement overlying both frontal lobes. (**c**) Noncontrast CT scan obtained 1 year later shows worsening lesion size and edema (*arrow*). The patient had been on low-dose prednisone and was symptomatically stable. (**d**) MR image obtained following high-dose prednisone therapy shows a decrease in edema but only partial resolution of the enhancing left frontal mass (*arrow*). There was no further decrease in size of the mass on serial scans during the next 2 years with the patient on immunosuppressive therapy (From Shah et al. [19]. Copyright permission obtained from American Society of Neuroradiology)

cell count (mononuclear pleocytosis) [>50 cells μL] and the presence of oligoclonal bands along with elevated IgG indices. In some cases CSF glucose level is low. A normal CSF panel (which may be present in one-third of patients even in the presence of contrast-enhancing MR lesions or biopsy-proven neurosarcoidosis or in

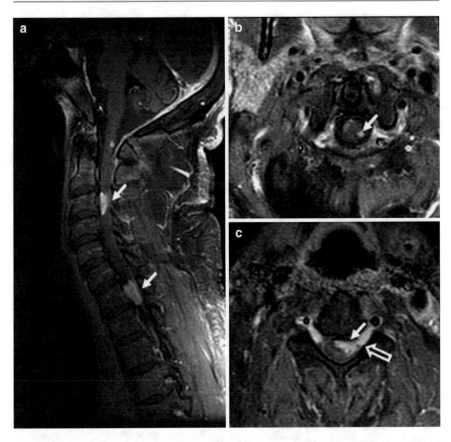

Fig. 5.8 Spinal cord involvement in sarcoidosis. (**a–c**) Enhanced parasagittal and axial T1-weighted images of the cervical cord show multiple enhancing parenchymal nodules (*arrows*). The peripheral distribution of these nodules, which are abutting the surface of the cord, suggests a leptomeningeal origin of these nodules. Note enhancement extending along the nerve roots (*open arrow*, **c**) (From Shah et al. [19]. Copyright permission obtained from American Society of Neuroradiology)

patients with isolated facial palsy) does not exclude such diagnosis. In all patients, the CSF examination should include search for malignant cells utilizing flow cytometry, serology for various infections, bacterial cultures, PCR assays for viral agents, and serologic studies for a number of infections. Angiotensin-converting enzyme (ACE), which is produced by granulomas, is increased in 24–55 % of patients, and while it is a nonsensitive marker of neurosarcoidosis, it is highly specific [19, 21].

Electromyography and nerve conduction studies enable clinicians to diagnose patients with neuromuscular diseases such as neuropathy, mononeuritis multiplex, and myopathy. This test also helps the neurophysiologist to determine whether the disease process is demyelinating versus axonal, how severe and widespread the neuropathic process is, and whether it is acute or chronic. Routine nerve conduction

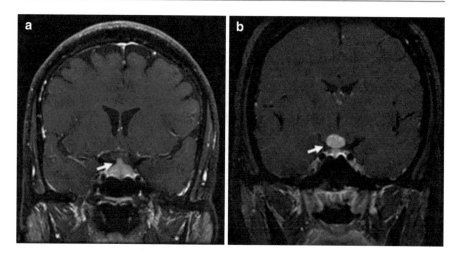

Fig. 5.9 Sellar-suprasellar involvement in sarcoidosis. (**a**) Enhanced coronal T1-weighted image shows an enlarged and enhancing pituitary infundibulum (*arrow*). This patient also had multiple enhancing parenchymal nodules in a perivascular distribution. (**b**) Enhanced coronal T1-weighted image from a different patient shows a homogeneously enhancing infundibular and hypothalamic mass (*arrow*) (From Shah et al. [19]. Copyright permission obtained from American Society of Neuroradiology)

Table 5.1 Proposed diagnostic criteria for neurosarcoidosis

Definite	Clinical presentation suggestive of neurosarcoidosis with exclusion of other possible diagnoses and the presence of positive nervous system histology
Probable	Clinical syndrome suggestive histology of neurosarcoidosis with laboratory support for CNS inflammation (elevated levels of CAF protein and/or cells, the presence of oligoclonal bands, and/or MRI evidence compatible with neurosarcoidosis) and exclusion of alternative diagnoses together with evidence of systemic sarcoidosis (either through positive histology, including Kveim test, and/or at least two indirect indicators from gallium scan, chest imaging and serum ACE)
Possible	Clinical presentation suggestive of neurosarcoidosis with exclusion of alternative diagnoses where the above criteria are not met

From Zajicek et al. [20] Copyright permission obtained

study with main concentration on large nerve fiber may miss a diagnosis of small fiber neuropathy. In cases where a systematic diagnosis approach fails to establish a diagnosis, the neurologist should consider muscle and nerve biopsy. In such cases the presence of epineural and perineural granulomas and granulomatous vasculitis may indicate a diagnosis of neurosarcoidosis. Accurate diagnosis of small fiber neuropathy is necessary since it causes disabling problems such as cardiac sympathetic denervation, periodic limb movement disorder, and restless leg syndrome. Evaluation of intraepidermal nerve fiber density along with other examinations such as quantitative sudomotor axon reflex testing and tilt table test are currently being utilized to accurately diagnose small fiber neuropathy [22].

Conjunctival, as well as tongue, biopsy is an informative, technically simple, and relatively safe procedure, which can demonstrate the presence of non-caseating granulomas in support of sarcoidosis. Real-time endobronchial ultrasound-guided transbronchial needle aspiration is utilized to examine the mediastinal and hilar lymphadenopathy in patients suspected of sarcoidosis.

In cases when the initial screening tests failed to provide adequate evidence in support of sarcoidosis, a pan-body fluorodeoxyglucose positron emission tomography (FDG-PET) scan should be considered. Studies have shown that FDG-PET is more sensitive than [67]gallium nuclear scan in detecting systemic sarcoidosis. In addition, FDG-PET helps visualize neurologic disease activity otherwise not evident on the MRI and when combined with CT (PET/CT) assists neurologist to assess disease activity and response to therapy [23]. [67]Gallium nuclear scan is used in clinical practice since it potentially can reveal elevated uptake at the sites of active inflammation (hot spots), which are appropriate for biopsy.

In patients with exclusive CNS sarcoidosis, a tissue biopsy of the region of interest is the most definitive diagnostic test. Biopsy also helps in ruling out alternative diagnoses in patients who do not respond well to immunosuppressive therapy or with worsening disease.

Treatment

There is no known cure for sarcoidosis and its treatment rests on immunosuppression as well as symptomatic treatment. Neurosarcoidosis is a devastating condition and carries a significant mortality and morbidity rate. In addition, there are not any randomized, controlled, and well-executed clinical trials to establish the superiority of one treatment over the other options. Therefore, most of the available treatment approaches are based on small case series and anecdotal case reports. In general, patients with neurosarcoidosis require aggressive treatment. Left untreated, neurosarcoidosis with brain and spinal cord involvement is potentially fatal, and rapid immunosuppression with corticosteroids is necessary to block such path. The most significant concept in treatment of neurosarcoidosis is profound immunosuppression. Presently, corticosteroids remain the foundation of its treatment. Patients with mild to moderate neurosarcoidosis can be treated with oral prednisone with doses in the range of 40–80 mg daily, and since this is a chronic ailment, patients need long-term treatment.

In many cases the dose of corticosteroid should be tapered slowly and systematically, over a course of 6–12 months. The authors treat neurosarcoidosis patients with pulse intravenous infusion of methylprednisolone (Solu-Medrol) 1000 mg daily for 5 days followed by oral maintenance dose of prednisone of 40–80 mg daily for at least 1 year. This pulse therapy should be followed by the use of oral prednisone. The treatment of neurosarcoidosis patients is also an individualized process and dosing and duration of therapy with corticosteroids vary across the patients. Corticosteroids work by suppressing lymphocyte and mononuclear phagocytic activity, suppression of transcription of pro-inflammatory cytokines, downregulation of cellular receptors, and repairing the disrupted blood-brain barrier.

In severe cases with severe myelitis or brain parenchymal involvement, or in unresponsive patients, combined therapy with a second immunosuppressant should be planned. Once clinical response and improvement are observed, the clinician should think about slow tapering of the corticosteroids. Treatment of neurosarcoidosis with corticosteroids is associated with a number of complications such as iatrogenic hyperglycemia, hypertension, hypokalemia, significant weight gain, myopathy, premature cataract and glaucoma, and uncommonly aseptic necrosis of femur head.

Certain immune-suppressant cytotoxic agents such as methotrexate (a folate analogue), azathioprine (a purine analogue), mycophenolate mofetil, cyclosporine, and cyclophosphamide have been utilized to treat patients with inadequate therapeutic response to corticosteroids or those with features of poor prognosis and elevated chance of disease recurrence. Each one of these agents does possess its own hematologic, hepatotoxic, gastrointestinal, or urologic complications and close monitoring of these patients is necessary. In addition, chronic treatment with these agents may cause uncommon malignancies. Some cases of neurosarcoidosis have been treated with anti-malarial drugs such as hydroxychloroquine. However, this medication does have toxic effects on the retina, liver, and skin.

Few case reports exist on CNS radiation for treatment of patients with neurosarcoidosis with widespread encephalopathy and vasculopathy. These patients have been treated with either total nodal or craniospinal irradiation. CNS radiation should be considered only for very severe cases since it does have its own adverse complications and is not curative.

In neurosarcoidosis patients with large parenchymal lesions, which cause hydrocephalus or increase the intracranial pressure, urgent neurosurgical debulking and cerebrospinal fluid diversion procedures such as ventriculo-peritoneal shunt implant should be considered.

Tumor necrosis factor-α (TNF-α) antagonists, such as monoclonal antibody known as infliximab, have been utilized for treating refractory cases of neurosarcoidosis. TNF-α, a potent pro-inflammatory cytokine, is released by macrophages and other immune cells during formation of granuloma. By binding to TNF-α, infliximab blocks its interaction with the TNF-α receptor. It is used as monotherapy or combined with corticosteroids and is effective for patients with severe leptomeningeal, brain, and spinal cord involvement. Other monoclonal antibodies such as adalimumab and rituximab have been utilized to treat neurosarcoidosis. Significant adverse effects of this group of new therapies include lymphoma, progressive multifocal leukoencephalopathy, and recrudescence of tuberculosis. Another interesting and more recent experimental monoclonal antibody, adalimumab, which also serves as an antagonist against TNF-α, has been utilized for treatment of patients with corticosteroid-resistant patients.

In patients with small fiber neuropathy and autonomic dysfunction that are refractory to corticosteroids, IV immunoglobulin and TNF-α antagonists have shown their potential in alleviating the symptoms to a significant extent.

Treatment of complications of neurosarcoidosis is also an interesting subject which requires more discussion. Patients with hydrocephalus and raised intracranial pressure need ventriculostomy with drainage and possibly shunt placement. Patients with epilepsy due to neurosarcoidosis should be treated with antiepileptics. Treatment of those with involvement of hypothalamic-pituitary axis with neurosarcoidosis requires consultation from endocrinologist, correction of water and electrolyte deficits, and hormone replacement treatment. Patients with peripheral neuropathy due to neurosarcoidosis should be treated with various agents such as antidepressants, antiepileptics, opioid or opioid agonists, and intravenous immunoglobulin. Those with ischemic stroke due to neurosarcoidosis should be treated with antiplatelets or anticoagulants. Depression and cognitive decline require psychiatric consult, treatment with antidepressants, and cognitive rehabilitation. Similar to other neurological diseases, once a diagnosis of neurosarcoidosis is established, the rehabilitation process with heavy emphasis on physical and occupational therapy begins to ascertain that patients will become independent as much as possible.

References

1. Spencer TS, Campellone JV, Maldonado I, Huang N, Usmani Q, Reginato AJ. Clinical and magnetic resonance imaging manifestations of neurosarcoidosis. Semin Arthritis Rheum. 2005;34(4):649–61.
2. Ricker W, Clark M. Sarcoidosis: a clinicopathologic review of 300 cases, including 22 autopsies. Am J Clin Pathol. 1949;19(8):725–49.
3. Iannuzzi MC, Rybicki BA, Teirstein AS. Sarcoidosis. N Engl J Med. 2007;357(21):2153–65.
4. Nozaki K, Scott TF, Sohn M, Judson MA. Isolated neurosarcoidosis: case series in 2 sarcoidosis centers. Neurologist. 2012;18:373–7.
5. Chapelon C, Ziza JM, Piette JC, Levy Y, Raguin G, Wechsler B, Bitker MO, Bletry O, Laplane D, Bousser MG. Neurosarcoidosis: signs, course and treatment in 35 confirmed cases. Medicine (Baltimore). 1990;69:261–76.
6. La Mantia L, Erbetta A. Headache and inflammatory disorders of the central nervous system. Neurol Sci. 2004;25(Suppl 3):S148–53.
7. Krumholz A, Stern BJ, Stern EG. Clinical implications of seizures in neurosarcoidosis. Arch Neurol. 1991;48:842–4.
8. Degardin A, Devos P, Vermersch P, de Seze J. Cerebrovascular symptomatic involvement in sarcoidosis. Acta Neurol Belg. 2010;110(4):349–52.
9. Caplan L, Corbett J, Goodwin J, Thomas C, Shenker D. Schatz n. neuro-ophthalmologic signs in the angiitic form of neurosarcoidosis. Neurology. 1983;33:1130–5.
10. Byrne JV, Lawton CA. Meningeal sarcoidosis causing intracranial hypertension secondary to dural sinus thrombosis. Br J Radiol. 1983;56:755–7.
11. Bihan H, Christozova V, Dumas JL, Jomaa R, Valeyre D, Tazi A, Reach G, Krivitzky A, Cohen R. Sarcoidosis: clinical, hormonal, and magnetic resonance imaging (MRI) manifestations of hypothalamic-pituitary disease in 9 patients and review of the literature. Medicine (Baltimore). 2007;86(5):259–68.
12. Polydefkis M, Allen RP, Hauer P, Earley CJ, Griffin JW, McArthur JC. Subclinical sensory neuropathy in late-onset restless legs syndrome. Neurology. 2000;55:1115–21.
13. May MC, Deng JC, Albores J, Zeidler M, Harper RM, Avidan AY. Hypocretin deficiency associated with narcolepsy type 1 and central hypoventilation syndrome in neurosarcoidosis of the hypothalamus. J Clin Sleep Med. 2015;11(9):1063–5.
14. Servan J, Marchand F, Garma L, Seilhean D, Hauw JJ, Delattre JY. Narcolepsy disclosing neurosarcoidosis. Rev Neurol (Paris). 1995;151:281–3.
15. Rubinstein I, Gray TA, Moldofsky H, Hoffstein V. Neurosarcoidosis associated with hypersomnolence treated with corticosteroids and brain irradiation. Chest. 1988;94:205–6.

16. Verbraecken J, Hoitsma E, van der Grinten CP, Cobben NA, Wouters EF, Drent M. Sleep disturbances associated with periodic leg movements in chronic sarcoidosis. Sarcoidosis Vasc Diff Lung Dis. 2004;21:137–46.
17. Turner GA, Lower EE, Corser BC, Gunther KL, Baughman RP. Sleep apnea in sarcoidosis. Sarcoidosis Vasc Diff Lung Dis. 1997;14:61–4.
18. Pihtili A, Bingol Z, Kiyan E, Cuhadaroglu C, Issever H, Gulbaran Z. Obstructive sleep apnea is common in patients with interstitial lung disease. Sleep Breath. 2013;17:1281–8.
19. Shah R, Roberson GH, Curé JK. Correlation of MR imaging findings and clinical manifestations in neurosarcoidosis. AJNR Am J Neuroradiol. 2009;30(5):953–61.
20. Zajicek JP, Scolding NJ, Foster O, et al. Central nervous system sarcoidosis – diagnosis and management. QJM. 1999;92(2):103–17.
21. Burke WM, Keogh A, Maloney PJ, Delprado W, Bryant DH, Spratt P. Transmission of sarcoidosis *via* cardiac transplantation. Lancet. 1990;336(8730):1579.
22. Bakkers M, Merkies IS, Lauria G, Devigili G, Penza P, Lombardi R, Hermans MC, van Nes SI, De Baets M, Faberm CG. Intraepidermal nerve fiber density and its application in sarcoidosis. Neurology. 2009;73:1142–8.
23. Prabhakar HB, Rabinowitz CB, Gibbons FK, O'Donnell WJ, Shepard JA, Aquino SL. Imaging features of sarcoidosis on MDCT, FDG PET, and PET/CT. AJR Am J Roentgenol. 2008 Mar;190(3 Suppl):S1–6.

Cell-Derived Microparticles/Exosomes in Neuroinflammation

6

Lawrence L. Horstman, Wenche Jy, and Yeon S. Ahn

Abbreviations of Diseases Are as Usual in Neurology

ALS   Amyotrophic lateral sclerosis
MS   Multiple sclerosis
PD   Parkinson's disease
TBI   Traumatic brain injury

Fundamentals and Terminology

Introduction

After long controversy, it is now recognized that essentially all neurodegenerative diseases have inflammatory components [1]. Many other neurological disorders are exacerbated by inflammation, including the progressive impairment following stroke or traumatic brain injury (TBI). It has been known that levels of circulating cell-derived microparticles (MP) are generally increased in inflammatory states, making them useful as biomarkers. More recently, certain species of MP or exosomes have been implicated as causative agents in neuroinflammation, to be reviewed.

L.L. Horstman, BS • W. Jy, PhD (✉) • Y.S. Ahn, MD
University of Miami, Department of Medicine (Wallace H. Coulter Platelet Laboratory),
1600 NW 10TH Ave., Mail Code R36A, Miami, FL 33136, USA
e-mail: wjy@med.miami.edu

© Springer International Publishing AG 2017
A. Minagar, J.S. Alexander (eds.), *Inflammatory Disorders of the Nervous System*, Current Clinical Neurology, DOI 10.1007/978-3-319-51220-4_6

Terminologies

In the peripheral circulation, MP are derived chiefly from platelets (PMP), red cells (RMP), endothelial cells (EMP), and leukocytes (LMP). Each can occur in multiple phenotypes, identified in flow cytometry by lineage-specific fluorescent monoclonal antibodies (mAb). They range in size from about 0.2–1.5 um diameter and carry protein markers of the parent cell. Proteomic studies and other evidence indicate that they derive from detergent-resistant regions of the cell membrane, known as *lipid rafts*.

Although "MP" is convenient and widely used, alternatives such as *extracellular vesicles* (ECV) or *microvesicles* (MV) are gaining currency, having the advantage of excluding nonbiological particles in literature searches. We use "MP" in this review because of long tradition in the field of blood coagulation and continuing use in neuroinflammation. The term, *exosomes*, came into use ca. 2000 [2, 3] to denote a class of very small (50–120 nm) MP, said to derive from endosomes rather than the plasma membrane. Until very recently, it was unclear if they were qualitatively distinct from MP. This question is important to this review because many recent advances in neuroinflammation concern exosomes, as reviewed [4].

Exosomes: Distinctly Different?

Initial doubts arose from markers said to be unique to exosomes but which are also found on MP in the larger size range. For example, the "canonical exosome proteins" are said to include CD63 and flotillin [5], but CD63 is also a marker of platelet MP (PMP), and flotillin is a marker of lipid rafts of the plasma membrane, including red blood cells (RBC) [6]. Similarly, lysosomal protein LAMP-1 (CD107a) is often listed as exosomes-specific but is also a marker of PMP [7]. In addition, if exosomes originate from multivesicular endosomes, one wonders how to explain their lipid raft proteins or the fact that 60 nm "nanovesicles" were described long ago from RBC, which lack endosomes [8], and more recently [9].

Only in the last few years have these uncertainties been acknowledged and addressed. Xu et al. compared proteomic profiles between exosomes and MP (aka ECV) from a cancer cell line and observe that a majority of about 180 proteins listed were absent from one but not the other particle type [10], showing qualitative difference. With respect to functional differences, it was shown that exosomes from RBC, but not the larger MP fraction, induced a T-cell response [9]. Kanada et al. demonstrate qualitative differences between exosomes vs. the larger vesicles in their respective ability to transport and deliver functional RNA or DNA to target cells, finding exosomes but not MP deliver RNA whereas MP but not exosomes deliver DNA [11].

These and other reports confirm a qualitative distinction. Some authors speak of *ectosomes* as opposed to *exosomes*, to indicate shedding from the plasma membrane, e.g., [12, 13]. However, this distinction is not easily made, partly because exosomes fuse with plasma membrane (lipid rafts) before release, explaining how they acquire markers of the plasma membrane, e.g., [14]. Some authors avoid the term, *exosomes*, using the more inclusive "extracellular vesicles" [11]. In practice, distinguishing exosomes is not simple, as shown by many papers on various isolation methods, [15–17], among others.

Functions, Old and New

Early interest in MP stemmed from their procoagulant activity (PCA), which remains relevant to this review for reasons noted below. Their PCA was attributed to the reversal of normal membrane asymmetry, meaning that normally in-facing and anionic phospholipids (PL) such as phosphatidylserine (PS) flip to the plasma side. These PL exhibit PCA by serving as sites for the assembly of the vitamin K-dependent clotting factors into active complexes, promoting coagulation via tissue factor (TF) pathway.

Recent work, however, calls for revision of this paradigm. It has been shown that MP exert PCA primarily by amplifying the contact pathway, not the TF pathway [18, 19], confirmed in our laboratory. The contact pathway is closely tied to the complement and kinin systems, suggesting involvement in previously unexpected pathways of inflammation.

The second major function to be recognized was a role in inflammation. There are two aspects to this role, the first being as biomarkers. It is generally observed that circulating MP of several lineages increases in response to inflammation induced experimentally by administration of lipopolysaccharide (LPS), zymosan, or overt infection. For example, we examined a variety of MP phenotypes in sepsis, especially endothelial MP (EMP) subtypes, and determined that a strong inflammatory response favored survival, concluding that inflammation was not associated with mortality [20]. In addition, MP can function to transport agents which can induce or modulate inflammation, e.g., cytokines and bioactive lipids. This topic, cell-cell signaling, was reviewed as of 2007 [21] and is updated in the following sections.

The third major function of MP has come to light only in the last decade, being the transport of functional RNA, DNA, and other functional transcripts, to be reviewed. Some key references in this area were cited in section "Exosomes: Distinctly Different?".

Formation and Fate

The biochemical details of these topics remain poorly understood. It is well known that a rise in cytoplasmic calcium will trigger release of MP, therefore, the use of calcium ionophores such as A23187 are often used to induce vesiculation ex vivo. With regard to mechanisms of clearance of MP, this topic has become very complex in recent years and will be reviewed separately in another forum. However, limited studies of several MP lineages find that all have short half-life in circulation,

<10 min, e.g., [15]. Progress in understanding biochemical mechanisms has been made [22–24]. A major advance has been the identification of the mechanism of membrane "flip-flop" causing reversal of membrane asymmetry, related to MP shedding [25, 26]. This was previously attributed to presumed enzymes called *flippase, floppase,* or *PL translocase,* now known to be an ion channel.

MP in Neuroinflammation: Findings from the Authors' Group

Introduction

This article explains how the authors became involved in studies of neuroinflammatory conditions. Although some of the references are now old, the findings of section "MP in Vascular Dementia" are not widely appreciated and may be important to future work.

MP in Vascular Dementia

It was observed by Y.S. Ahn that patients with immune thrombocytopenia (ITP) were protected against bleeding symptoms by high levels of circulating platelet MP [27], later extended to include red cell-derived MP (RMP). Furthermore, he observed that a number of patients with long-term chronic elevation of PMP exhibited slowly progressing cognitive decline, which in some cases progressed to dementia. Imaging with MRI showed periventricular and subcortical white matter hyperintensities consistent with ischemic small-vessel disease. We suggested that antiplatelet antibodies activate platelets to enhance shedding of procoagulant PMP, promoting thrombotic occlusions of small vessels. In a follow-up study, it was observed that cognitive impairment progressed more rapidly in splenectomized patients [28]. This further supports a causative link of PMP with cognitive impairment since splenectomy retards clearance of PMP [29]. Of note, patients with cognitive impairment had significantly higher platelet-associated IgM (but not IgG) compared to patient controls ($p < 0.02$) [28].

A related study found that the association between PMP and cognitive decline was not limited to ITP patients [30]. Alzheimer's disease (AD) was ruled out. Recent work from other laboratories tends to confirm the main findings mentioned above [31]. Recent proteomic study of MP in patients with lacunar infarcts suggests MP assay as a diagnostic aid and for insight into the disease process [32].

Also of related interest was a study of the electrophoretic mobility of patient platelets in which it was observed that the patients with cognitive impairments had the highest mobility [33]. It was not possible at that time to measure zeta potentials of the MP but it is expected that MP will have electric charge related to that of the parent cell. This leads us to conjecture that high negative charge on MP could predispose to vascular dementia. Others have shown that electric charge can be crucial to the functional properties of MP [34]. These observations may bear on postoperative cognitive impairment, since surgical procedures entail extensive disruption of endothelia and activation of platelets and other cells, inducing release of MP [35, 36].

Early Findings on MP in Multiple Sclerosis (MS)

The first clear evidence of an association between MP in circulation and MS disease activity was found by A. Minagar et al. [37]. They found that endothelial MP (EMP) bearing CD31 (PECAM-1) were elevated significantly during exacerbations of RR-MS compared to remissions. In follow-up studies, they observed that MS plasma, but not control plasma, induced formation of EMP-monocyte complexes [38] and that these complexes are a good biomarkers of disease activity in MS [39, 40]. The same group subsequently showed that treatment with interferon 1beta induced reduction of MS-associated EMP in patients [41].

Since autoimmunity may contribute to the etiology of MS, it is of interest that MP-associated autoantigens can form immune complexes with inflammatory potential [42]. Antiphospholipid antibodies (APLA) were reported in MS, leading to a more systematic study of APLA in a series of MS patients, with the unexpected finding that APLA in MS were exclusively IgM class [43].

Evidence of platelet activation in MS was also reported by that group [44]. Since platelet activation is always accompanied by release of PMP, it is likely that the "missing PMP" are being consumed or sequestered in MS or bind to leukocytes. This may apply to Alzheimer's disease (AD) as well since platelet activation was observed in AD but not elevation of free PMP [45].

MP-Associated Bioactive Agents in Neuroinflammation

Micro-RNA (miRNA)

A giant step in neuroscience, cancer research, and other fields was the discovery that MP can transport active RNA oligomers from cell to cell, both naturally and by therapeutic design. Among these are small interfering RNA (siRNA) which can silence or modulate the expression of specific genes.

For example, it was demonstrated that expression of MiR-155 in microglial cells regulated replication of the Japanese encephalitis virus and modulated aspects of innate immunity such as complement [46]. Nucleotides bound to MP/exosomes are protected against degradation by plasma enzymes. Cell-to-cell transfer of miRNA via MP has been shown to exert major modulation of neuroinflammatory responses, as in brain infection [47].

The several phenotypes of MP/exosome that arise from a single lineage, such as monocytes, exhibit varying RNA content and transcripts: MP-bearing transcripts of pro-inflammatory cytokines (such as TNF, IL-6, IL-8) when incubated with human brain endothelial cells (EC) led to the uptake of the MP and, unexpectedly, promoted tightness of EC monolayer junctions in tissue culture, measured by impedance and directly by permeability [48]. Frohlich et al. observed a variety of effects of MP transferred from stimulated oligodendrocytes to neurons [49].

Pusic and Kraig, after commenting on myelination in MS, report isolating exosomes from old vs. young animals with enriched environment and found that the latter but not the former promoted myelination when administered intranasally; this effect was attributed to MiR-219 [50]. In a similar vein, oxidized LDL particles were observed to "epigenetically reprogram" monocytes [51].

As earlier noted, MP can also transport DNA fragments, e.g., [11]. Patients with MS on natalizumab therapy are prone to polyomavirus; the MP/exosomes from plasma or urine, and from mononuclear cells, all contained transcripts of the virus in infected subjects [52]. It is beyond the scope of this review to consider the role of MP in viral infections but a large literature on this subject exists. Very recently, the first known instance of DNA interference in an animal was reported [52b], leading us to expect more on this in the future.

Cytokines

It is usually assumed that cytokines/chemokines are released as soluble agents. However, as we have pointed out in earlier reviews, at least some are known to be MP associated and many others probably are, because cell-free plasma and serum contain MP unless centrifuged at 100,000 xg. More recent direct evidence supporting this vie is the report by Konadu et al. of at least 21 cytokines found associated with MP/exosomes in plasma of HIV-positive subjects [53]. Mullen et al. have shown that several important inflammatory mediators, including IL-1beta and HMGB1, are actually released on exosomes via a novel pathway [54]. Indeed, MP-associated secretion of IL-1beta was shown in 2001 [55].

Matrix Metaloproteinases (MMPs)

The importance of MMPs in neuroinflammation is widely appreciated in many specific conditions, such as ischemic stroke [56]. Most frequently implicated are MMP-2 and MMP-9 [57, 58]. They are released from many cell types, including from astrocytes [59] and from stem cells [60] and are transported on MP.

For example, McColl et al. studied the effect of prior inflammatory state (induced by IL-1beta) on postischemic brain injury in mice and observed that neutrophil-derived MMP-9 was a major culprit in the exacerbation of injury by the inflammatory state, since inhibition of MMP-9 ameliorated the damage [61]. Of note, MMPs are often released together with their inhibitors [59], suggesting a delicate balance. The above-cited references and related others [62–65] suggest that many or most of the MMPs are released bound to MP of the "ecto-MP" type. A recent clinical study documented clear correlations between MMP-3, MMP-9, and disease status in MS patients [66].

Heat Shock Proteins (HSP)

These constitute a large family of immunomodulatory agents [67]. Their traditional function is to serve as protein-folding chaperones, and as hallmarks of exosomes, being found in nearly all proteomic studies of MP, especially HSP-70. Several appear to have neuron-specific functions. For example, antibodies to HSP-90beta interfered with remyelination [68].

The small HSP, alphaB crystallin, elevations of which are associated with a range of inflammatory neurodegenerative disease, was shown to be secreted in exosomes [69], as discussed also by vanNoort [67]. Pinocytic uptake of exosomes has been found to depend on an HSP called ERK1/ERK2 (HSP27) [70].

MP as Immune Complex (IC) and Complement

Several neuroinflammatory disorders are known or suspected to involve autoimmunity. Practically all proteomic studies of MP/exosomes detect substantial amounts of IgG, IgM, and complement (C) fragments on MP. It has long been known that MP-associated antibody-antigen (Ab:Ag) complexes (IC) are released on MP by the action of C. Recently, it was shown that MP-IC exert significant neuroinflammatory action [42]. The cause of shedding of IC from cell surfaces is often C-mediated attack on the opsonized cells, resulting in the release of Ab/Ag/C complex MP. A specific protein, mortalin, has been identified as instrumental in this process [71]. Mortalin belongs to the HSP family ("stress chaperones") and has been implicated in Parkinson's disease (PD) [72]. Additional related references are given in the review by Robbins et al. [73], covering also cytokines on MP and their surface expression of PAMPs/DAMPs ("pathogen-associated molecular patterns" and "danger-associated molecular patterns"), which should include also "altered-self" proteins. The C system plays versatile roles in neuroinflammation, including beneficial ones [74].

Bioactive Lipids

Many bioactive lipids are available on MP, and oxidized phospholipids (oxPL) on them are also pro-inflammatory [75]. However, if inflammatory lipids are critical in neurodegenerative diseases, the question arises, why do they not respond well to NSAIDs? i.e., to cyclooxygenase (COX) inhibitors? To answer that, Fiebich et al. propose a novel "two-hit" cycle involving prostaglandin and ATP released from injured cells [76]. MP-associated bioactive lipids in neuroinflammation were discussed in our earlier review.

Cell-Cell Signals ("Cross Talk")

All of the above agents can be transferred from cell to cell via MP, such as neuron-glia "cross talk" [77]. Evidence shows that lipid raft regions of the cell are crucial in cell-cell signal functions [78–80], consistent with evidence that MP are released from lipid rafts. An emerging paradigm is the central role of lipid rafts in the release of MP/exosomes, in cell-cell signaling, in transmission of viral and other microbial infections, and in prion/prion-like diseases, as cited in following sections.

Recent Advances: MP in Selected Neuroinflammatory States

Foreword

Some of the disorders in this article are considered from more than one perspective; continue in the next section (protein-misfolding diseases).

MP in Brain Injury and Neurovascular Dysfunction

Some sources on this were earlier cited, regarding infection in section "Micro-RNA (miRNA)" [47] and ischemic brain injury in section "Matrix Metaloproteinases (MMPs)" [61]. Brain injury of several causes such as stroke or trauma present similar neuroinflammatory profiles in the progressive worsening of disability for up to 7 days following the initial insult. This progressive deterioration is attributed to inflammatory responses such as oxidative stress. Traumatic brain injury (TBI), ischemic stroke, and hemorrhagic stroke have similar post-event sequelae in the neurovascular unit [81].

The review of Terasaki et al. [81] prominently cites evidence supporting a causative role for MP in the progressive decline following brain injury. Taylor advocates MP as useful biomarkers for monitoring TBI [82]. Rivero et al. provide an up-to-date account of exosome-mediated inflammatory signaling pathways and demonstrate that administration of exosomes loaded with selected siRNA improves indicators of recovery in an animal model with spine injury [83]. Sanborn et al. have characterized the rise and fall of some MP subtypes post-subarachnoid hemorrhage [84].

MP and Infectious Diseases of the CNS

A great many infectious agents, especially virus, selectively bind to lipid rafts of the host cell to gain entry, and conversely, new virions are released in MP, such as retrovirus [85]. Biochemical details of the budding process are now better understood, as given, for example, by Nabhan et al. [86]. Release of the virions may be prompted by immune mechanisms responding to immune complex (IC) and can be complement-mediated. Examples include pseudorabies virus, cholera, rotavirus, shigella, HIV, and Newcastle disease virus [87–92]. These facts suggest inhibiting MP release might be a therapeutic target in slowing the dissemination of virions; see 6.

Tantalizing evidence for a viral trigger in the etiology of several neurodegenerative diseases (MS, ALS, AD, PD, others) is well known. Mechanisms of brain damage by virus-induced neuroinflammation were recently reviewed [93], as was HIV-associated dementia [94]. However, the latter paid little attention to a possible role of MP, although several studies have shown correlations of MP to HIV (HTLV-1) progression, including from our laboratory [95].

Viral theories of neurodegenerative diseases have recently shifted focus to human endogenous retroviruses (HERV), for example, in amyotrophic lateral sclerosis (ALS) [96]. A number of papers have shown that HERV transcripts occur on MP, e.g., [97]. Several other reports of HERV transport by MP are in the field of reproductive medicine and as cited above [85].

Multiple Sclerosis (MS)

The significance of MP in MS has been recently reviewed [98]. Therefore, we here review only some recent work that strikes us as seminal. Among the most intensive studies of MP in MS is that by Verderio et al. [99], a technical tour de force by 20 authors, using two EAEs (animal models of MS). The MP species studied were mainly from microglia/macrophages measured in CSF. Results demonstrate elevation of MP in close association with the evolution of inflammation in the animal models, consistent with results in patients in that report and with an earlier study cited above [37].

A most interesting finding in that report is that a mouse strain (A-SMase KO) known to be resistant to EAE was also deficient in ability to release MP and was also resistant to the inflammatory effects of injecting inflammatory MP [99]. This is persuasive evidence that MP play a decisive role in MS. However, others have shown that MP/exosomes derived from oligodendrocytes can have widely differing effects, suggesting caution in attributing adverse vs. beneficial effects to any given MP phenotype [49]; see also [100]. Nevertheless, it may be interesting to test the effect of inhibitors of MP release on the progression of disease in EAE animal models.

Another highlight concerns the known tendency of progressive MS to remit during pregnancy. Working with an animal model, Gatson et al. initially demonstrated that the active component of this effect was a factor in serum [101] and, in a follow-up work, identified the serum factor as exosome associated [102]. This discovery could have therapeutic impact, if and when the specifics are delineated. It was recently observed that chronic infection with *Staph. aureus* also abated progression of EAE (animal model of MS), and the mechanism of benefit was identified [103].

Miscellaneous Others

Neuropsychiatric systemic lupus (NPSLE) was recently shown to be characterized by unusual pattern of MP lineages, of which only monocyte MP were distinctive, others being reduced [104]. The authors do not know if the reduced levels of some phenotypes result in reduced shedding, or increased consumption, possibly sequestered in the brain.

MP in Protein-Misfolding Diseases

Background

Expert opinion increasingly favors the view that most of the neurodegenerative disease (AD, PD, ALS, others), without definite known cause, share in expressing aberrant proteins in the brain not cleared by normal mechanisms, forming insoluble aggregates or plaques. This is generally attributed to misfolded proteins. They are also known as "prion-like" diseases [105] on the model of kuru, scrapie (in sheep), and other prion-mediated spongiform encephalopathies, notably, Creutzfeldt-Jakob disease [106]. It was recently shown that AD is likely transmissible [107]. In Huntington's disease (HD), the aberrant protein is polyglutamine [108, 109]. Like many viruses, these self-propagating misfolded proteins are selectively associated with lipid raft domains of the cells [110, 111] and may be attacked by the complement system [112]. It is known that prion protein occurs in circulating endothelial MP [113]. The main source of circulating amyloid precursor protein (APP), implicated in AD, is platelets [114] and more recently, that it is carried on platelet MP (PMP) [115]. It appears that protein misfolding can be transmitted and "spread" on MP, as further commented below.

Amyotrophic Lateral Sclerosis (ALS)

A virus link to ALS has long been suspected, as reviewed [96]. However, promising new work suggests that ALS is a protein-misfolding disease. Evidence for involvement of MP/exosomes in the transport of these toxic proteins is given by Bellingham et al. [116]. Mutant superoxide dismutase-1 (SOD-1) was proposed as a candidate culprit in ALS [117], and very recent experiments offer further support in that direction [118]. It is believed that the complement (C) system normally acts to eliminate such aberrant proteins [112]. It is believed that aggregated misfolded protein is the cause of neurodegeneration but Lee et al. question this assumption in ALS [119].

MP, α-Synuclein, and Parkinson's Disease (PD)

The neuron-specific protein, α-synuclein, is recognized as a major player in PD [120, 121]. Plasma exosomes containing α-synuclein likely originate in the CNS and increase in PD [122]. Plasma exosomes were found to accelerate aggregation of α-synuclein [123]. Exosomes isolated from CSF of patients with PD or AD were tested for several miRNA and other markers, including α-synuclein, with significant differences between AD, PD, and normal controls, suggesting use as a diagnostic aid, and involvement in pathogenesis [124]. Most encouraging was the administration of exosomal siRNA against α-synuclein on a murine model, resulting in reduction of α-synuclein aggregates, the presumed cause of neurodegeneration [125]. Related work purports to elucidate the secretion of toxic exosomal [125]. These papers are only a small sampler of literature found on this topic for their review. For example, search of PubMed using "amyloid precursor protein and extracellular vesicles" yields 80 papers on this alone. Thus, MP/exosomes are recognized as major players in these diseases.

Therapeutic Strategies Involving MP

Therapeutic MP/Exosomes Crossing the Blood-Brain Barrier (BBB)

Properties of MP which govern their ability to cross the BBB are important for three reasons:

(i) Design or selection of MP for purposes of delivering drug therapy
(ii) For use as vectors of gene therapy
(iii) For insight on pathological aspects of certain MP types

Our readings indicate growing interest in using cell-derived MP/exosomes as vectors for gene therapy, avoiding risks of virus vectors. In reviewing literature on MP crossing the BBB, we identified at least five variables which appear to govern this capability:

1. The presence of specific promoters of endocytosis. An example was cited in section "Heat Shock Proteins": surface expression of ERK1/2, also called HSP27 [70].
2. The presence of agent tending to disrupt endothelial integrity, increasing vascular permeability, for example, semaphorin3A [126] and the Nef protein of HIV [127].
3. Pre-existing partial compromise of the BBB, such as by traumatic brain injury (TBI), facilitating crossing [128]. This may pertain to increased risk of neurodegenerative disorders in subjects with history of TBI and to the life-threatening "coagulopathy of trauma" which is prevalent in TBI [129].
4. Electric charge (zeta potential) on MP is another determinant of passage across the BBB [130].
5. Smaller size also favors passage, other factors being equal, as shown for nonbiological MP engineered for drug delivery [131, 132].

Much promising work in this direction is ongoing. Haney et al. developed exosomes for delivery of catalase to PD patients [133]. Sampey et al. discuss the effect of viral infections on exosomes and suggest that viral mechanisms of crossing the

BBB might be engineered into exosomes [134]. de Rivero showed that neuron-derived exosomes delivered cargo of siRNA across the BBB of spine-injured animals [83]. Work of L. Alvarez et al. on exosomal delivery of siRNA to the mouse brain is often cited as pioneering [135]. Related work by Frolich et al. was earlier cited [49].

Statin Therapy and Hypothesis

Many studies led to a major clinical trial of simvastatin for MS, with finding of significant benefits [136], as discussed [137, 138]. However, the explanation for the benefit was not clear. In view of work cited above, it is possible that the benefit results from reduced release of MP. Release of MP is strongly dependent on ample cellular cholesterol [139], thus one of the pleiotropic effects of statins [140] is reduction of MP release [141, 142]. This may also bear on the anti-inflammatory action of statins. For example, in a rat model of hemorrhagic stroke, simvastatin reduced post-injury mortality [143], attributed to mitigation of inflammation. Release of some virions has similar lipid raft dependence [92]. On the other hand, mounting evidence indicates that statins applied to neuroinflammatory disorders can have adverse effects [140]. The adverse effects may be explained in the same terms, insofar as MP/exosomes constitute a network of signals, many of which are neuroprotective and regenerative [144]. Incidentally, it is interesting that measles virus impairs cholesterol biosynthesis [145], possibly to avoid easy shedding in MP, thus evading innate immunity.

Stem Cell-Derived MP/Exosomes

It was shown that administration of exosomes derived from multipotent mesenchymal stromal cells promoted recovery following stroke in a rat model [146]. In a related study, the benefit was attributed to the presence of a micro-RNA (MiR-133b) bound to the exosomes [147]. Others had previously shown the presence of MMP-9 and FGF-2 on mouse MP derived from angioblast stem cells [60]. Most recently, it was reported that MP from endothelial progenitor cells protected against complement-mediated glomerulonephritis [148]. Also recently, traumatic brain injury (TBI) was found to respond very favorably to administration of exosomes derived from mesenchymal stem cells [149]. MP-mediated inflammatory signaling is well summarized by de Rivero et al., in terms of the inflammasome [83].

Conversely, it was shown that MP from ischemic mice induce apoptosis of endothelial cells (EC); this effect was not caused by oxidative stress but instead involved caspase3, since inhibition of caspase reduces cell death [150]. This experimental design could be applied to evaluate harm from MP in neurodegenerative diseases. Those authors define MP as <400 nm in size and demonstrate activation of TNF-a and TRAIL pathways. Hayon et al. provide a broadly informative summary of the role of MP in rehabilitation of ischemic brain [151], with emphasis on factors from platelets and their PMP. Camussi et al. discuss transfer of genetic information via MP/exosomes to result in "epigenetic reprogramming" of cells [152].

Inhibition of Complement (C) System

The C system is the core of innate immunity and is capable of inducing release of MP, especially in immune mediated disorders [153–155]. It can also degrade otherwise healthy cells expressing antibodies or damaged self-proteins and plays a major role in the clearance of many MP phenotypes. Accordingly, the C system may be a target of therapy in selected neurological disorders.

Fluitier et al., using a mouse model of traumatic brain injury (TBI) and an inhibitor of C6 made in their laboratory, were able to significantly promote neurological recovery and reduce secondary neuronal injury post-TBI by inhibiting the terminal membrane attack complex (MAC) [156]. At least three C inhibitors are approved for humans: compstatin [157, 158], the C1 inhibitor (C1-INH) [159], and eculizumab, approved for paroxysmal nocturnal hemoglobinuria (PNH) [160]. PNH can have neurological complications [161]. However, that the C system is also known to exert many effects favorable to tissue repair and recovery.

Pilzer et al. provide new insight on C-mediated MP generation, showing that a specific cellular protein, mortalin/GRP75, is responsible for shedding of MP with bound MAC, this being a mechanism for eliminating MAC from the cell surface [71, 155]. Sims et al. had earlier shown that cells can recover their membrane potentials after shedding MAC [153]. Mortalin is also known as the heat shock protein, HSPA9.

Elward et al. cast new light on C-mediated clearance of senescent cells and MP and underlying mechanisms which may in future allow manipulation of MP levels in blood or CSF. Their main finding was a key role for clustering of CD46, which then binds C1q or C opsonins [162]. (CD46 is also known as "membrane cofactor protein," a C regulator, along with CD55 and CD59.)

Concluding Comments

It is seen in this review that MP/exosomes are now regarded as fundamental in neuroinflammatory conditions. Because of the unexpectedly large literature on these matters, and length restrictions, many fine papers could not be cited, and discussion of several additional specific disorders had to be dropped.

Among topics not covered are the intracellular vesicles known as clathrin-coated pits, which may be released from the plasma membrane in exosomes to transmit prion infection [*Eur. J. Cell Biol.*, 2009, 88(1): 45–63]. Intracellular trafficking via MP is a related field with important new developments, such as intracellular transport across the nuclear membrane and to the plasma membrane. As stated in a recent issue of *Cell*: "Vesicular nucleo-cytoplasma transport is becoming recognized as a general cellular mechanism for translocation of large cargos across the nuclear envelope" [C. Hagen, K.C. Dent, et al., Dec. 17, 2015; Cell, v163, p1692–1701]. These particles are the likely source of exosomal genetic transcripts.

It is clear that better understanding of detailed mechanisms of MP formation, cargo sorting, release, clearance, and targeting hold great promise for gaining new insights into many devastating neurological conditions. Those insights, some of which are seen in this review, hold the promise of effective new therapies.

Acknowledgment   For their support, the Wallace H. Coulter Foundation

References

1. McGeer PL, McGeer EG. History of innate immunity in neurodegenerative disorders. Front Pharmacol. 2011;2 (Dec., Art. #77):1–5.
2. Zitvogel L, Regnault A, Lozier A, et al. Eradication of established murine tumors using a novel cell-free vaccine: dendritic cell-derived exosomes. Nat Med. 1998;4(5):594–600.
3. Wolfers J, Lozier A, Raposo G, et al. Tumor-derived exosomes are a source of shared tumor rejection antigens for CTL cross priming. Nat Med. 2001;7(3):297–303.
4. Tsilioni I, Panagiotidou S, Theoharides TC. Exosomes in neurologic and psychiatric disorders. Clin Ther. 2014;36(6):882–8.
5. Lobb RJ, Becker M, En SW, et al. Optimized exosome isolation protocol for cell culture supernatants and human plasma. J Extracell Vesicles. 2015;17(4):27031.
6. Salzer U, Zhu R, Luten M, et al. Vesicles generated during storage of red cells are rich in the lipid raft marker stomatin. Transfusion. 2008;48:451–62.
7. Flaumenhaft R, Dilks JR, Richardson J, et al. Megakaryocyte-derived microparticles: direct visualization and distinction from platelet-derived microparticles. Blood. 2009;113(5):1112–21.
8. Allan D, Thomas P, Limbrick AR. The isolation and characterization of 60 nm vesicles ("nanovesicles") produced during ionophore A23187-induced budding of human erythrocytes. Biochem J. 1980;188:881–7.
9. Danesh A, Inglis HC, Jackman RP, et al. Exosomes from red blood cell units bind to monocytes and induce proinflammatory cytokines, boosting T-cell responses in vitro. Blood. 2014;123(5):687–96.
10. Xu X, Greening DW, Rai A, et al. Highly-purified exosomes and shed microvesicles isolated from human colon cancer cell line LIM1863 by sequential centrifugal ultrafiltration are biochemically and functionally distinct. Methods Inf Med. 2015;87:11–25.
11. Kanada M, Bachmann MH, Hardy JW, et al. Differential fates of biomolecules delivered to target cells via extracellular vesicles. Proc Nat Acad Sci USA. 2015;112(12):E1433–42.
12. Choi DS, Kim DK, Kim YK, et al. Proteomics, transcriptomics and lipidomics of exosomes and ectosomes [Review]. Proteomics. 2013;13(10–11):1554–71.
13. Sadallah S, Eken C, Schifferli JA. Erythrocyte-derived ectosomes have immunosuppressive properties. J Leukoc Biol. 2008;84(5):1316–25.
14. Valapala M, Vishwanatha J. Lipid raft endocytosis and exosomal transport facilitate extracellula trafficking of annexin A2. J Biol Chem. 2011;286(35):30911–25.
15. Yamashita T, Takahashi Y, Nishikiwa M, et al. Effect of exosome isolation methods on physicochemical properties of exosomes and clearance of exosomes from circulation. Eur J Pharm Biopharm. 2016;98(Jan):1–8.
16. Wang J, Yao Y, Wu J, et al. Identification and analysis of exosomes secreted from macrophages extracted by different methods. Int J Clin Exp Pathol. 2015;8(6):6135–42.
17. Zarovni N, Corrado A, Gluzzi P, et al. Integrated isolation and quantitative analysis of exosome shuttled proteins and nucleic acid using immunocapture approaches. Methods Inf Med. 2015;87:46–58.

18. VanDerMeijden PE, VanSchilfgaard M, VanOerle R, et al. Platelet- and erythrocyte-derived microparticles trigger thrombin generation via FXIIa. J Thromb Haemost. 2012;10:1355–62.
19. Rubin O, Delobel J, Prudent M, et al. Red blood cell-derived microparticles isolated from blood units initiate and propagate thrombin generation. Transfusion. 2013;53(8):1744–55.
20. Soriano AO, Jy W, Chirinos JA, et al. Levels of endothelial and platelet microparticles and their interactions with leukocytes correlate with organ dysfunction and predict mortality in severe sepsis. Crit Care Med. 2005;33(11):2540–6.
21. Horstman LL, Minagar A, Jy W, et al. Cell-derived microparticles and exosomes in neuroinflammatory conditions. Int Rev Neurobiol. 2007;79:229–68.
22. Johnson BL, Goetzman HS, Prakash PS, et al. Mechanisms underlying mouse TNF-alpha stimulated neutrophil derived microparticle generation. Biochem Biophyis Res Commun. 2013;437(4):591–6.
23. Koseoglu S, Dilks JR, Peters CG, et al. Dynamin-related protein-1 controls fusion pore dynamics during platelet granule exocytosis. Arterioscl Thromb Vasc Biol. 2013;33(3):481–6.
24. O'Connell DJ, Rozenvayn N, Flaumenhaft R. Phosphatidylinositol 4,5-bisphosphate regulates activation-induced platelet microparticle formation. Biochem. 2005;44:6361–70.
25. Fujii T, Sakata A, Nishinura S, et al. TMEM16F is required for phosphatidylserine and microparticle release in activated mouse platelets. Proc Nat Acad Sci USA. 2015;112(41):12800–7.
26. Brooks MB, Catalfamo JL, MacNguyen R, et al. A TMEM16F point mutation causes an absence of canine platelet TMEM16F and inefficient activation and death-induced phospholipid scrambling. J Thromb Haemost. 2015;13:2240–52. PRE-PUB(tba):tba
27. Jy W, Horstman LL, Arce M, et al. Clinical significance of platelet microparticles in autoimmune thrombocytopenias [with Editorial pg 321]. J Lab Clin Med. 1992;119:334–45.
28. Ahn YS, Horstman LL, Jy W, et al. Vascular dementia in patients with immune thrombocytopenic purpura (ITP). Thromb Res. 2002;107:337–44.
29. Sewify EM, Sayed D, Abdel ARF, et al. Increased circulating red cell microparticles (RMP) and platelet microparticles (PMP) in immune thrombocytopenic purpura. Thromb Res. 2013;131(2):e59–63.
30. Lee YJ, Horstman LL, Janania J, et al. Elevated platelet microparticles in transient ischemic attacks, lacunar infarcts, and multiinfarct dementias. Thromb Res. 1993;72:295–304.
31. Lavallee PC, Labreuche J, Faille D, et al. Circulating markers of endothelial dysfunction and platelet activation in patients with severe symptomatic cerebral small vessel disease. Cerebrovasc Dis. 2013;36(2):131–8.
32. Datta A, Chen CP, Sze SK. Discovery of prognostic biomarker candidates of lacunar infarction by quantitative proteomics of microparticles enriched plasma. PloS One. 2014;9(4):e94663.
33. Jy W, Horstman LL, Homolak D, et al. Electrophoretic properties of platelets from normal, thrombotic and ITP patients by doppler electrophoretic light scattering analysis. Platelets. 1995;6:354–8.
34. London F, Walsh PN. The role of electrostatic interaction in the assembly of the factor X activating complex on both activated platelets and negatively-charged phospholipid vesicles. Biochemistry. 1996;35(37):12146–54.
35. VanDijk D, Jansen EWL, Hijman R, et al. Cognitive outcomes after off-pump and on-pump coronary artery bypass graft surgery. JAMA. 2002;287(11):1405–12.
36. Humphries S, Harrison MJ. Cognitive change 5 years after coronary artery bypass surgery. Health Psychol. 2003;22(6):579–86.
37. Minagar A, Jy W, Jimenez JJ, et al. Elevated plasma endothelial microparticles in multiple sclerosis. Neurology. 2001;56(10):1319–24.
38. Jimenez JJ, Jy W, Mauro L, et al. Elevated endothelial microparticle-monocyte complexes induced by multiple sclerosis plasma and the inhibitory effects of interferon-beta 1b on release of endothelial microparticles, formation and transendothelial migration of monocyte-endothelial microparticle complexes. Multiple Sclerosis. 2005;11(3):310–5.

39. Jy W, Jimenez JJ, Minagar A, et al. Endothelial microparticles (EMP) enhance adhesion and transmigration of monocytes: EMP-monocyte conjugates as a marker of disease activity in multiple sclerosis (MS). Blood. 2002;100(11):460a Ab 1783.
40. Jy W, Minagar A, Jimenez JJ, et al. Endothelial microparticles (EMP) bind and activate monocytes: Elevated EMP-monocyte complexes in multiple sclerosis. Frontiers Biosci. 2004;9:3137–44.
41. Sheremata WA, Jy W, Delgado S, et al. Interferon-beta1a reduces plasma CD31+ endothelial microparticles (CD31+ EMP) in multiple sclerosis. J Neuroinflammation. 2006;3:23–4.
42. Cloutier N, Tan S, Boudreau LH, et al. The exposure of autoantigens by microparticles underlies the formation of potent inflammatory components: the microparticle-associated immune complexes. EMBO Mol Med. 2013;5(2):235–49.
43. Bidot CJ, Horstman LL, Jy W, et al. Clinical and neuroimaging correlates of antiphospholipid antibodies in multiple sclerosis. JCM Neurol. 2007;7:36.
44. Sheremata WA, Jy W, Horstman LL, et al. Evidence of platelet activation in multiple sclerosis. J Neuroinflammation. 2008;5:27.
45. Sevush S, Jy W, Horstman LL, et al. Platelet activation in Alzheimer's disease. Arch Neurol. 1998;55(4):530–6.
46. Pareek S, Roy S, Kumari B, et al. MiR-155 induction in microglial cells suppresses Japanese encephalitis virus replication and negatively modulates innate immune response. J Neuroinflammation. 2014;11:97.
47. Hill JM, Zhang Y, Clement C, et al. HSV-1 infection of human brain cells induces miRNA-146a and Alzheimer-type inflammatory signaling. Neuroreport. 2009;20(16):1500–6.
48. Wen B, Combes V, Bonhoure A, et al. Endotoxin-induced monocytic microparticles have contrasting effects on endothelial inflammatory response. PloS One. 2014;9(3):e91597.
49. Frohlich D, Kuo WP, Fruhbeis C. Multifaceted effects of oligodendroglial exosomes on neurons: impact on neuronal firing rate, signal transduction and gene regulation. Philos Trans R Soc Lond B Biol Sci. 2014;369:1652.
50. Pusic AD. Youth and environmental enrichment generate serum exosomes containing miR-219 that promotes CNS myelination. Glia. 2014;62(2):284–99.
51. Bekkering S, Quintin J, Joosten LA, et al. Oxidized low-density lipoprotein induces long-term proinflammatory cytokine production and foam cell formation via epigenetic reprogramming of monocytes. Atheroscler Thromb Vasc Biol. 2014;34(8):1731–8.
52. Giovannelli I, Martelli F, Repice A, et al. Detection of JCPyV micro RNA in blood and urine samples of multiple sclerosis patients undergoing natalizumab therapy. J Neurovirol. 2015;21:666–70. EPUB PREPRINT
52b. Omotezako T, Onuma TA, Noshida H. DNA interference: DNA-induces gene silencing in the appendicularian Oikop. Proc Biol Sci. 2015;282(1807):20150435.
53. Konadu KA, Chu J, Huang MB, et al. Association of cytokines with exosomes in the plasma of HIV-1-seropositive individuals. J Infect Dis. 2014;211:1712–6. E Pub Pre-Print
54. Mullen L, Hanschman EM, Herzenberg CHL, et al. Cysteine oxidation targets peroxiredoxins 1 and 2 for exosomal release through a novel mechanism of redox-dependent secretion. Mol Med. 2015;21:98–108. PrePub(Feb13):TBA
55. MacKenzie A, Wilson HL, Kiss-Toth E, et al. Rapid secretion of interleukin-1ß by microvesicle shedding. Immunity. 2001;8:825–35.
56. Lenglet S, Montecucco F, Mach F. Role of matrix metalloproteinases in animal models of acute ischemic stroke. Curr Vasc Pharmacol. 2013;13:161–6. EPub PrePrint
57. Sporer B. UKoedel, Paul R, et al.: Human immunodeficiency virus type-1 Nef protein induces blood-brain barrier disruption in the rat: role of matrix metalloproteinase-9. J Neuroimmunol. 2000;102:125–30.
58. Muraski ME, Roycik MD, Newcomer RG, et al. Matrix metalloproteinase-9/gelatinase B is a putative therapeutic target of chronic obstructive pulmonary disease and multiple sclerosis. Curr Pharm Biotech. 2009;9(1):24–46.
59. Shai O, Ould-Yahoui A, Ferhat L, et al. Differential vesicular distribution and trafficking of MMP-2, MMP-9, and their inhibitors in astrocytes. Glia. 2010;58(3):344–66.

60. Candela ME, Geraci E, Turturrici G, et al. Membrane vesicles containing matrix metallopro-
    teinase-9 and fibroblast growth factor 2 are released into the extracellular space from mouse
    mesoangioblast stem cells. J Cell Physiol. 2010;224(1):144–51.
61. McColl BW, Rothwell NJ, Allan SM. Systemic inflammation alters the kinetics of cerebro-
    vascular tight junction disruption after experimental stroke in mice. J Neurosci.
    2008;28(38):9451–62.
62. Justice PA, Sun W, Li Y, et al. Membrane vesiculation function and exocytosis of wild type
    and mutant matrix proteins of vesicular stomatitis virus. J Virol. 1995;69(5):3156–60.
63. Hakulinen J, Sankkila L, Sugiyama N, et al. Secretion of active membrane type 1 matrix
    metalloproteinase (MMP-14) into extracellular space in microvesicular exosomes. J Cell
    Biochem. 2008;105(5):1211–8.
64. Lozito TP, Tuan RS. Endothelial cell microparticles act as centers of matrix metalloprotein-
    ase-2 (MMP-2) activity and vascular matrix remodeling. J Cell Physiol.
    2012;227(2):534–49.
65. Hanania R, Sun HS, Xu K, et al. Classically activated macrophages use stable microtu-
    bules for matrix metalloproteinase-9 (MMP-9) secretion. J Biol Chem. 2012;287(11):
    8468–83.
66. Liubisavlievic S, Stojanovic I, Basic J, et al. The role of matrix metalloproteinase 3 and 9 in
    the pathogenesis of acute neuroinflammation. Implications for disease modifying therapy.
    J Mol Neurosci. 2015;56:840–7. EPub PrePrint(Feb22):TBA
67. van Noort JM, Bsibsi M, Nacken P, et al. The link between small heat shock proteins and the
    immune system. Int J Biochem Cell Biol. 2012;44(10):1670–9.
68. Cid C, Alvaerez-Cermeno JC, Salinas M, et al. Anti-heat shock protein 90beta antibodies
    decrease pre-oligodendrocyte population in perinatal and adult cell cultures: Implications for
    remyelination in multiple sclerosis. J Neurochem. 2005;95:349–60.
69. Gangalum RK, Atanasov IC, Zhou ZH, et al. AlphaB-crystallin is found in detergent-resistant
    membrane microdomains and is secreted via exosomes from human retinal pigment cells.
    J Biol Chem. 2011;286(5):3261–9.
70. Sevennson K, Christianson HC, Wittrup A, et al. Exosome uptake depends on ERK1/2-heat
    shock protein 27 signaling and lipid-raft mediated endocytosis negatively regulated by cave-
    olin-1. J Bio Chem. 2013;288(24):17713–24.
71. Pilzer D, Fishelson Z. Mortalin/GRP75 promotes release of membrane vesicles from immune
    attacked cells and protection from complement-mediated lysis. Int Immunol.
    2005;17(9):1239–48.
72. Wadhwa R, Ryu J, Ahn HM, et al. Functional significance of point mutations in stress chap-
    erone mortalin and their relevance to Parkinson disease. J Biol Chem. 2015;290:8447–56.
    ePub Pre-print
73. Robbins PD, Morelli AE. Regulation of immune responses by extracellular vesicles. Nat Rev
    Immunol. 2014;14(3):195–208.
74. Orsini F, DeBlasion D, Zangari R, et al. Versatility of the complement system in neuroinflam-
    mation, neurodegeneration, and brain homeostasis. Front Cell Neurosci. 2014;8:380.
75. Bochkov VN. Inflammatory profile of oxidized phospholipids. Thromb Haemost.
    2007;97(3):348–54.
76. Fiebich BL, Akter S, Akundi RS. The two-hit hypothesis for neuroinflammation: role of
    exogenous ATP in modulating inflammation in the brain. Front Cell Neurosci. 2014;8:260.
77. Fruhbeis C, Frolich D, Kramer-Albers EM. Emerging roles of exosomes in neuron-glia com-
    munication. Front Physiol. 2012;30(3):119.
78. Bodin S, Viala C, Ragab A, et al. A critical role of lipid rafts in the organization of a key
    Fc-gamma-RIIa-mediated signaling pathway in human platelets. Thromb Haemost.
    2003;89:318–30.
79. Simons K, Toomre D. Lipid rafts and signal transduction. Nat Rev Molec Cell Biol.
    2000;1:31–9.
80. Foster LJ. deHoog CL, Mann M: Unbiased quantitative proteomics of lipid rafts reveals high
    specificity for signaling factors. Proc Nat Acad Sci USA. 2003;100(10):5813–8.

81. Terasaki Y, Liu Y, Hawakawa K, et al. Mechanisms of neurovasculation dysfunction in acute ischemic brain. Curr Med Chem. 2014;21(18):2035–42.
82. Taylor DD, Gercel-Taylor C. Exosome platform for diagnosis and monitoring of traumatic brain injury. Philos Trans R Soc Lond B Biol Sci. 2014;369:1652.
83. de Rivero JP, Brand 3rd F, Adamczak S, et al. Exosome-mediated inflammasome signaling after central nervous system injury. J Neurochem. 2015;136:39–48. Pre-pub(Jan27):TBA
84. Sanborn MR, Thom SR, Bohman LE, et al. Temporal dynamics of microparticle elevation following subarachnoid hemorrhage. J Neurosurg. 2012;117(3):579–86.
85. Demirov DG, Freed EO. Retroviral budding. Virus Res. 2004;106(2):87–102.
86. Nabhan JF, Hu R, Oh RS, et al. Formation and release of arrestin domain-containing protein 1-mediated microvesicles (ARMMs) at plasma membrane by recruitment of TSG101 protein. Proc Natl Acad Sci USA. 2012;109(11):4146–51.
87. Lyman MG, Curanovic D, Enquist LW. Targeting of pseudorabies virus structural proteins to axons requires association of the viral Us9 protein with lipid rafts. PloS Pathog. 2008;4(5):e1000065.
88. Deng GM, Tsokos GC. Cholera toxin B accelerates disease progression in lupus-prone mice by promoting lipid raft aggregation. J Immunol. 2008;181(6):4019–26.
89. Cuadras MA, Greenberg HB. Rotavirus infectious particles use lipid rafts during replication for transport to the cell surface in vitro and in vivo. Virology. 2003;313(1):308–21.
90. Lafont F, Tran VNG, Hanada K, et al. Initial steps of Shigella infection depend on the cholesterol/sphingolipid raft-mediated CD44-IpaB interaction. EMBO J. 2002;21(17):4449–57.
91. Carter GC, Bernstone L, Sangani D, et al. HIV entry in macrophages is dependent on intact lipid rafts. Virology. 2009;386(1):192–202.
92. Laliberte JP, McGinnes LW, Peeples NE, et al. Integrity of membrane lipid rafts is necessary for the ordered assembly and release of infectious Newcastle disease virus particles. J Virol. 2006;80(21):10652–62.
93. Karim S, Mirza Z, Kamal MA, et al. The role of viruses in neurodegenerative and neurobehavioral diseases. CNS Neurol Disord Drug Targets. 2014;13(7):1213–23.
94. Hong S, Banks WA. Role of the immune system in HIV-associated neuroinflammation and neurocognitive implications. Brain Behav Immun. 2015;45C:1–12.
95. Corrales-Medina VF, Simkins J, Chirinos JA, et al. Increased levels of platelet microparticles in HIV-infected patients with good response to highly active antiretroviral therapy. J Acquir Immune Defic Syndr. 2010;54(2):217–8.
96. Alfahad T, Nath A. Retroviruses and amyotrophic lateral sclerosis. Antiviral Res. 2013;99(2):180–7.
97. Wordinger T, Gatson NN, Balai L, et al. Extracellular vesicles and their convergence with viral pathways. Adv Virol. 2012;2012:767694.
98. Saenz-Cuesia M, Osorio-Quereiata I, Otaequi D. Extracellular vesicles in multiple sclerosis: what are they telling us? [Reviewl]. Front Cell Neurosci. 2014;28(8):100.
99. Verderio C, Muzio M, Turola E, et al. Myeloid microvesicles are a marker and therapeutic target for neuroinflammation. Ann Neurol. 2012;72:610–24.
100. Peferoen L, Kipp M, VanDerValk P, et al. Oligodendrocyte-microglia cross-talk in the central nervous system [review]. Immunology. 2014;141(3):302–13.
101. Gatson NN, Williams JL, Powell ND, et al. Induction of pregnancy during established EAE halts progression of CNS autoimmune injury via pregnancy-specific serum factors. J Neuroimmunol. 2011;230(1–2):105–13.
102. Williams JL, Gatson NN, Smith KM, et al. Serum exosomes in pregnancy-associated immune modulation and neuroprotection during CNS autoimmunity. Clin Immunol. 2013;149(2):236–43.
103. Kumar R, Kretzschmar B, Herold S, et al. Beneficial effect of chronic Staphylococcus aureus infection in a model of multiple sclerosis is mediated through secretion of extracellular adherence protein. J Neuroinflammation. 2015;12:22. PrePub PrePrint(Feb3):TBA
104. Crookston KP, Sibbitt WL, Chang WL, et al. Circulating microparticles in neuropsychiatric systemic lupus erythematosus. Int Rheum Dis. 2013;16(1):72–80.

105. Grad LI, Fernando SM, Cashman NR. From molecule to molecule and cell to cell: Prion-like mechanisms in amyotrophic lateral sclerosis. Neurobiol Dis. 2015;77:257–65. Epub PrePrint
106. Singh J, Udgaonkar JB. Molecular mechanism of the misfolding and oligomerization of the prior protein: Current understanding and its implications. Biochemistry. 2015;54(29):4431–42.
107. Jaunmuktane Z, Meade S, Ellis M, et al. Evidence for human transmission of amyloid-beta pathology and cerebral amyloid angiopathy. Nature. 2015;525(7568):247–50.
108. Lupton CJ, Steer DL, Wintrode PL, et al. Enhanced molecular mobility of ordinarily structured regions drives polyglutamine disease. J Biol Chem. 2015;290(40):24190–200.
109. Scherzinger E, Lurz R, Turmaine M, et al. Huntingtin-encoded polyglutamine expansions form amyloid-like protein aggregates in vitro and in vivo. Cell. 1997;90(3):549–58.
110. Taylor DR, Hooper NM. Role of lipid rafts in the processing of the pathogenic prion and Alzheimer's amyloid-beta proteins. Semin Cell Dev Biol. 2007;18(5):638–48.
111. Taylor DR, Hooper NM. The prion proteins and lipid rafts. Mol Membr Biol. 2006;23(1):89–99.
112. Erlich P, Dumestre-Perard C, Ling WL, et al. Complement protein C1q forms a complex with cytotoxic prion protein oligomers. J Biol Chem. 2010;285(25):19267–76.
113. Simak J, Holada K, D'Agnillo F, et al. Cellular prion protein is expressed on endothelial cells and is released during apoptosis on membrane microparticles found in human plasma. Transfusion. 2002;42:334–42.
114. Chen M, Inestrosa NC, Ross GS, et al. Platelets are the principal source of amyloid beta peptide in human blood. Biochem Biophyis Res Commun. 1995;213(1):96–103.
115. Pienimaeki-Roemer A, Kuhlmann K, Bottcher A, et al. Lipidomic and proteomic characterization of platelet extracellular vesicle subfractions from senescent platelets. Transfusion. 2015;55(3):507–21.
116. Bellingham SA, Guo BB, Coleman BM, et al. Exosomes: vehicles for the transport of toxic proteins associated with neurodegenerative disease? Front Physiol. 2012;3:124. 3 EPUB PREPRINT
117. Munch C, O'Brien J, Bertolotti A. Prion-like propagation of mutant superoxide dismutase-1 misfolding in neuronal cells. Proc Natl Acad Sci USA. 2011;108(9):3548-ILLEG.
118. Liu KX, Edwards B, Lee S, et al. Neuron-specific antioxidant OXR1 extends survival of a mouse model of amyotrophic lateral sclerosis. Brain. 2015;138:1167–81. PrePub PrePrint
119. Lee JY, Quaguchi Y, Li M, et al. Uncoupling of protein aggregation and neurodegeneration in a mouse amyotrophic lateral sclerosis model. Neurodegen Dis. 2015;15:339–49. TBA(Pre-Print)
120. Gallegos S, Pacheco C, Peters C, et al. Features of alpha-synuclein that could esxplain progression and irreversibility of Parkinson's disease. Front Neurosci. 2015;9:59.
121. Dettmer U, Selkoe D, Bartels T. New insights into cellular alpha-synuclein homeostasis in health and disease. Curr Opin Neurobiol. 2015;15(36):15–22.
122. Shi M, Liu C, Cook TJ, et al. Plasma exosomal alpha-synuclein is likely CNS-derived and increased in Parkinson's disease. Acta Neuropathol. 2014;128(5):639–50.
123. Grey M, Dunning CJ, Gaspar R, et al. Acceleration of alpha-synuclein aggregation by exosomes. J Biol Checm. 2015;290(5):2969–82.
124. Gui YX, Liu H, Zhang LS, et al. Altered microRNA in cerebrospinal fluid exosomes in Parkinson disease and Alzheimer disease. Oncotarget. 2015;6:37043–53. TBA(Pre-Pub):tba
125. Cooper JM, Wiklander PB, Nordin JZ, et al. Systemic exosomal siRNA delivery reduced alpha-synuclein aggregates in brains of transgenic mice. Mov Disord. 2014;29(12):1476–85.
126. Treps L, Edmond S, Harford-Wright E, et al. Extra-cellular vesicle-transported Semaphorin3A promotes vascular permeability in glioblastoma. Oncogene. 2015;35:2615–23. PrePrint(in press):tba
127. Raymond AD, Diaz P, Chevelon S, et al. Microglia-derived HIV Nef+ exosome impairment of the blood-brain barrier is treatable by nanomedicine-based delivery of Nef peptides. J Neurovirol. 2015;22:129–39. PrePub(TBA):tba

128. Hay JR, Johnson VE, Young AM, et al. Blood-brain barrier disruption is an early event that may persist for many years after traumatic brain injury in humans. J Neuropathol Exp Neurol. 2015;74(12):1147–57.
129. Tian Y, Salsbery B, Wang M, et al. Brain-derived microparticles induce systemic coagulation in a murine model of traumatic brain injury [editorial pg 2015-6]. Blood. 2014;125(13):2151–9.
130. Lockman PR, Mumper JMKJ, Allen DD. Nanoparticles surface charges alter blood-brain barrier integrity and permeability. J Drug Targeting. 2004;12(9–10):635–41.
131. Joachim E, Il-Doo K, Yinchuan J, et al. Gelatin nanoparticles enhance the neuroprotective effects of intranasally administered osteopontin in rat ischemic stroke model. Drug Delivery and Translational Res. 2014;4(5):395–9.
132. Cutler JI, Auyeung EA, Mirkin CA. Spherical nucleic acids [gold core]. J Am Chem Soc. 2012;134:1376–91.
133. Haney MJ, Klyachko NL, Zhao Y, et al. Exosomes as drug delivery vehicles for Parkinson's disease therapy. J Control Release. 2015;207:18–30. Epub(InPrewss):tba
134. Sampey GC, Meyering SS, Asad-Zadeh M, et al. Exosomes and their role in CNS viral infections. J Neurovirol. 2014;20(3):199–208.
135. Alvarez-Erviti L, Seow Y, HaiFang Y, et al. Delivery of siRNA to the mouse brain by systemic injection of targeted exosomes [see online supplement for details]. Nat Biotech. 2011;29(4):341–5.
136. Chataway J, Schuerer N, Alsanousi A, et al. Effect of high-dose simvastatin on brain atrophy and disability in secondary progressive multiple sclerosis (MS-STAT): a randomised, placebo-controlled, phase 2 trial [See issue Sept. 13 for letters]. Lancet. 2014;383(9936):2213–21.
137. Malkki H. Could simvastatin slow down secondary progressive MS? [Comment on Chataway et al., in Lancet, June 28, 2014]. Nat Rev Neurol. 2014;10:241.
138. Ulivieri C, Baldari CT. Statins: from cholesterol-lowering drugs to novel immunomodulators for the treatment of Th17-mediated autoimmune diseases. Pharmacol Res. 2014;88:41–52.
139. Krisanova N, Sivko R, Kasatkina L, et al. Neuroprotection by lowering cholesterol: a decrease in the membrane cholesterol content reduces transporter-mediated glutamate release from brain nerve terminals. Biochim Biophys Acta. 2012;1822(10):1553–61.
140. Lei O, Peng WN, You H, et al. Statins in nervous system-associated diseases: angels or devils? Pharmazie. 2014;69(6):448–54.
141. Tramontano AF, O'Leary J, Black AD, et al. Statin decreases endothelial microparticle release from human coronary artery endothelial cells: implication for the Rho-kinase pathway. Biochem Biophys Res Com. 2004;320:34–8.
142. Suades R, Padro T, Alonso R, et al. Lipid-lowering therapy with statins reduces microparticle shedding from endothelium, platelets, and inflammatory cells. Thromb Haemost. 2013;119(2):366–77.
143. Relja B, Lehnert M, Seyboth K, et al. Simvastatin reduces mortality and hepatic injury after hemorrhage/resuscitation in rats. Shock. 2009;34:46–54. Epub preprint
144. Kalani A, Tyagi A, Tyagi N. Exosomes: mediators of neurodegeneration, neuroprotection and therapeutics. Mol Neurobiol. 2014;49(1):590–600.
145. Robinzon S, Dafa-Berger A, Dyer MD, et al. Impaired cholesterol biosynthesis in a neuronal cell line persistently infected with measles virus. J Virol. 2009;83(11):5495–504.
146. Xin H, Li Y, Cui Y, et al. Systemic administration of exosomes released from mesenchymal stromal stem cells promotes functional recovery and neurovascular plasticity after stroke in rats. J Cereb Blood Flow Metab. 2013;33(11):1711-ILLEG.
147. Xin H, Li Y, Liu Z, et al. MiR-133 promotes neural plasticity and functional recovery after treatment of stroke with multipotent mesenchymal stromal stem cells in rats via transfer of exosome-enriched extracellular particles. Stem Cells. 2013;31(12):2737–46.
148. Cantaluppi V, Medica D, Mannari C, et al. Endothelial progenitor cell-derived extracellular vesicles protect from complement-mediated mesangial injury in experimental anti-Thy1.1 glomerulonephritis. Nephrol Dial Transplant. 2015;30(3):410–22.
149. Zhang Y, Chopp M, Meng Y, et al. Effect of exosomes derived from multipluripotent mesenchymal stromal cells on functional recovery and neurovascular plasticity in rats after traumatic brain injury. J Neurosurg. 2015;122:856–67. EpubPrePrint(TBA):TBA

150. Schock SC, Edrissi H, Burger D, et al. Microparticles generated during chronic cerebral ischemia deliver proapoptotic signals to cultured endothelial cells. Biochem Biophyis Res Commun. 2014;450:912–7. PrePub PrePrint(TBA)
151. Hayon Y, Shai E, Varon D, et al. The role of platelets and their microparticles in rehabilitation of ischemic brain tissue. CNS Neurol Disord Drug Targets. 2012;11(7):921–5.
152. Camussi G, Deregibus MC, Bruno S, et al. Exosome/microvesicle-mediated epigenetic reprogramming of cells. Am J Cancer Res. 2011;1(1):98–110.
153. Sims PJ, Wiedmer T. Repolarization of the membrane potential of blood platelets after complement damage: Evidence for a Ca2+−dependent exocytotic elimination of C5b-9 pores. Blood. 1986;68(2):556–61.
154. Horstman LL, Jy W, Schultz DR, et al. Complement mediated fragmentation and lysis of opsonized platelets: gender differences in sensitivity. J Lab Clin Med. 1994;123:515–25.
155. Pilzer D, Gasser O, Moskcovitch O, et al. Emission of membrane vesicles: roles in complement resistance, immunity and cancer. Sprig Semin Immunopath. 2005;27(3):375–87.
156. Fluiter K, Opperhuizen AL, Morgan BP, et al. Inhibition of the membrane attack complex of the complement system reduces secondary neuronaxonal loss and promotes neurologica recovery after traumatic brain injury in mice. J Immunol. 2014;192(5):2339–48.
157. Sahu A, Morikis D, Labris JD. Compstatin, a peptide inhibitor of complement, exhibits species-specific binding to complement component C3. Mol Immunol. 2008;39(10):557–66.
158. Risitano A, Ricklin D, Huang Y, et al. Peptide inhibitors of C3a activation as a novel strategy of complement inhibition for the treatment of paroxysmal nocturnal hemoglobinuria [with Commentary, pg 1975]. Blood. 2014;123(13):2094–101.
159. Davis AE, Mejia P, Lu F. Biological activities of C1 inhibitor. Mol Immunol. 2008;45(16):4057–63.
160. Hill A, Hillman P, Richards SJ, et al. The complement inhibitor eculizumab in paroxysmal nocturnal hemoglobinuria. New Engl J Med. 2006;355:1233–43.
161. Samadder NJ, Casaubon L, Silver F, et al. Neurological complications of paroxysmal nocturnal hemoglobinuria. Can J Neurol Sci. 2007;34(3):368–71.
162. Elward K, Griffiths M, Mizumo M, et al. CD46 plays a key role in tailoring innate immune recognition of apoptotic and necrotic cells. J Biol Chem. 2005;280(43):36342–54.

Acute Disseminated Encephalomyelitis: Clinical Features, Pathophysiology, and Clinical Management

7

Omar Hussein and Alireza Minagar

Introduction

ADEM is a presumably immune-mediated multifocal or diffuse inflammatory demyelinating disease of the brain and the spinal cord that, often but not always, occurs para-infection or postvaccination. It affects children more commonly than adults but that might be attributed to the more clearly defined diagnostic criteria available for children more than adults who might also have pre-existing white matter lesion(s) secondary to a different pathology leading to underscoring adult ADEM [1]. From certain viewpoints, ADEM resembles MS and other demyelinating diseases; however, significant differences do exist. ADEM occurs worldwide and usually males and females are affected equally, unlike relapsing-remitting MS that is more common among females. However few studies suggested slight male predominance [2–4]. A cornerstone landmark for the diagnosis of ADEM, especially in children, is encephalopathy in the absence of fever along with other manifestation [1]. This is attributed to the early involvement of the cortical gray matter in the course of the disease unlike most other demyelinating conditions in which cortical involvement usually occurs latter as the disease progresses. Gray matter involvement also causes dystonia and other movement disorders [3]. ADEM rarely exists in multiphasic and recurrent forms, but if occurred, encephalopathy remains the cornerstone. To date, there is no unique biomarker that exists to distinguish ADEM from other demyelinating or non-demyelinating conditions making it mostly a diagnosis of exclusion [3]. Pathological differences also do exist between the different autoimmune demyelinating conditions according to biopsy and postmortem tissue analysis [5]. Neuroimaging is, somehow, helpful as ADEM usually presents as multifocal larger lesions or less commonly as a single large confluent white and deep

O. Hussein, MD • A. Minagar, MD (✉)
Department of Neurology, LSU Health Sciences Center,
1501 Kings Highway, Shreveport, LA 71130, USA
e-mail: aminag@lsuhsc.edu

© Springer International Publishing AG 2017
A. Minagar, J.S. Alexander (eds.), *Inflammatory Disorders of the Nervous System*, Current Clinical Neurology, DOI 10.1007/978-3-319-51220-4_7

gray matter bilateral symmetrical lesion involving the basal ganglia and the thalami that, sometimes but not always, enhance. Despite of this, tumefactive MS and different brain tumors especially gliomas can mimic this presentation making the diagnosis and early initiation of treatment a dilemma. Recently, advances in neuroimaging including MR perfusion, spectroscopy, and susceptibility images have been used to try to differentiate between these conditions. Large randomized studies still lack regarding these attempts. The cornerstone in the treatment of ADEM is early initiation of pulse steroid therapy followed by oral taper. It is crucial to differentiate ADEM from other autoimmune demyelinating conditions as usually ADEM does not require long-term immune modulation or immune suppression, but in some cases, this remains difficult and thus requires close follow-ups for any relapses or new lesions to appear. In some mimicking conditions like lymphoma, early pulse steroid therapy without reaching a definite diagnosis might create a real challenge as this might mask the diagnosis of lymphoma even if brain biopsy is performed later on. Thus, in such challenging suspicious cases, brain biopsy is recommended.

Clinical Features

ADEM is usually a monophasic disease with acute onset. However, hyperacute and subacute cases as well as multiphasic and recurrent cases have been described [1–4]. Patients with ADEM are mostly children with mean age between 5 and 8 years old [2, 3]. The clinical manifestations depend on the location, severity, and extent of the lesions. Clinical feature usually commences 1–4 weeks following the infection. Encephalopathy, defined as altered sensorium ranging from drowsiness to coma or just behavioral changes in the absence of fever, systemic illness, or seizure, is the key manifestation required for the diagnosis of ADEM [1]. Other neurologic presentations including headache, fever, and seizures (35%) are among the common clinical manifestations. Uncommonly and depending on the location of the demyelinating lesions, optic neuritis, myelitis, ataxia, weakness and sensory abnormalities, abnormal involuntary movements, ataxia, falls, aphasia (uncommonly), cranial nerve palsies (apart from optic nerves), and general presentations of meningitis and encephalitis can occur. Respiratory compromise can occur if brain stem is affected. A number of patients with ADEM also develop neuropsychiatric syndrome. Signs of long tract involvement such as hyperactive reflexes as well as the presence of clonus and extensor plantar responses are also commonly present. Nevertheless, peripheral nervous system demyelination is not unusual in pediatric and adult patients [3]. The neurological manifestations of ADEM tend to fluctuate and evolve during the first 3 months of onset; thus, recurrence should not be considered before 3 months. According to the revised International Pediatric Multiple Sclerosis Study Group (IPMSSG) criteria in 2012, this is irrespective of corticosteroid use (Table 7.1) [1]. A key exclusionary criterion is the lack of clinical or imaging evidence of prior CNS lesions [6].

Table 7.1 Comparison of 2007 and 2012 definitions for pediatric acute demyelinating disorders of the central nervous system (CNS)

Disorder	2007	2012
CIS	A first monofocal or multifocal CNS demyelinating event; encephalopathy absent	A first monofocal or multifocal CNS demyelinating event; encephalopathy is absent, *unless due to fever*
Monophasic ADEM	A first polysymptomatic clinical event, with presumed inflammatory cause that affects multifocal areas of the CNS Encephalopathy is present MRI typically shows large, ≥1–2 cm white matter lesion; gray matter involvement (thalamus or basal ganglia) is frequent New or fluctuating symptoms, signs, or MRI findings within 3 months of the incident ADEM are part of the acute event	A first polyfocal clinical CNS event with presumed inflammatory cause Encephalopathy that *cannot be explained by fever* is present MRI typically shows *diffuse, poorly demarcated, large, 1–2 cm* lesions involving predominantly the cerebral white matter; *TI hypointense white matter lesions are rare*; deep gray matter (e.g., thalamus or basal ganglia) can be present No new symptoms, signs, or MRI findings after 3 months of the incident ADEM
Recurrent ADEM	New event of ADEM with a recurrence of the initial symptoms and signs, three or more months after the first ADEM event	*Now subsumed under multiphasic ADEM*
Multiphasic ADEM	New event of ADEM, but involves new anatomic areas of the CNS and must occur at least 3 months after the onset of the initial ADEM event and at least 1 month after completing steroid therapy	New event of ADEM 3 months or more after the initial event that can be associated with *new or reemergence of prior clinical and MRI findings. Timing in relation to steroids is no longer pertinent*
MS	Any of the following: Multiple clinical episodes of CNS demyelination separated in time and space Single clinical event which is associated with 2001 McDonald Brain MRI criteria[a] for DIS and subsequent changes on MRI consistent with criteria 2001 McDonald criteria for DIT [4] An episode consistent with the clinical features of ADEM cannot be considered as the first event of MS	Any of the following: Two or more nonencephalopathic CNS clinical events separated by more than 30 days, involving more than one area of CNS Single clinical event and MRI features rely on 2010 Revised McDonald criteria[b] for DIS and DIT [4] (but criteria relative for DIT for a single attack and single MRI only apply to children ≥12 years and only apply to cases without an ADEM onset) ADEM followed 3 months later by a nonencephalopathic clinical event with new lesions on brain MRI consistent with MS

(continued)

Table 7.1 (continued)

Disorder	2007	2012

NMO	All are required:
	  Optic neuritis
	  Acute myelitis
	  At least one of two supportive criteria
	  Contiguous spinal cord MRI lesion ≥3 vertebral segments
	  Anti-aquaporin-4 IgG seropositive status
		All are required:
		  Optic neuritis
		  Acute myelitis
		  At least two of three supportive criteria
		  Contiguous spinal cord MRI lesion ≥3 vertebral segments
		  Brain MRI not meeting diagnostic criteria for MS
		  Anti-aquaporin-4 IgG seropositive status

ADEM acute disseminated encephalomyelitis, *CIS* clinically isolated syndrome, *CNS* central nervous system, *DIS* dissemination in space, *DIT* dissemination in time, *MRI* magnetic resonance imaging, *MS* multiple sclerosis, *NMO* neuromyelitis optica

[a]The 2001 McDonald MRI criteria for DIS require three of the following four MRI features: ≥9 T2 lesions or 1 gadolinium-enhancing lesions, ≥3 periventricular lesions, ≥1 infratentorial lesion(s), and ≥1 juxtacortical lesion(s). The DIT criteria require subsequent white matter lesions whose timing depends on the temporal relation of the initial MRI with the onset of the clinical symptoms

[b]The 2010 Revised McDonald MRI criteria for DIS require the presence of at least two of the following four criteria: ≥1 lesion in each of the four locations; periventricular, juxtacortical, infratentorial, and spinal cord. The 2010 Revised McDonald MRI criteria for DIT can be satisfied either by the emergence of newT2 lesions (with or without enhancement) on serial scan(s) or can be met on a single baseline scan if there exists simultaneous presence of a clinically silent gadolinium-enhancing lesion and a nonenhancing lesion

While ADEM is generally considered a monophasic disease, patients with ADEM and multiphasic course or recurrent attacks exist as mentioned above [1]. According to the revised IPMSSG criteria, recurrent ADEM is now subsumed under multiphasic ADEM. Thus, multiphasic ADEM is now defined as new event of ADEM 3 months or more after the initial event that can be associated with new or reemergence of prior clinical and MRI findings [1].

After publishing the initial IPMSSG in 2007, few prospective studies are conducted to evaluate the predictive value of such criteria in predicting relapse of the first episode of ADEM to MS. For this to occur, the second episode was defined as nonencephalopathic event with new MRI finding consistent with dissemination in space occurring at least 3 months after the first episode. A second relapse consistent with MS rather than multiphasic ADEM was detected in 2–18%. Of all relapses, 80% occurred with 2 years of the first event [2, 4].

Acute hemorrhagic leukoencephalitis (AHLE) is rare variant of ADEM (< 2%) commonly presenting with fever, neck stiffness, seizures, and/or focal neurological deficits following upper respiratory infection with more rapid progression within days leading to coma and death in some cases due to increased cerebral edema and herniation if untreated urgently. It is considered the most aggressive of all demyelinating diseases. Areas of hemorrhage and necrosis along a massive white matter involvement are evident on the MRI. Many cases are diagnosed on postmortem autopsy [7].

Immunopathogenesis and Neuropathology

The exact pathophysiology of ADEM remains only partially understood, and the issue becomes more complicated when neurologists review the potential relationship between ADEM and MS as why most patients with ADEM will not progress to clinically definite MS. Most experts concur that ADEM is an immune-mediated disease and the similarities between ADEM and experimental allergic encephalomyelitis also raise interesting questions about ADEM being an autoimmune condition (RRERRRRR) [8–11].

Presently, the prevailing hypotheses about the pathophysiology of ADEM include "molecular mimicry theory versus inflammatory theory," and both share the fundamental tenet that the patient's immune system has been exposed to an antigenic challenge (viral or bacterial antigens) and this in turn precipitates a massive immune response which clinically manifests as ADEM. Based on the molecular mimicry hypothesis, certain CNS molecules such as myelin basic protein, proteolipid protein, and myelin oligodendrocyte protein share certain structural features with antigenic infrastructure and determinants of invading microorganism, and as a result the provoked immune response, particularly antiviral or antibacterial antibodies, cross-reacts with some or all of the abovementioned CNS natural molecules, and this translates into a formidable autoimmune response and initiation of ADEM. Of note, viruses implicated in ADEM include influenza virus, enterovirus, measles, mumps, rubella, VZV, EBV, CMV, HSV, hepatitis A, and coxsackievirus. Bacteria linked to pathophysiology of ADEM are *Mycoplasma pneumoniae*, *Borrelia burgdorferi*, *Leptospira*, and group A beta-hemolytic streptococcus [12]. In addition, potent anti-myelin basic protein antibodies have been detected in patients with post-vaccinial ADEM after being vaccinated with Semple rabies vaccine [13, 14].

According to the inflammatory hypothesis of ADEM, the patient's CNS is injured secondary to the offensive viral infection. As a result of this and due to disruption of the blood-brain barrier, CNS antigens such as myelin-based epitopes are released into the peripheral circulation [9]. The released antigens are exposed to the T lymphocytes which in turn cause a new cascade of inflammation targeted against the patient's CNS. This infection-based hypothesis originates from another animal model of inflammatory demyelination, Theiler murine encephalomyelitis virus (TMEV), which generates a two-stage disease: the initial CNS viral infection followed by a second autoimmune response with more destruction to the patient's CNS. A number of chemokines and cytokines such as IL-6 and TNF-α have been proposed in pathophysiology of ADEM; however, Based on their analysis Franciotta et al. [15] analyzed the cytokine and chemokine profile in the CSF of patients with ADEM versus MS and noticed that compared to healthy controls, CSF of patients with ADEM contained significantly higher levels of chemokines with attractant/activating properties toward neutrophils (CXCL1 and CXCL7), monocytes/T lymphocytes (CCL3 and CCL5), Th1 lymphocytes (CXCL10), and Th2 lymphocytes (CCL1, CCL22, CCL17). Based on their analysis, they noticed that within the CSF, mean levels of CXCL7, CCL1, CCL22, and CCL17 were more elevated in patients with ADEM than those with MS. The CSF levels of CCL11 were lower in MS patients than those with ADEM. The authors concluded that increased expression of chemokines active on neutrophils and Th2 lymphocytes can separate ADEM from MS.

The most salient and the neuropathological hallmark of ADEM (which is also recognized as perivenous encephalomyelitis) is the presence of peri-venular (perivenous) inflammation with penetration and presence of macrophages and areas of demyelination which affect various and large areas of cerebral hemispheres, brain stem, cerebellum, subcortical gray matter, and spinal cord in a sleeve like fashion. While perivenous inflammatory demyelination also occurs in the context of MS, demyelination in MS consists more obviously of confluent layers of macrophages mixed with reactive astrocytes. In ADEM, it is presumed that such immune cell-mediated inflammatory demyelination stems from or is triggered by infection or immunization. Other less common abnormalities consist of the presence of lymphocytes and neutrophils outside the Virchow-Robin space, infiltration of the vascular wall by the inflammatory cells, perivascular edema, and swelling of the endothelium. Chronologically, ADEM lesions appear to be of similar oldness and more prominently affect the small vessels of the white matter; however, they also affect the deeper layers of the cerebral cortex, thalami, hypothalamus, and basal ganglia as well as the vessels in walls of the lateral and third ventricle. Interestingly, the neuropathology of ADEM shares certain similarities with monophasic EAE.

Regarding AHLE, influenza, HSV, mycoplasma pneumonia, and EBV have been reported to precede the condition. It is hypothesized that AHLE results from direct viral neuro-invasion, neurotoxin production, and immune-mediated demyelination. Pathologically it consists of deep white matter fine vacuolation, perivascular demyelination associated with areas of ring and ball hemorrhages, and fibrinoid vascular necrosis along with neutrophil and monocyte infiltrates [16]. Although nonspecific, when incorporated with in the clinical context, AHLE diagnosis can be made.

Diagnosis

Diagnostic criteria for ADEM both from 2007 to 2012 are cited in Table 7.1 [1]. In patients with ADEM, certain nonspecific markers such as platelet counts and sedimentation rate can be increased as in most other autoimmune diseases. Examination of CSF may be unremarkable; however, it usually demonstrates elevated protein concentration (usually between 0.5 and 1.0 g/dL) and lymphocytic pleocytosis (between 50 and 200 cells/mm^3). The oligoclonal bands are less commonly observed than in MS and are more frequently found in adults than children with ADEM. In a minority of patients with ADEM, increases in CSF immunoglobulins can be detected. Serum anti-aquaporin-4 IgG antibody is absent, while serum anti-MOG (myelin oligodendrocyte glycoprotein) antibodies may be present transiently. Certain nonspecific markers of inflammation such as elevated IgG index and increased myelin basic protein level are occasionally detected. In some patients with ADEM, virologic investigation of the CSF and/or serum may reveal the presence of certain viral protein and other viral biomarkers, which have been associated with development of ADEM.

Neuroimaging is one of the most significant diagnostic tests for ADEM. CT scan of the brain may be unremarkable or at best demonstrates areas of nonspecific low attenuation involving subcortical white matter. These affected areas may or may not enhance following infusion of the CT contrast. MRI of the brain and spinal cord with and without contrast is a more informative diagnostic tool and plays a major role in establishing the diagnosis of ADEM and excluding some of its differential diagnoses. Indeed, observing giant and disseminated demyelinating lesions on brain and spinal MR imaging strongly supports a diagnosis of ADEM; however, brain tumors and tumefactive MS can also present similarly.

According to the IPMSSG, typically, MRI shows diffuse or multifocal, poorly demarcated, large, (>1–2 cm) hyperintense lesion(s) on T2-weighted as well as fluid-attenuated inversion recovery (FLAIR) sequences involving predominantly the cerebral white matter as well as deep gray matter lesions, and infratentorial structures (mainly thalami and basal ganglia) can be detected (Figs. 7.1, 7.2, 7.3, and 7.4) [12]. White matter lesions which manifest as hypointense signals on T1-weighted images

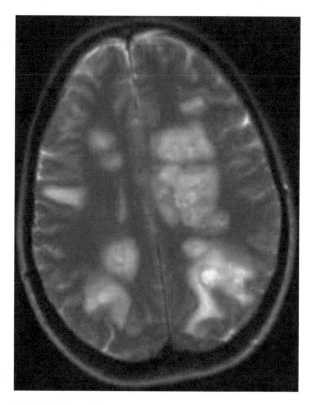

Fig. 7.1 T2-weighted axial view of brain of a patient with ADEM which demonstrates multiple large hyperintense lesions involving mainly the white matter (From Dale [8] Copyright permission obtained)

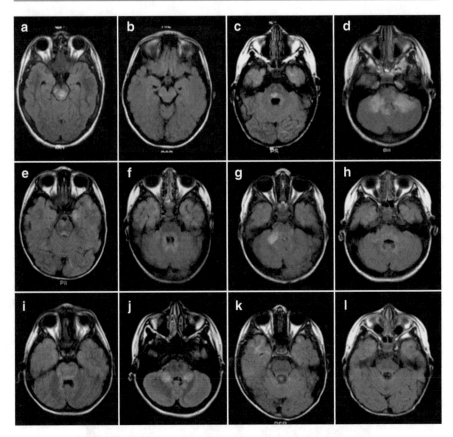

Fig. 7.2 (a–l) Axial fluid-attenuated inversion recovery (FLAIR) images through the infratentorial regions of 12 children with ADEM (From Marin and Callen [12] Elsevier, Inc. Copyright permission obtained)

are uncommon but not unheard of. A single diffuse bilateral symmetric large lesion involving the deep gray matter is occasionally present. Infrequently, these can exert mass effect. In such cases, neurosurgical biopsy should be considered to exclude glioma and other primary or metastatic brain tumors, infective processes, and other inflammatory diseases. The presence of hypointense lesions on T1-weighted images, particularly if persistant, with the presence of two or more periventricular lesions should suggest a diagnosis of MS rather than ADEM [1].

Based on our observations of our patients with ADEM, these MRI abnormal signals are often larger than MS lesions, more symmetric, lack well-defined margins, and can involve the subcortical gray matter – the basal ganglia and thalami (Fig. 7.5). Some of the ADEM lesions reveal enhancement on post-contrast T1-weighted sequence (14–30%), and usually their pattern of enhancement is more homogeneous than MS lesions. Following treatment, repeat MRI of the brain does not show development of new lesions and only reveals significant resolution of old lesions. Interestingly, MRI of the brain also assists neurologists to search for certain features

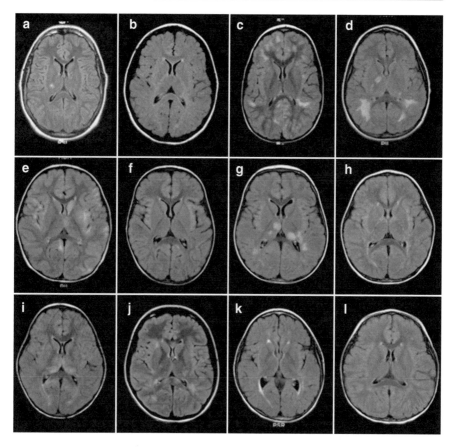

Fig. 7.3 (a–l) Axial FLAIR images at the level of the basal ganglia and thalamus of 12 children with ADEM (From Marin and Callen [12] Elsevier, Inc. Copyright permission obtained)

such as location and symmetry of distribution of the demyelinating lesions with the relative absence of periventricular lesions and presence of deep gray matter lesions, which are not typically seen in MRI of MS patients.

Proton MR spectroscopy (H-MRS) is an advanced neuroimaging technique which has been utilized to study patients with ADEM. In acute stage of ADEM, H-MRS reveals increase in lipid with decrease in myoinositol/creatinine ratio with unchanged N-acetylaspartate (NAA) or choline concentrations [17, 18]. With further underlying disease progression, decline in NAA and increase of choline concentrations in regions, where hyperintense T2-weighted abnormal signals are present, are detected [17, 19].

The differential diagnoses of ADEM consist of long list of acute diseases or disorders which cause leukoencephalopathy and either clinically or neuroradiologically imitate ADEM. The differential diagnoses of AHLE include ADEM, tumefactive MS, acute necrotizing encephalitis of childhood, Leigh syndrome, vanishing white matter disease, or toxic meningoencephalitis.

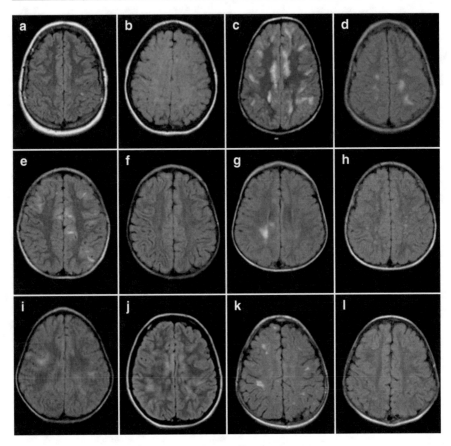

Fig. 7.4 (**a–l**) Axial FLAIR images through the cerebral convexities of 12 children with ADEM (From Marin and Callen [12] Elsevier, Inc. Copyright permission obtained)

Clinical Management

ADEM is relatively uncommon and in many occasions spontaneously improves and is self-limiting. Therefore, no double-blinded placebo-controlled clinical trial to establish the best treatment or superiority of one treatment over the other exists. Most of existing literature on treatment of ADEM heavily stems from personal observations and experience, small care series, care reports, and certain retrospective studies. The existing therapies for ADEM, heavily, rely on immunosuppression, and once a diagnosis of ADEM is made, a neurologist should treat the patient with intravenous pulse corticosteroid therapy (usually methylprednisolone 10–30 mg/kg/day for children less than 30 kg and 1000 mg iv daily for 5 days for those heavier than 30 kg). Some neurologists use intravenous dexamethasone (1 mg/kg/day) instead of methylprednisolone. Most neurologists follow this pulse steroid therapy with a tapering oral prednisone regimen.

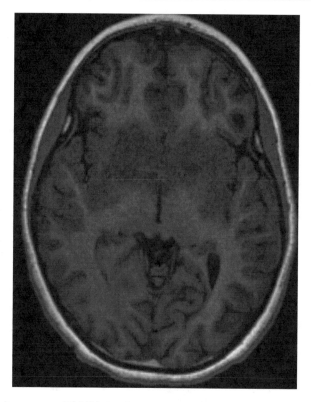

Fig. 7.5 Axial pre-contrast T1 MRI showing symmetrical hypodense lesion across the basal ganglia, the corpus callosum, and the internal capsule bilaterally

While most patients improve with treatment patients who fail to improve, should receive a course of plasma exchange. In a milestone clinical study, Weinshenker et al. [20] examined the efficacy of plasma exchange in treatment of patients with severe demyelinating diseases of CNS unresponsive to corticosteroids in the course of a randomized controlled crossover trial of genuine versus sham plasma exchange. The investigators performed this trial on a cohort of 22 patients who qualified. They detected that 42% of the patients have experienced moderate or significant progress of their neurologic status compared to the 6% of the patients in the sham therapy and the result of this study was statistically significant. This study included one patient with ADEM, and it practically paved the path for more common use of this procedure for treatment of severe demyelinating diseases of CNS. Various experts may do five or seven rounds of plasma exchange. Intravenous immunoglobulin (IVIG) has also been used for treatment of these patients. Plasma exchange has been superior over IVIG in some case reports and small studies. Usually failure of one measure leads to the initiation of the other.

Regarding AHLE, this is considered a medical emergency requiring aggressive immune suppression with combined pulse steroid therapy and plasma exchange or IVIG together with close continuous monitoring and medical and/or surgical treatment of increased intracranial pressure due to edema. AHLE is a grave disease but cases that are treated early and aggressively may recover with minimal deficits.

MS Versus ADEM

It is a great dilemma to many neurologists whether a first demyelinating attack is in fact a clinically isolated syndrome, that requires an immunomodulatory agents to delay the onset of second attack or it is a monophasic form of ADEM not requiring further immunomodulation or suppression. The underlying immunopathogenesis of MS and ADEM is different, and patients with ADEM are expected to have complete or significant recovery without developing further attacks. In certain patients the line between MS and ADEM is blurry, and such determination is difficult. Certain relative features assist neurologists to separate these two diseases. Patients with ADEM are generally much younger (younger than 10 years), and there is no gender difference, while the peak age for MS is 29 years, and females are more predisposed than males. In certain cases, ADEM follows viral infections or happens after vaccination. Such prior events are usually absent in MS patients. Patients with ADEM develop meningoencephalitis with seizures, while these features are scarce among MS population. Neuroimaging of the brain in ADEM reveals giant contrast-enhancing lesions with involvement of white and gray matter, while the MS lesions are smaller, patchy, and ovoid. Longitudinal MR imaging in ADEM demonstrates resolution of demyelinating lesions, while in MS the neurologists encounter development of more lesions. Examination of CSF shows much higher number of lymphocytes in ADEM, while in MS the number of lymphocytes is typically less than $50/mm^3$. Oligoclonal bands may or may not be present in the CSF of ADEM patients, while they are present in the CSF of up to 94% of patients with relapsing MS. Both diseases show a favorable therapeutic response to corticosteroids.

References

1. Krupp LB, Tardieu M, Amato MP, Banwell B, Chitnis T, Dale RC, Ghezzi A, Hintzen R, Kornberg A, Pohl D, Rostasy K, Tenembaum S, Wassmer E, International Pediatric Multiple Sclerosis Study Group. International pediatric multiple sclerosis study group criteria for pediatric multiple sclerosis and immune-mediated central nervous system demyelinating disorders: revisions to the 2007 definitions. Mult Scler. 2013;19(10):1261–7.
2. Anlar B, Basaran C, Kose G, Guven A, Haspolat S, Yakut A, Serdaroglu A, Senbil N, Tan H, Karaagaoglu E, Karli OK. Acute disseminated encephalomyelitis in children: outcome and prognosis. Neuropediatrics. 2003;34(4):194–9.
3. Steiner I, Kennedy PG. Acute disseminated encephalomyelitis: current knowledge and open questions. J Neurovirol. 2015;21(5):473–9.
4. Tenembaum S, Chamoles N, Fejerman N. Acute disseminated encephalomyelitis: a long-term follow-up study of 84 pediatric patients. Neurology. 2002;59(8):1224–31.
5. Young NP, Weinshenker BG, Parisi JE, Scheithauer B, Giannini C, Roemer SF, Thomsen KM, Mandrekar JN, Erickson BJ, Lucchinetti CF. Perivenous demyelination: association with clinically defined acute disseminated encephalomyelitis and comparison with pathologically confirmed multiple sclerosis. Brain. 2010;133(Pt 2):333–48.

6. Wingerchuk DM, Weinshenker BG. Continuum. Minneap Minn. 2013;19(4):944–67.
7. Lann MS, Lovell MA, Kleinschmidt-DeMasters BK. Acute hemorrhagic leukoencephalitis. A critical entity for forensic pathologists to recognize. Am J Forensic Med Pathol. 2010;31(1):7–11.
8. Dale RC. Acute disseminated encephalomyelitis. Semin Pediatr Infect Dis. 2003;14(2):90–5.
9. Rossi A. Imaging of acute disseminated encephalomyelitis. Neuroimaging Clin N Am. 2008;18:149–61.
10. Rivers TM, Sprunt DH, Berry GP. Observations on attempts to produce acute disseminated encephalomyelitis in monkeys. J Exp Med. 1933;58(1):39–53.
11. Rivers TM, Schwentker FF. Encephalomyelitis accompanied by myelin destruction experimentally produced in monkeys. J Exp Med. 1935;61(5):689–702.
12. Marin SE, Callen DJA. The magnetic resonance imaging appearance of monophasic acute disseminated encephalomyelitis. An update post application of the 2007 consensus criteria. Neuroimaging Clin N Am. 2013;23(2):245–66.
13. Ubol S, Hemachudha T, Whitaker JN, Griffin DE. Antibody to peptides of human myelin basic protein in post-rabies vaccine encephalomyelitis sera. J Neuroimmunol. 1990;26(2):107–11.
14. O'Connor KC, Chitnis T, Griffin DE, Piyasirisilp S, Bar-Or A, Khoury S, Wucherpfennig KW, Hafler DA. Myelin basic protein-reactive autoantibodies in the serum and cerebrospinal fluid of multiple sclerosis patients are characterized by low-affinity interactions. J Neuroimmunol. 2003;136(1–2):140–8.
15. Franciotta D, Zardini E, Ravaglia S, Piccolo G, Andreoni L, Bergamaschi R, Romani A, Tavazzi E, Naldi P, Ceroni M, Marchioni E. Cytokines and chemokines in cerebrospinal fluid and serum of adult patients with acute disseminated encephalomyelitis. J Neurol Sci. 2006;247(2):202–7.
16. Kuperan S, Ostrow P, Landi MK, Bakshi R. Acute hemorrhagic leukoencephalitis vs ADEM: FLAIR MRI and neuropathology findings. Neurology. 2003;60(4):721–2.
17. Balasubramanya KS, Kovoor JM, Jayakumar PN, Ravishankar S, Kamble RB, Panicker J, Nagaraja D. Diffusion-weighted imaging and proton MR spectroscopy in the characterization of acute disseminated encephalomyelitis. Neuroradiology. 2007;49(2):177–83.
18. Ben Sira L, Miller E, Artzi M, Fattal-Valevski A, Constantini S, Ben BD. 1H-MRS for the diagnosis of acute disseminated encephalomyelitis: insight into the acute-disease stage. Pediatr Radiol. 2010;40(1):106–13.
19. Bizzi A, Uluğ AM, Crawford TO, Passe T, Bugiani M, Bryan RN, Barker PB. Quantitative proton MR spectroscopic imaging in acute disseminated encephalomyelitis. AJNR Am J Neuroradiol. 2001;22(6):1125–30.
20. Weinshenker BG, O'Brien PC, Petterson TM, Noseworthy JH, Lucchinetti CF, Dodick DW, Pineda AA, Stevens LN, Rodriguez M. A randomized trial of plasma exchange in acute central nervous system inflammatory demyelinating disease. Ann Neurol. 1999;46(6):878–86.

Autoimmune Encephalitis: Clinical Features, Pathophysiology, and Treatment

8

Ramin Zand

Autoimmune encephalitis represents a group of disorders characterized by various immunologic mechanisms, clinical manifestations, and therapeutic outcomes. They can be associated with paraneoplastic syndromes or nonneoplastic autoimmune processes. Autoimmune encephalitis is usually associated with antibodies that can acutely or subacutely affect any part of the central or peripheral nervous system including neuromuscular junctions and muscles. Antibody-associated encephalitis can be divided into two main categories: (1) encephalopathy associated with antibodies against intracellular antigens and (2) encephalopathy associated with antibodies directed against the neuronal surface and synaptic antigens [1, 2]. The discovery of various antibodies related to autoimmune encephalitis has given us a new insight into pathogenic mechanisms and treatment of these syndromes. That is important since many patients with autoimmune encephalopathy are children and young adults, and they may respond well to immunosuppressive treatment if diagnosed without delay. In this chapter, we review the epidemiology, pathophysiology, clinical characteristics, diagnosis, and treatment of different syndromes associated with autoimmune encephalitis.

History

In 1934, Greenfield initially described two cases of subacute cerebellar degeneration occurring with carcinoma outside the nervous system [3]. Thirteen years later in 1947, Denny-Brown reported two patients with primary sensory neuropathy and muscular changes associated with bronchial carcinoma [4].

R. Zand, MD
Department of Neurology, University of Tennesse, Geisinger Health System,
100 North Academy Avenue, Danville, PA 17822, USA
e-mail: ramin.zand@gmail.com

© Springer International Publishing AG 2017
A. Minagar, J.S. Alexander (eds.), *Inflammatory Disorders of the Nervous System*, Current Clinical Neurology, DOI 10.1007/978-3-319-51220-4_8

In 1954, Henson et al. [5] published a series of 19 cases with various types of carcinomatous neuropathy and myopathy. Eight of these patients had proximal atrophic weakness of limbs and involvement of ocular and bulbar muscles. Four patients also exhibited myasthenic features with a favorable response to neostigmine in some cases. Later in 1956, Chartan et al. [6] described episodes of severe mental disturbance in three male patients with bronchial carcinoma. In all of those, the mental disorder either preceded or overshadowed the presence of cancer.

In 1968, Corsellis et al. [7] reported autoimmune limbic encephalitis associated with small-cell lung cancer. For years, it was believed that "limbic encephalitis" was almost always associated with a form of neoplasia mainly lung, thymic, or testicular tumors. In 2001, it was shown that voltage-gated potassium channels (VGKC) were associated with reversible limbic encephalitis [8]. Four years later, other antibodies to the cell surface or synaptic proteins were detected in six patients with subacute limbic encephalitis and involvement of additional brain regions [9]. Further studies of those patients with immunotherapy-responsive encephalitis resulted in the characterization of the antigen as the NR1 subunit of the N-methyl-D-aspartic acid receptor (NMDA receptor) and the definition of its clinical characteristics [10–12], since many other neuronal cell surface antigens have been detected and introduced in patients with autoimmune encephalitis.

Epidemiology

The California Encephalitis Project was established in 1998 to identify the etiologic agents and to study epidemiology and clinical characteristics of encephalitis. In 2009, they reported ten cases of NMDA receptor antibodies and concluded that unlike classic paraneoplastic encephalitis, anti-NMDA receptor encephalitis affects younger patients [13]. Since, an increasing number of cases have been reported to the California Encephalitis Project, making NMDA receptor antibodies a significant cause of encephalitis among young patients. Between 2007 and 2011, 761 cases of encephalitis of uncertain etiology in individuals aged ≤30 years were reported to the California Encephalitis Project. Of these, 32 patients were tested positive for anti-NMDAR encephalitis; however, viral encephalitis was diagnosed in only 42 patients [14]. Although anti-NMDAR encephalitis was initially thought to affect young women, often with teratomas, it can affect men and children, with or without any identifiable tumor [15]. Overall, 75% of patients with anti-NMDAR encephalitis can significantly recover when diagnosed promptly [10].

Among paraneoplastic syndrome, Lambert-Eaton myasthenic syndrome, which affects approximately 3% of patients with small-cell lung cancer, and myasthenia gravis, which affects 15% of patients with thymoma, are common [16]. Up to 9% of patients with small-cell lung cancer have at least one form of paraneoplastic syndrome (commonly Lambert-Eaton myasthenic syndrome, sensory neuronopathy, or limbic encephalitis) [16]. γ-Aminobutyric acid (GABA-B) receptor antibodies are also responsible for paraneoplastic limbic encephalitis in patients with small-cell lung cancer [17].

Pathophysiology and Clinical Presentation

Antibodies in autoimmune encephalitis can target intracellular antigens or antigens on neuronal surface/synaptic space. Among those, antibodies which target intracellular antigens are usually associated with paraneoplastic syndromes and a poor prognosis. Antibodies to intracellular antigens include anti-Hu (also known as anti-neuronal nuclear antibody, type 1, ANNA-1), anti-Ma2 (also called anti-Ta), collapsin-responsive mediator protein-3, protein-4, and protein-5 (CRMP3–5), anti-amphiphysin, anti-Yo, anti-Ri, adenylate kinase 5, and BR serine/threonine kinase (BRSK2) antibodies. Table 8.1 summarizes the antibodies to intracellular antigens and their clinical presentation.

Antibodies to neuronal surface/synaptic antigens can also be associated with cancer; however, they are more responsive to immunotherapy. Antibodies to neuronal surface/synaptic antigens are often related to limbic encephalitis. In this group, anti-N-methyl-D-aspartate (NMDA) receptor encephalitis and anti-leucine-rich glioma-inactivated 1 (LGI1) comprise 85% of patients [1]. Anti-NMDA receptor encephalitis has become one of the most frequently recognized autoimmune encephalitides since its discovery. The disease is more frequent among women (80%) and adults younger than 45 years old [39]. Almost half of the patients initially present with a headache and a viral-like process, followed by psychiatric manifestations, altered mental status, in addition to language and memory dysfunction [15, 40]. Seizure is frequent among pediatric patients [39]. More than two-third of the patients suffer from seizures [39]. Table 8.2 summarizes the antibodies to intracellular antigens, their associated syndromes.

More than half of patients with autoimmune encephalitis present with symptoms of limbic encephalopathy including memory deficits, altered mental status, seizures, and neuropsychiatric syndrome. Refractory seizures and status epilepticus have also been reported [59, 60, 68]. Other common features of autoimmune encephalitis include headache, tremor, language difficulties, ataxia, and sleep disorders.

Diagnostic Approach

The diagnosis of autoimmune encephalitis can be challenging because symptoms usually precede the diagnosis of cancer or resemble other neurological or psychological disorders. An international panel of experts has identified diagnostic criteria for paraneoplastic neurological syndromes (Table 8.3) [69].

Patients with clinical presentations of encephalitis should have a full workup including neuroimaging, cerebrospinal fluid (CSF) examination, electroencephalography (EEG), pertinent laboratory and serological studies, and, in some cases, electromyography (EMG). Many other conditions (Table 8.4) are more frequent than autoimmune etiologies of encephalopathies. They should be considered and excluded.

Magnetic resonance imaging (MRI) of the brain is neither sensitive nor specific for the diagnosis of autoimmune encephalitis. However, it is essential to exclude

Table 8.1 Summary of antibodies to intracellular antigens, their mechanisms, and related syndromes

Antibody	Associated tumor	Affected areas	Clinical syndromes

Type 1 antineuronal nuclear antibody (ANNA-1/anti-Hu)	Adults: [18–20]
	  Small-cell lung cancer
	  Other tumors (rare)
	  No cancer (15%)
	Pediatrics:
	  No cancer (six out of eight cases) [21]
		Multifocal, central, and peripheral nervous systems [18–20]	Sensory neuropathy – dorsal root ganglia involvement [22]
			Limbic encephalitis [22]
			Brain stem encephalitis and paraneoplastic cerebellar degeneration [23, 24]

Type 2 antineuronal nuclear antibody (ANNA-2/anti-Ri)	Breast, adnexal tumor [25]	Central nervous system neuronal nuclei [25]	Opsoclonus, ataxia [25] Ophthalmoplegia [26]
Purkinje cell cytoplasmic antibody type 1 (PCA-1/anti-Yo)	Ovarian, uterus, adnexal, or breast tumor [27]	Cerebellum – Purkinje cell cytoplasmic antigens [27]	Paraneoplastic cerebellar degeneration [23]
Anti-Ma proteins (Ma1, Ma2)	Testicular cancer (more common in germ cell tumors) [28]	Limbic system, cerebellum, brain stem [28, 29]	Limbic encephalitis (differs from classic limbic encephalitis) [29] Brain stem encephalopathy and myelopathy [29] Ophthalmoplegia, atypical parkinsonism, hypokinetic syndrome [29] Progressive muscular atrophy (a case report) [30]
Anti-amphiphysin	Breast, small-cell lung, ovarian cancer [31, 32]	A nerve terminal protein with a putative role in endocytosis [33]	Stiff-man syndrome [31] Sensory neuronopathy, encephalomyelitis, limbic encephalitis, Lambert-Eaton myasthenic syndrome [32]
Anti-CV2/CRMP5	Thymoma, small-cell lung cancer [34] Renal cell carcinoma and lymphoma [35]	Central and peripheral neurons, including synapses [34]	Basal ganglia abnormalities [35] Cranial, peripheral, and autonomic neuropathy [34] Cerebellar ataxia, dementia, and neuromuscular junction disorders [34]
Others (only a few cases reported): Anti-CRMP3–4 [36] Anti-adenylate kinase 5 [37] Anti-BRSK2 [38]	CRMP3–4: thymoma Anti-adenylate kinase 5: no cancer detected Anti-BRSK2: small-cell lung cancer	Limbic system	Limbic encephalitis (progressive short-term memory deficits, confusion, seizures, and psychosis)

Table 8.2 Summary of antibodies to neural surface, their clinical syndrome, and associated tumors

Antigens	Clinical syndrome	Associated tumor	Miscellaneous
N-methyl-D-aspartate receptor (NMDAR)	Prodromal syndrome (a headache, fever, or viral-like symptoms) Psychiatric disorders (anxiety, bizarre behavior, hallucinations, delusions, etc.) Amnesia Seizure Altered mental status Movement disorders Catatonia Autonomic Instability (hyperthermia, fluctuations of blood pressure, tachycardia, bradycardia) [10, 12, 15, 41–43]	Ovarian teratoma (10–50%, age dependent) Other rare tumors: Testicular germ cell tumor [1] Teratoma of the mediastinum, small-cell lung cancer [10] Hodgkin's lymphoma [44] Neuroblastoma [45]	Also reported in children less than one year old Four times more frequent among women
Leucine-rich glioma-inactivated 1 (LGI1)	Seizures (faciobrachial dystonic) Myoclonus Memory and cognitive deficits Rapid eye movement, sleep behavior disorders [46–49] Chorea [50]	Thymoma Small-cell lung cancer (only 20% are associated with a tumor)	Extracellularly secreted LGI1 links two epilepsy-related receptors (ADAM22 and ADAM23) [51] This syndrome was previously attributed to voltage-gated potassium channels [52]
A-amino-3-hydroxy-5-methyl-4-isoxazolepropionic acid (AMPA) receptor	Limbic encephalitis: progressive short-term memory deficits, confusion, and seizures Psychosis with bipolar features [53]	Two-thirds of patients: lung, thymoma, breast, ovarian teratoma [53]	Relapse is common
Contactin-associated protein-like 2 (CASPR2)	Encephalitis Peripheral nerve hyperexcitability [54] Morvan syndrome (neuromyotonia, pain, hyperhidrosis, weight loss, severe insomnia, and hallucinations) [55]	Lung, thymoma (<20%)	Can be mistaken for a motor neuron disease

(continued)

Table 8.2 (continued)

Antigens	Clinical syndrome	Associated tumor	Miscellaneous
Gamma-aminobutyric acid A (GABA-A) receptor	Refractory status epilepticus or epilepsia partialis (reported as 100%) [56]	Thymoma (rare) [56]	Diffuse fluid-attenuated inversion recovery (FLAIR) and T2 signal abnormalities [56]
Gamma-aminobutyric acid B (GABA-B) receptor	Limbic encephalitis: progressive short-term memory deficits, confusion, and seizures Ataxia Opsoclonus-myoclonus syndrome [57]	Small-cell lung cancer (50%) [57]	
IgLON5	Unique non-rapid eye movement (REM) and REM parasomnia Obstructive sleep apnea Gait instability followed by dysarthria, dysphagia, ataxia, or chorea [58]	Not paraneoplastic	Pathological features may suggest a tauopathy [58]
Voltage-gated potassium channel (VGKC)	Sleep disturbances, severe insomnia Limbic encephalitis Morvan syndrome Seizure, status epilepticus [59, 60]	Thymoma, prostate adenothymoma, prostate adenocarcinoma, colon adenocarcinoma, and melanoma [61]	Sleep disorders are diagnostic hallmark [61]
Glycine receptor (GlyR) α1 subunit	Progressive encephalomyelitis with rigidity and myoclonus (PERM) [61] Atypical stiff-person syndrome Seizure Behavioral changes [62]	Thymoma (10%) [63]	Only a few cases reported
Dipeptidyl-peptidase-like protein-6 (DDPX)	Agitation, confusion, myoclonus, tremor, and seizures [64] Weight loss, psychosis, depression, movement disturbances [65]	B-cell neoplasms (10%) [65]	
Metabotropic glutamate receptor 5 (mGluR5)	Limbic encephalitis Headache Involuntary movements [66, 67]	Hodgkin's lymphoma [66]	Only a few cases reported

Table 8.3 Diagnostic criteria for paraneoplastic neurological syndromes

Criteria for *definite* paraneoplastic neurological syndromes
1. A classical syndrome and cancer that develops within 5 years of the diagnosis of the neurological disorder
2. A nonclassical syndrome that resolves or significantly improves after cancer treatment without concomitant immunotherapy, provided that the syndrome is not susceptible to spontaneous remission
3. A nonclassical syndrome with onconeural antibodies (well characterized or not) and cancer that develops within 5 years of the diagnosis of the neurological disorder
4. A neurological syndrome (classical or not) with well-characterized onconeural antibodies (anti-Hu, Yo, CV2, Ri, Ma2, or amphiphysin) and no cancer
Criteria for *possible* paraneoplastic neurological syndromes
1. A classical syndrome, no onconeural antibodies, no cancer but at high risk to have an underlying tumor
2. A neurological syndrome (classical or not) with partially characterized onconeural antibodies and no cancer
3. A nonclassical neurological syndrome, no onconeural antibodies, and cancer present within 2 years of diagnosis

Table 8.4 Differential diagnosis of autoimmune encephalitis

Viral encephalitis, e.g., human herpesvirus 6 (HHV-6), human immunodeficiency virus (HIV), herpes simplex virus (HSV), varicella zoster virus (VZV)	Creutzfeldt-Jakob disease
Primary CNS tumor or metastatic disease	Whipple disease
Ischemic and hemorrhagic cerebrovascular disease	Wernicke encephalopathy
Psychiatric disorders	Chronic CNS infections with atypical bacteria, e.g., *Treponema pallidum*, *Listeria*, tuberculosis
Toxic-metabolic encephalopathy	Other neuroinflammatory diseases, e.g., lupus cerebritis, Behcet's disease, primary angiitis of the central nervous system (PACNS)
Multiple sclerosis	Nonconvulsive status epilepticus
Rapidly progressive dementia	Motor neuron disease

other conditions such as ischemic infarction or tumors. Among patients with encephalitis, signal hyperintensities on fluid-attenuated inversion recovery (FLAIR) and T2-weighted images can be seen in the mesiotemporal lobe, cortical and subcortical regions, or brain stem. Contrast enhancement can be variable, and leptomeningeal enhancement has been reported [70]. The extent of abnormal findings on the MRI is different for each syndrome. For instance, MRI in GABA-A receptor encephalitis often shows multifocal and widespread FLAIR and T2 signal abnormalities [56]. Encephalitic syndromes associated with LGI1 and AMPA receptor antibodies also always cause FLAIR hyperintensity in the mesiotemporal lobe. In a study on 50 patients with paraneoplastic limbic encephalitis, researchers observed that 57% of patients with MRI studies had signal abnormalities in the limbic system [20]. There is also a report of cortical ribboning similar to that seen in Creutzfeldt-Jakob disease

(CJD) among patients with voltage-gated potassium channel (VGKC) autoantibody-associated encephalopathy [71]. Brain MRI is often normal or shows transient FLAIR hyperintensity with or without contrast enhancement in anti-NMDAR encephalitis [10, 72].

Several autoimmune encephalitis syndromes are associated with seizure or status epilepticus [59, 60]. Diffuse slowing or epileptiform abnormalities in the temporal lobe on EEG are the most common findings in patients with encephalitis. EEG is also important to exclude other etiologies for encephalopathy such as subclinical seizures.

Although CSF examination can be normal especially in the initial phase, a mild elevation of protein (<100 mg/dL) and lymphocytic pleocytosis or oligoclonal bands can be an indicator of autoimmune encephalitis [10, 13, 15, 17, 46, 73]. More than 90% of patients with antibodies against NMDA, AMPA, and GABA-B receptors have pleocytosis or oligoclonal bands on CSF examination [10, 53, 56, 57]. CSF analysis is also essential to exclude other etiologies of encephalopathy including infectious and neoplastic causes.

Pertinent antibody testing should be performed in both serum and CSF. Antibodies to cell surface/ synaptic proteins can be detected primarily in CSF. In a multiinstitutional observational study, detection of NMDA receptor antibodies was compared in 250 paired serum and CSF samples. It showed that the screening test is significantly more sensitive in CSF than serum (100% vs. 85%) [39]. A positive serum antibody testing, when CSF is negative for the antibody, raises the possibility of a false positive diagnosis. Although many tests for autoimmune encephalitis are commercially available, a number of autoimmune encephalitis cases can be caused by other, still unavailable or unknown antibodies. Therefore, a negative test result does not rule out autoimmune encephalitis.

All patients with autoimmune encephalitis should be screened for the presence of a tumor. The detected antibody type can also guide the type and extent of screening. On the other hand, detection of a tumor could also assist in the diagnosis of paraneoplastic encephalitis variants and guide the antibody screening plan.

Treatment and Outcome

Autoimmune encephalitis is often associated with a favorable outcome after tumor removal and antineoplastic treatment (if applicable), as well as immunotherapy. In general, steroids, intravenous immunoglobulin, and plasmapheresis are the first line of immunotherapy especially when a tumor is detected and treated [9, 39]. Rituximab and cyclophosphamide comprise the second-line immunotherapy when the first-line treatment fails. Although seizures must be addressed aggressively during the acute phase of the disease, patients often do not require long-term antiepileptic medication.

In a large multiinstitutional observational study, over 500 patients with anti-NMDA receptor encephalitis were treated and monitored up to 2 years. Out of 501 patients, 94% received first-line immunotherapy (steroids, intravenous immunoglobulin, plasmapheresis) or tumor removal, resulting in improvement within

4 weeks in 53% of patients. More than half of patients who failed first-line therapy received second-line immunotherapy (rituximab, cyclophosphamide), resulting in better outcome than those who did not. During the first 24 months, almost 80% of patients reached a good outcome, where relapses occurred in approximately 12% of the patients. About 6% of patients died [39].

Predictors of poor outcome in anti-NMDA receptor encephalitis are a delay in diagnosis and treatment, the need for intensive care, high titer of antibody in CSF and serum, and the presence of teratoma [39, 74]. The overall prognosis for patients with autoimmune encephalitis is variable. Some patients have a complete recovery, while others die or develop a permanent neurologic disability.

Summary

Autoimmune encephalitis has different immunologic mechanisms, clinical manifestations, and therapeutic outcomes. It can be divided into two categories: antibodies against intracellular antigens or antibodies against neuronal surface/synaptic antigens. More than half of patients with autoimmune encephalitis present with symptoms of limbic encephalopathy including memory deficits, altered mental status, seizures, and neuropsychiatric syndrome. Patients with the clinical presentation of encephalitis should have a complete workup including neuroimaging, EEG, lumbar puncture, and serologic testing. Other etiologies of encephalitis are more common and should be excluded. Patients often respond favorably to immunotherapy. Delay in diagnosis and treatment has been associated with a worse prognosis.

References

1. Lancaster E, Martinez-Hernandez E, Dalmau J. Encephalitis and antibodies to synaptic and neuronal cell surface proteins. Neurology. 2011;77:179–89.
2. Tüzün E, Dalmau J. Limbic encephalitis and variants: classification, diagnosis and treatment. Neurologist. 2007;13:261–71.
3. Greenfield JG. Subacute spino-cerebellar degeneration occurring in elderly patients. Brain. 1934;57:161–76.
4. Denny-Brown D. Primary sensory neuropathy with muscular changes associated with carcinoma. J Neurol Neurosurg Psychiatry. 1948;11:73–87.
5. Henson RA, Russell DS, Wilkinson M. Carcinomatous neuropathy and myopathy a clinical and pathological study. Brain. 1954;77:82–121.
6. Charatan FB, Brierley JB. Mental disorder associated with primary lung carcinoma. Br Med J. 1956;1:765–8.
7. Corsellis JA, Goldberg GJ, Norton AR. 'Limbic encephalitis' and its association with carcinoma. Brain. 1968;91:481–96.
8. Buckley C et al. Potassium channel antibodies in two patients with reversible limbic encephalitis. Ann Neurol. 2001;50:73–8.
9. Ances BM et al. Treatment-responsive limbic encephalitis identified by neuropil antibodies: MRI and PET correlates. Brain. 2005;128:1764–77.
10. Dalmau J et al. Anti-NMDA-receptor encephalitis: case series and analysis of the effects of antibodies. Lancet Neurol. 2008;7:1091–8.

11. Dalmau J et al. Paraneoplastic anti-N-methyl-D-aspartate receptor encephalitis associated with ovarian teratoma. Ann Neurol. 2007;61:25–36.
12. Lau CG, Zukin RS. NMDA receptor trafficking in synaptic plasticity and neuropsychiatric disorders. Nat Rev Neurosci. 2007;8:413–26.
13. Gable MS et al. Anti-NMDA receptor encephalitis: report of ten cases and comparison with viral encephalitis. Eur J Clin Microbiol Infect Dis. 2009;28:1421–9.
14. Gable MS, Sheriff H, Dalmau J, Tilley DH, Glaser CA. The frequency of autoimmune N-methyl-D-aspartate receptor encephalitis surpasses that of individual viral etiologies in young individuals enrolled in the California encephalitis project. Clin Infect Dis. 2012;54:899–904.
15. Dalmau J, Lancaster E, Martinez-Hernandez E, Rosenfeld MR, Balice-Gordon R. Clinical experience and laboratory investigations in patients with anti-NMDAR encephalitis. Lancet Neurol. 2011;10:63–74.
16. Gozzard P et al. Paraneoplastic neurologic disorders in small cell lung carcinoma: a prospective study. Neurology. 2015;85:235–9.
17. Boronat A, Sabater L, Saiz A, Dalmau J, Graus F. GABA(B) receptor antibodies in limbic encephalitis and anti-GAD-associated neurologic disorders. Neurology. 2011;76:795–800.
18. Graus F et al. Anti-Hu-associated paraneoplastic encephalomyelitis: analysis of 200 patients. Brain. 2001;124:1138–48.
19. Sillevis Smitt P et al. Survival and outcome in 73 anti-Hu positive patients with paraneoplastic encephalomyelitis/sensory neuronopathy. J Neurol. 2002;249:745–53.
20. Gultekin SH et al. Paraneoplastic limbic encephalitis: neurological symptoms, immunological findings and tumour association in 50 patients. Brain. 2000;123(Pt 7):1481–94.
21. Honnorat J et al. Autoimmune limbic encephalopathy and anti-Hu antibodies in children without cancer. Neurology. 2013;80:2226–32.
22. Dalmau J, Graus F, Rosenblum MK, Posner JB. Anti-Hu--associated paraneoplastic encephalomyelitis/sensory neuronopathy. A clinical study of 71 patients. Medicine (Baltimore). 1992;71:59–72.
23. Shams'ili S et al. Paraneoplastic cerebellar degeneration associated with antineuronal antibodies: analysis of 50 patients. Brain. 2003;126:1409–18.
24. Saiz A et al. Anti-Hu-associated brainstem encephalitis. J Neurol Neurosurg Psychiatry. 2009;80:404–7.
25. Luque FA et al. Anti-Ri: an antibody associated with paraneoplastic opsoclonus and breast cancer. Ann Neurol. 1991;29:241–51.
26. Kim H, Lim Y, Kim K-K. Anti-ri-antibody-associated paraneoplastic syndrome in a man with breast cancer showing a reversible pontine lesion on MRI. J Clin Neurol. 2009;5:151–2.
27. Greenlee JE et al. Association of anti-Yo (type I) antibody with paraneoplastic cerebellar degeneration in the setting of transitional cell carcinoma of the bladder: detection of Yo antigen in tumor tissue and fall in antibody titers following tumor removal. Ann Neurol. 1999;45:805–9.
28. Voltz R et al. A serologic marker of paraneoplastic limbic and brain-stem encephalitis in patients with testicular cancer. N Engl J Med. 1999;340:1788–95.
29. Dalmau J et al. Clinical analysis of anti-Ma2-associated encephalitis. Brain. 2004;127:1831–44.
30. Waragai M et al. Anti-Ma2 associated paraneoplastic neurological syndrome presenting as encephalitis and progressive muscular atrophy. J Neurol Neurosurg Psychiatry. 2006;77:111–3.
31. Saiz A et al. Anti-amphiphysin I antibodies in patients with paraneoplastic neurological disorders associated with small cell lung carcinoma. J Neurol Neurosurg Psychiatry. 1999;66:214–7.
32. Antoine JC et al. Antiamphiphysin antibodies are associated with various paraneoplastic neurological syndromes and tumors. Arch Neurol. 1999;56:172–7.
33. David C, McPherson PS, Mundigl O, de Camilli P. A role of amphiphysin in synaptic vesicle endocytosis suggested by its binding to dynamin in nerve terminals. Proc Natl Acad Sci U S A. 1996;93:331–5.

34. Yu Z et al. CRMP-5 neuronal autoantibody: marker of lung cancer and thymoma-related auto-immunity. Ann Neurol. 2001;49:146–54.
35. Vernino S et al. Paraneoplastic chorea associated with CRMP-5 neuronal antibody and lung carcinoma. Ann Neurol. 2002;51:625–30.
36. Knudsen A et al. Antibodies to CRMP3-4 associated with limbic encephalitis and thymoma. Clin Exp Immunol. 2007;149:16–22.
37. Tüzün E, Rossi JE, Karner SF, Centurion AF, Dalmau J. Adenylate kinase 5 autoimmunity in treatment refractory limbic encephalitis. J Neuroimmunol. 2007;186:177–80.
38. Sabater L, Gómez-Choco M, Saiz A, Graus F. BR serine/threonine kinase 2: a new autoantigen in paraneoplastic limbic encephalitis. J Neuroimmunol. 2005;170:186–90.
39. Titulaer MJ et al. Treatment and prognostic factors for long-term outcome in patients with anti-NMDA receptor encephalitis: an observational cohort study. Lancet Neurol. 2013;12:157–65.
40. Kayser MS, Titulaer MJ, Gresa-Arribas N, Dalmau J. Frequency and characteristics of isolated psychiatric episodes in anti–N-methyl-d-aspartate receptor encephalitis. JAMA Neurol. 2013;70:1133–9.
41. Hacohen Y et al. Paediatric autoimmune encephalopathies: clinical features, laboratory investigations and outcomes in patients with or without antibodies to known central nervous system autoantigens. J Neurol Neurosurg Psychiatry. 2013;84:748–55.
42. Iizuka T et al. Anti-NMDA receptor encephalitis in Japan: long-term outcome without tumor removal. Neurology. 2008;70:504–11.
43. Shimazaki H, Ando Y, Nakano I, Dalmau J. Reversible limbic encephalitis with antibodies against the membranes of neurones of the hippocampus. J Neurol Neurosurg Psychiatry. 2007;78:324–5.
44. Pillay N, Gilbert JJ, Ebers GC, Brown JD. Internuclear ophthalmoplegia and 'optic neuritis': paraneoplastic effects of bronchial carcinoma. Neurology. 1984;34:788–91.
45. Lebas A, Husson B, Didelot A, Honnorat J, Tardieu M. Expanding spectrum of encephalitis with NMDA receptor antibodies in young children. J Child Neurol. 2010;25:742–5.
46. Wingfield T et al. Autoimmune encephalitis: a case series and comprehensive review of the literature. QJM. 2011;104:921–31.
47. Andrade DM, Tai P, Dalmau J, Wennberg R. Tonic seizures: a diagnostic clue of anti-LGI1 encephalitis? Neurology. 2011;76:1355–7.
48. Irani SR et al. Faciobrachial dystonic seizures precede Lgi1 antibody limbic encephalitis. Ann Neurol. 2011;69:892–900.
49. Sen A et al. Pathognomonic seizures in limbic encephalitis associated with anti-LGI1 antibodies. Lancet (London/England). 2014;383:2018.
50. Tofaris GK et al. Immunotherapy-responsive chorea as the presenting feature of LGI1-antibody encephalitis. Neurology. 2012;79:195–6.
51. Fukata Y et al. Disruption of LGI1-linked synaptic complex causes abnormal synaptic transmission and epilepsy. Proc Natl Acad Sci U S A. 2010;107:3799–804.
52. Lai M et al. Investigation of LGI1 as the antigen in limbic encephalitis previously attributed to potassium channels: a case series. Lancet Neurol. 2010;9:776–85.
53. Höftberger R et al. Encephalitis and AMPA receptor antibodies: Novel findings in a case series of 22 patients. Neurology. 2015;84:2403–12.
54. Klein CJ et al. Insights from LGI1 and CASPR2 potassium channel complex autoantibody subtyping. JAMA Neurol. 2013;70:229–34.
55. Irani SR et al. Morvan syndrome: clinical and serological observations in 29 cases. Ann Neurol. 2012;72:241–55.
56. Petit-Pedrol M et al. Encephalitis with refractory seizures, status epilepticus, and antibodies to the GABAA receptor: a case series, characterisation of the antigen, and analysis of the effects of antibodies. Lancet Neurol. 2014;13:276–86.
57. Höftberger R et al. Encephalitis and GABAB receptor antibodies: novel findings in a new case series of 20 patients. Neurology. 2013;81:1500–6.

58. Sabater L et al. A novel non-rapid-eye movement and rapid-eye-movement parasomnia with sleep breathing disorder associated with antibodies to IgLON5: a case series, characterisation of the antigen, and post-mortem study. Lancet Neurol. 2014;13:575–86.
59. Suleiman J et al. VGKC antibodies in pediatric encephalitis presenting with status epilepticus. Neurology. 2011;76:1252–5.
60. Cornelius JR et al. Sleep manifestations of voltage-gated potassium channel complex autoimmunity. Arch Neurol. 2011;68:733–8.
61. Hutchinson M et al. Progressive encephalomyelitis, rigidity, and myoclonus: a novel glycine receptor antibody. Neurology. 2008;71:1291–2.
62. Mas N et al. Antiglycine-receptor encephalomyelitis with rigidity. J Neurol Neurosurg Psychiatry. 2011;82:1399–401.
63. Clerinx K et al. Progressive encephalomyelitis with rigidity and myoclonus: resolution after thymectomy. Neurology. 2011;76:303–4.
64. Boronat A et al. Encephalitis and antibodies to dipeptidyl-peptidase-like protein-6, a subunit of Kv4.2 potassium channels. Ann Neurol. 2013;73:120–8.
65. Tobin WO et al. DPPX potassium channel antibody: frequency, clinical accompaniments, and outcomes in 20 patients. Neurology. 2014;83:1797–803.
66. Prüss H et al. Limbic encephalitis with mGluR5 antibodies and immunotherapy-responsive prosopagnosia. Neurology. 2014;83:1384–6.
67. Lancaster E et al. Antibodies to metabotropic glutamate receptor 5 in the Ophelia syndrome. Neurology. 2011;77:1698–701.
68. Johnson N, Henry C, Fessler AJ, Dalmau J. Anti-NMDA receptor encephalitis causing prolonged nonconvulsive status epilepticus. Neurology. 2010;75:1480–2.
69. Graus F et al. Recommended diagnostic criteria for paraneoplastic neurological syndromes. J Neurol Neurosurg Psychiatry. 2004;75:1135–40.
70. Flanagan EP et al. Autoimmune dementia: clinical course and predictors of immunotherapy response. Mayo Clin Proc. 2010;85:881–97.
71. Geschwind MD et al. Voltage-gated potassium channel autoimmunity mimicking creutzfeldt-jakob disease. Arch Neurol. 2008;65:1341–6.
72. Florance NR et al. Anti-N-methyl-D-aspartate receptor (NMDAR) encephalitis in children and adolescents. Ann Neurol. 2009;66:11–8.
73. Lawn ND, Westmoreland BF, Kiely MJ, Lennon VA, Vernino S. Clinical, magnetic resonance imaging, and electroencephalographic findings in paraneoplastic limbic encephalitis. Mayo Clin Proc. 2003;78:1363–8.
74. Gresa-Arribas N et al. Antibody titres at diagnosis and during follow-up of anti-NMDA receptor encephalitis: a retrospective study. Lancet Neurol. 2014;13:167–77.

Neuromyelitis Optica: Immunopathogenesis, Clinical Manifestations, and Treatments

9

Shin C. Beh, Teresa C. Frohman, and Elliot M. Frohman

Neuromyelitis optica (NMO) is an autoimmune inflammatory disease of the central nervous system (CNS), typically characterized by severe recurrent attacks of acute optic neuritis (AON) and transverse myelitis (TM). The initial description of the disease we recognize today as NMO was attributed to Eugene Devic (hence the eponymous term Devic's disease) and Ferdinand Gault in the nineteenth century, although numerous antecedent case reports that underscore highly reminiscent facets of this disorder strongly suggest that Devic and colleagues were not in fact the first to have codified the highly conspicuous and typically catastrophically disabling syndrome that characterizes this disorder [1].

Immunopathophysiology

Although initially thought to be a severe variant of multiple sclerosis (MS), the discovery of complement-fixing antibodies directed against aquaporin-4 (AQP4), also referred to as NMO-IgG, proved that NMO was a distinct disease entity [2–6].

S.C. Beh, MD (✉)
Department of Neurology and Neurotherapeutics, Multiple Sclerosis & Neuroimmunology Program, University of Texas Southwestern School of Medicine,
5323 Harry Hines Blvd, Dallas, TX 75390, USA
e-mail: scjbeh@gmail.com

T.C. Frohman, PA-C
Department of Neurology and Neurotherapeutics, University of Texas Southwestern School of Medicine, Dallas, TX, USA

E.M. Frohman, MD, PhD
Department of Neurology and Neurotherapeutics, University of Texas Southwestern School of Medicine, Dallas, TX, USA

Department of Ophthalmology, University of Texas Southwestern School of Medicine, Dallas, TX, USA

© Springer International Publishing AG 2017
A. Minagar, J.S. Alexander (eds.), *Inflammatory Disorders of the Nervous System*, Current Clinical Neurology, DOI 10.1007/978-3-319-51220-4_9

AQP4 is the most abundant water channel in the CNS and is predominantly located on astrocytic foot processes that form the glia limitans of the blood-brain barrier (BBB), ependyma, and around the synapses at the nodes of Ranvier [7]. Corresponding with the usual distribution of lesions in NMO, AQP4 is concentrated in the hypothalamus, diencephalon, brainstem (particularly within the floor of the IV ventricular tegmentum), optic nerves, and spinal cord [8].

The binding of NMO-IgG to the AQP4 epitope results in astrocytic damage via activation of the classical complement pathway and antibody-dependent, cell-mediated cytotoxicity [9–11]. As such, NMO can be considered as an autoimmune astrocytopathy, as opposed to MS, which is now widely recognized as a highly complex autoimmune disorder of the CNS, and characterized by histopathological and pathophysiologic heterogeneity, affecting both white and gray matter, and now considered both a demyelinating and neurodegenerative disorder [12].

Two pathologic subtypes of NMO lesions have been described. The classic NMO lesion is characterized by confluent and/or focal demyelination, infiltration of myelin-laden macrophages, severe axonal loss, necrosis of both gray and white matter in the cord, and pronounced astrocytic loss. The second NMO lesion is characterized by vacuolated myelin in the relative absence of frank demyelination, reactive astrocytes, microglial activation, limited axonal injury, and variable, typically granulocytic inflammation [11]. Remyelination is sometimes present at the edge of NMO lesions. Interestingly, peripheral Schwann cells have been observed to enter the spinal cord to drive remyelination; this observation provides further evidence of astrocytic dysfunction in NMO, since astrocytes normally prevent Schwann cells from entering the CNS [11].

B-cell dysregulation lies at the immunoetiopathological center of NMO, as evidenced by increased levels of circulating plasmablasts and intrathecal B-cells expressing NMO-IgG antibodies during NMO attacks [13, 14], as well as the efficacy of rituximab in treating the disease (further discussed later). Plasmablasts, the likely precursor of NMO-IgG producing plasma cells, rely on interleukin-6 (IL-6) for survival [13]. Other B-cell cytokines that play an important role in NMO include IL-5, IL-17, nitric oxide, tumor necrosis factor-alpha (TNF-alpha), a proliferation-inducing ligand (APRIL), and B-cell-activating factor (BAFF) [15]. Interestingly, suppressive B-cell activity may also be impaired in NMO, as evidenced by lower IL-10 and IL-35 levels [15].

There is also evidence that T-cell dysfunction contributes to the immunopathogenesis of the disease. Peripheral AQP4-specific T-cells are needed to drive the production of NMO-IgG from B-cells [16]. Increased circulating Th1 and Th17 subsets have also been observed in NMO [16]. While T-cells most likely play an important pathogenic role in NMO, their precise significance in initiating and accelerating the disease is unclear.

Eosinophils have also been implicated in NMO immunopathogenesis. In the bone marrow, eosinophils are the main source of APRIL and IL-6. Eosinophil infiltration of the CNS may help support plasma cell survival and NMO-IgG production within NMO lesions. The role of eosinophils in NMO may also explain why two MS disease-modifying agents have been observed to exacerbate NMO disease activity – fingolimod (which promotes retention of eosinophils in the bone marrow) and natalizumab (which increases the levels of circulating eosinophils) [15].

Clinical Features

The incidence of NMO is highest during the third to fourth decade of life, with a very strong female preponderance. Interestingly, the female/male ratio is 1:1 in monophasic NMO (no evidence of recurrence within 3 years of the index events of bilateral AON and TM), but 5:1 in the relapsing form of NMO. Compared to MS, which has a predilection for Caucasian patients, NMO appears to affect all racial groups [17–23]. On average, NMO patients are 10 years older than MS patients, with a median age of onset of 39 years [23, 24].

Various autoimmune diseases often coexist with NMO, the most common of which are systemic lupus erythematosus (SLE), autoimmune thyroid disease, and Sjogren's syndrome (SS) [23]. The frequency of concomitant autoimmune disease ranges from 10 to 40% [23]. Since patients with NMO may experience symptoms of a concomitant systemic autoimmune disease (e.g., sicca symptoms, rash, alopecia, photosensitive rash, arthritis), the presence of such symptoms does not militate against, but, in fact, supports the diagnostic suspicion of NMO. Furthermore, it is important to note that CNS complications of systemic autoimmune diseases are infrequent (e.g., seizures and psychosis in SLE). Therefore, in patients with typical neurologic manifestations of NMO, and who exhibit NMO-IgG seropositive, the "working" diagnosis of NMO can be confirmed expeditiously, with a high degree of confidence, and most particularly in the patient with a second, concomitant autoimmune disease. In such circumstances, moving rapidly (after achieving full control of the acute inflammatory "ictus") to implement an appropriate disease-modifying strategy is strongly encouraged ("time is tissue").

Severe AON or recurrent isolated AON should raise suspicion for NMO, particularly in the absence of brain MRI lesions typical of MS [23]. MS-related AON typically causes central visual blurring associated with impaired color vision (dyschromatopsia), retrobulbar pain that is exacerbated by eye movement, phosphenes, and visual deterioration with heat exposure (Uhthoff's phenomenon) [25, 26]. Bilateral simultaneous AON is exceedingly rare in MS and is strongly suggestive of NMO; conversely, unilateral AON is less common with (but does not rule out) NMO [27–29]. NMO-associated AON also typically results in more severe visual loss with a poor prognosis for recovery, compared to MS [25, 30, 31]. In fact, at 5 years from disease onset, 41% of NMO patients will suffer monocular or binocular blindness [29].

In MS, acute TM typically results in sensory manifestations [32, 33]. Acute TM in NMO commonly culminates in more devastating neurologic deficits, including paralysis, sensory loss, and bladder and bowel involvement below the level of the lesion [32]. Furthermore, the MRI often reveals longitudinally extensive TM (LETM) in NMO that involves most of the axial thickness of the spinal cord, in contradistinction to the longitudinally limited lesions in MS that only affect part of the spinal cord (typically the dorsal columns) [32]. The spinal cord MRI character-istics of NMO are discussed later. Lhermitte's phenomenon and paroxysmal tonic spasms are common manifestations of NMO and, interestingly, portend a relapsing rather than monophasic course of the disease [23, 34]. Radicular pain is also much more common in NMO compared to MS [35].

Intractable vomiting or hiccups (resulting from medullary lesions affecting the area postrema and nucleus tractus solitarius) are a common brainstem syndrome of NMO, affecting about 20% of patients [36, 37]. About 17% of NMO patients have been reported to suffer from persistent hiccups [36]. In our experience, this so-called area postrema syndrome often compels referrals to the gastroenterology ser-vice and is often mistakenly diagnosed as gastroparesis, despite unremarkable gastric emptying studies.

A far more ominous and potentially lethal manifestation of medullary involve-ment in NMO is neurogenic respiratory failure [34]; respiratory failure is distinctly rare in MS and almost always occurs in the setting of advanced MS with severe disability rather than in the acute or early phases of the disease [23].

Various brainstem ocular motor abnormalities (including upbeat nystagmus, downbeat nystagmus, vestibular nystagmus, and opsoclonus-myoclonus syndrome) have been reported in NMO; consistent with a brainstem localization, these patients also experienced concomitant pyramidal tract dysfunction as well as other cranial neuropathies [38]. Sensorineural hearing loss has also been reported in NMO, most probably due to brainstem involvement [39].

Diencephalic lesions can often lead to manifestations like the syndrome of inap-propriate antidiuretic hormone secretion (SIADH), narcolepsy, thermodysregula-tion, anorexia or other eating disorders [8, 40–43]. In contradistinction, such lesions in MS are infrequent [44].

NMO may also cause other manifestations, albeit rarely. Myopathy with elevated creatine kinase levels and muscle pain and nonspecific fatigue have been reported [45, 46]. Encephalopathy (which may be part of the posterior reversible encepha-lopathy syndrome [PRES]) has also been described in the disease [23, 47].

Investigations

An MRI of the spinal cord and brain is mandatory in any patient presenting with suspected NMO. The location and length of the spinal cord lesion on MRI can pro-vide vital clues about the diagnosis. Based on clinical and radiologic data, trans-verse myelitis can be categorized as longitudinally limited or longitudinally extensive [32]. Longitudinally limited partial TM with purely or predominantly sen-sory manifestations is more typical of MS [32]. In MS, the lesions often affect the cervicothoracic spinal cord and are typically located in the posterolateral or lateral portions of the spinal cord on axial sections [32]. On the other hand, LETM (which refers to a contiguous lesion that extends over three or more vertebral segments and involves more than two-thirds of the spinal cord thickness on axial sections) is dis-tinctly rare in MS and strongly indicates NMO [32]. Furthermore, T1 hypointensity of the central gray of the spinal cord is more suggestive of NMO [48, 49]. Lumbosacral myeloradiculitis has also been described in NMO [50].

A brain MRI is critical to differentiate MS from NMO and is part of the supportive criteria for the diagnosis of NMO (discussed later). The presence of lesions typical of MS would argue against, but not completely exclude, the diagnosis of NMO. Brain lesions occur in 60% of patients of NMO and may affect areas typical for the disease (discussed above), appear nonspecific, or, in rare cases, mimic MS lesions [8]. However, the presence of any lesion adjacent to the lateral ventricle and inferior temporal lobe, a subcortical U-fiber lesion, or a lesion reminiscent of a Dawson's finger could distinguish MS from NMO with 92% sensitivity and 96% specificity [51]. Diencephalic lesions are distinctly rare in MS and, if present, are more indicative of the diagnosis of NMO [8]. MRI changes suggestive of PRES have also been observed in NMO patients, although it is unclear if PRES was the result of NMO or a complication of therapy [47]. Kim et al. [52] described five categories of brain MRI lesions in NMO patients: (1) corticospinal tract lesions that were often related to LETM and likely represent Wallerian degeneration; (2) extensive, tumefactive, hemispheric white matter lesions with vasogenic edema; (3) periependymal lesions surrounding the cerebral aqueduct, third ventricle, or fourth ventricle; (4) periependymal lesions surrounding the lateral ventricles; and (5) medullary lesions, which were often contiguous with cervical cord lesions.

In patients with suspected AON, it is important to obtain an MRI of the orbits with and without gadolinium. Compared to MS, NMO-related AON often results in abnormal signal and gadolinium enhancement extending to the posterior portions of the optic nerves and even involves the optic chiasm (which some have termed this more extensive distribution along the anterior visual axis "longitudinally extensive optic neuritis") [53, 54].

NMO-IgG remains the most specific serologic marker of NMO and is one of the supportive criteria in the revised 2006 NMO diagnostic criteria [55]. Improved laboratory techniques have enhanced the sensitivity of NMO-IgG detection. NMO-IgG can be detected in almost three-quarters of recurrent NMO and predicts higher relapse rates [2, 56]. However, NMO-IgG titers are not reliable indicators of disease activity or prognosis [57].

Approximately 20–30% of patients who meet the criteria for NMO are NMO-IgG seronegative [57]. Antibodies against myelin oligodendrocyte glycoprotein (MOG-IgG) have been identified in a subset of NMO-IgG seronegative patients with NMO [58, 59]. MOG-IgG seropositivity has been strongly associated with bilateral relapsing AON, as well as simultaneous and sequential AON and TM [60, 61]. Interestingly, MOG-IgG seropositive AON is typically associated with corticosteroid-responsive papillitis on fundoscopic examination [60], a clinical finding that is distinctly atypical in MS-related AON.

NMO is often associated with organ-specific and nonspecific autoantibodies (e.g., antinuclear antibodies, SS-A, SS-B, ribonucleoprotein antibodies), often in the absence of corresponding disease [34, 62, 63]. The presence of autoantibodies does not militate against, but rather strengthens the evidence for a diagnosis of NMO.

Cerebrospinal fluid (CSF) should be obtained when evaluating a patient for possible NMO. CSF pleocytosis (>50 WBC/mm^3) may occur in NMO, particularly during an acute attack [34]; when present, a neutrophilic (>5 neutrophils/mm^3) and eosinophilic preponderance is usually detected [34]. CSF oligoclonal bands are infrequent in NMO (20–30%) [17, 24, 34, 55] and may only be detected during attacks [63] but are present in 85–90% of patients with MS [32]. In fact, in patients with TM and normal brain MRIs, the presence of CSF oligoclonal bands and an increased IgG index portend a higher risk of developing MS [32]. Other promising potential CSF biomarkers of NMO include glial fibrillary acidic protein (a marker of astrocytic destruction) [64] and IL-6 levels [13, 65, 66].

Diagnosis and Prognosis

The diagnosis of NMO can be made with confidence if patient's clinical, radiologic, and/or serologic findings meet the revised 2006 NMO diagnostic criteria (Box 9.1).

Box 9.1 The Revised 2006 Criteria for the Diagnosis of NMO [55]
1. Acute transverse myelitis
2. Acute optic neuritis
3. At least two of the following supportive criteria:
   (a) Longitudinally extensive transverse myelitis (contiguous MRI spinal cord lesion spanning at least three vertebral segments)
   (b) Brain MRI not meeting the McDonald criteria for the diagnosis of multiple sclerosis
   (c) NMO-IgG seropositivity

Diagnostic confusion may arise in patients who only manifest only limited forms of the disease, like isolated recurrent AON, TM, and diencephalic or brainstem syndromes; the term NMO spectrum disorder (NMOSD) has been applied to this subset of patients if they are seropositive for NMO-IgG [24].

However, under recently proposed guidelines (Box 9.2) [67], NMO would be subsumed into the single descriptive term NMOSD since the clinical behavior, immunopathogenesis, and treatment of patients with NMOSD and NMO are not demonstrably different. The new criteria allow the diagnosis of NMOSD to be made if the patient has at least one of six core clinical characteristics and are NMO-IgG seropositive. In those who are NMO-IgG seronegative, the diagnosis of NMOSD can be made if they meet a specific set of clinical (at least two core clinical characteristics, with at least one of these being AON, TM, or an area postrema syndrome) and MRI criteria. Furthermore, these guidelines strongly recommended that cell-based serum assays (quantitative fluorescence-activated cell-sorting assay [FACS]) be used to test for NMO-IgG, given the best current sensitivity and specificity of this method, compared to indirect immunofluorescence assays and enzyme-linked immunosorbent assays (ELISAs) [67].

Box 9.2 2015 NMO Spectrum Disorder (NMOSD) Diagnostic Criteria [67]
For NMO-IgG seropositive patients:

1. At least one core clinical characteristic
2. Alternate diagnoses excluded

For NMO-IgG seronegative patients:
At least two core clinical characteristics and meets all the following requirements:

1. At least one core clinical characteristic must be optic neuritis, LETM, or area postrema syndrome.
2. Dissemination in space (i.e., at least two core clinical characteristics).
3. Fulfillment of all MRI criteria (see below).
4. Alternate diagnoses excluded

Core clinical characteristics:

1. Acute optic neuritis
2. Acute myelitis
3. Area postrema syndrome
4. Acute brainstem syndrome
5. Symptomatic narcolepsy or acute diencephalic syndrome with NMOSD-typical diencephalic MRI lesions
6. Symptomatic cerebral syndrome with NMOSD-typical MRI lesions

MRI criteria for NMOSD in NMO-IgG seronegative patients:

1. Acute optic neuritis:
   (a) Normal or nonspecific brain MRI white matter lesions
   (b) Longitudinally extensive optic neuritis (i.e., abnormal T2 signal or gadolinium enhancement extending over half the optic nerve length *or* involves the chiasm)
2. Acute myelitis:
   (a) Longitudinally extensive transverse myelitis
   (b) Focal spinal atrophy extending over at least three contiguous vertebral segments in patients with a history consistent with myelitis
3. Area postrema syndrome: dorsal medullary lesion in the region of the area postrema
4. Acute brainstem syndrome: periependymal brainstem lesions

The outcome of NMO attacks is generally poor; only 21.6% of attacks show full clinical recovery, and 6% do not improve at all [68]. The presence of TM or bilateral AON tends to predict an unfavorable outcome; on the other hand, the absence of TM, as well as isolated unilateral AON, predicts a favorable outcome [68]. Following the initial attack, NMO can remit permanently (monophasic) or pursue a relapsing course [34]. The majority of NMO cases (approximately 90%) follow a relapsing course [23, 55, 67]. Near simultaneous bilateral AON and TM tend to favor monophasic disease; on the other hand, AON and TM attacks separated by weeks or months are more indicative of relapsing disease [23]. However, it is important to note that NMO can follow an unpredictable course, and mistakenly declaring the disease as "monophasic" could result in devastating consequences. As such, we strongly recommend that all patients with NMO/NMOSD be managed with immunotherapy aimed at curtailing future attacks (discussed below).

Treatment

Acute attacks of NMO can be treated with high-dose corticosteroid therapy (intravenous methylprednisolone 1000 mg daily for five consecutive days) [68, 69]. A recent study showed that only 17% of NMO relapses completely resolve following high-dose corticosteroid therapy; the majority of attacks demonstrate partial response (65.4%) [68], thereby suggesting that we once again emphasize the emerging adage that "time is tissue," and as such, the concomitant employment of corticosteroids and other treatment modalities, as close to the inception of the "ictus" as possible, likely has the best chance to accelerate recovery.

With respect to combining corticosteroids with other treatment strategies germane to both limiting the magnitude of tissue injury and the corresponding compromise in the patient's neurologic repertoire of capabilities. Another principal objective for the application of combination regimens is the prospect that particular measures may be effective in also accelerating the process of attenuating mechanisms that foment further inflammation, the vasogenic edematous burden within CNS tissue compartments that are inherently at greater risk of permanent damage and disorganization of their complex tissue architecture, at least in part, by virtue of their conspicuously limited compliance characteristics (i.e., small, perhaps even negligible changes in augmented tissue edema can result in escalation in compartment pressure, thereby resulting in altered flow characteristics with respect to fluid clearance and water homeostasis, both intracellularly as well as extracellularly).

Perhaps the neuroradiologic features of greatest conspicuity are those that also carry important prognostic ramifications, most specifically as they relate to the burden of residual physical disability, as a derivative of NMO-associated syndromes. Specifically, the longitudinally extensive spinal cord distribution of neuropathology associated with NMO reflects, in part, the movement of tissue water, both along and across tissue barriers.

As vasogenic edematous processes continue unabated, there is a dangerous and rapidly converging phenomenon that brings the expansion of spinal cord tissue water on a "collision course" with autoregulatory mechanisms that maintain adequate blood perfusion both across the transverse and caudal-rostral extent of the spinal axis.

Without rapid intervention to control the expansion of the vasogenic edema burden, the dynamic range of such compensatory responses is exceeded, with the potentially catastrophic consequence of embarrassed blood flow dynamics, including the failure of the circumferentially organized vascular arborization of the well-recognized vasocorona (which represents a final common vascular pathway for collateralizing ischemic changes across the transverse and longitudinal spinal axis).

Plasmapheresis (typically five full volume exchanges) has been shown to be an effective treatment for NMO relapses (as a first-line treatment or in treating steroid-refractory patients) [34, 70–76]. Since NMO is a humoral complement-mediated astrocytopathy, plasmapheresis is hypothesized to ameliorate attacks by removing pathogenic antibodies, activated complement, and cytokines from the circulation. Escalating therapy with plasmapheresis has been shown to significantly improve remission in corticosteroid-refractory patients [68]. In fact, early plasmapheresis has been shown to produce a better clinical outcome [34, 75]; in NMO patients with TM, early plasmapheresis is critical since TM is associated with a poor outcome [68]. In a small cohort of ten patients, intravenous immunoglobulin was shown to be beneficial in treating those who failed to stabilize with corticosteroids with or without plasmapheresis [77].

Once the acute attack of NMO has been stabilized, immunotherapy aimed at preventing further attacks should be instituted as soon as possible, since NMO relapses are potentially devastating. The importance of distinguishing MS from NMO is underscored by the fact that disease-modifying agents employed in MS, like interferon-beta, natalizumab, and fingolimod, are not only ineffective in NMO, but have been shown to aggravate NMO disease activity [78–81].

In MS, over time, the vast majority of patients will eventually transition from a predominantly relapsing-remitting course of both clinical and radiographic exacerbations, into the more insidious, often even imperceptible, recalcitrant, and, until recently, treatment-resistant phase of disease progression, the highly stereotyped signature of irreversible compromise (or even complete abolishment) of critical functional neurologic capabilities. In contradistinction, NMO has not been associated with a similar "progressive" course, but rather, the exacerbations themselves represent the principal corpus of activities, and the incomplete recovery from them, that drive the accrual of disability [23]. The rapid identification of the NMO clinical syndromes, followed by the expeditious employment of intensive and often combination therapy, is in keeping with accelerated cessation of the attack and its associated mechanisms. Without equivocation, immunosuppressive therapy to reduce humoral immune activity constitutes the mainstay for NMO disease-modifying treatment.

Azathioprine (AZA) was the first agent shown to be effective in preventing attacks and is typically used at doses of 2–3 mg/kg/day, often in combination with oral prednisone (1 mg/kg/day) [23, 82]. Potential adverse effects of AZA include transaminitis, leukopenia, gastrointestinal upset, recurrent infections, myelosuppression, and increased risk of lymphoma [82–85]. Although successful in reducing relapses, the majority of patients are unable to tolerate this regime; furthermore, many relapse when prednisone is tapered below 5–15 mg/day [69, 82]. In such cases, it would be better to consider alternative therapy to avoid the complications of chronic corticosteroid use. It is also important to remember that AZA should be avoided in patients with low thiopurine methyltransferase activity since this population is at risk of myelotoxicity [86].

In a retrospective study of 24 NMO patients, treatment with mycophenolate mofetil (MMF) has been shown to reduce relapses and stabilize the disease course [87]. A median dose of 2000 mg/day was used [87]. In our experience, MMF is a useful oral immunosuppressive agent to control disease activity in NMO and is far better tolerated than AZA. Potential adverse effects of MMF include gastrointestinal upset, photosensitivity, recurrent infections, and myelosuppression [83]. We recommend checking blood counts, renal function, and liver function every 3 months in patients on MMF to monitor for these potential adverse reactions.

Rituximab, a chimeric anti-CD20 monoclonal antibody that depletes B-cell and plasmablast levels, has been shown to be very effective in treating NMO [83, 88–94], underscoring the role of B-cell dysregulation in NMO etiopathogenesis. Rituximab is well tolerated; typical adverse reactions are infusion related (fever, chills, rash, angioedema, bronchospasm, and hypotension) and, infrequently, cardiac arrhythmias [23]. One important safety consideration before commencing rituximab therapy is to test for hepatitis B and C since rituximab has been associated with reactivation of these diseases [95–97].

While the precise rituximab-dosing interval in NMO is not clear, our center monitors monthly CD19 cell counts, and when cell counts begin to recover (i.e., when the percent of CD19 cells approaches 1%), we initiate re-treatment. While rituximab is an antibody against CD20 localized upon pre-B-cells, we employ the monthly surveillance strategy of specifically ascertaining when the CD19+ fraction is returning and approaching 1–2% [92]. The rationale for emphasizing the utilization of the CD19+ fraction of B-cells is related to the observation that this cell surface antigen is expressed earlier and persists later than CD20. As such, our surveillance strategy has allowed us to "bracket" our treatment in order to avoid "being late" in the re-treatment with the disease-modifying agent for NMO and to thereby avoid additional exacerbations.

It is important to underscore that beyond the 1–2% circulating composition of the CD19 fraction, the reconstitution curve (for CD19+ cells) becomes sigmoidal and thereby reflects the accelerated return of the B-cell fraction, along with the propensity to develop new exacerbations. Our group has investigated the role of rituximab dose magnitude and the duration of CD19 suppression. In essence, a 100 mg dose of rituximab administered intravenously is associated with a mean reduction (i.e., below 1%) of about 3 months, whereas a 1000 mg dose may suppress the CD19 fraction for about 9–12 months [92]. The next generation of anti-CD20 monoclonal antibodies (ocrelizumab and ofatumumab) is currently being studied in MS [98] and would also be potentially useful for treating NMO.

Mitoxantrone, which is approved for the treatment of MS, is also effective in NMO, but carries significant safety risks (including cardiotoxicity and hematogenous malignancies) [90, 99–101]. Cyclophosphamide is somewhat effective but is poorly tolerated, carcinogenic, and gonadotoxic [83, 102, 103]. Other therapies that have been described in small cohort of NMO patients include oral methotrexate [104], low-dose periodic oral corticosteroids [105], cyclosporine in combination with oral corticosteroids [106], preventive plasmapheresis [107, 108], and glatiramer acetate with [109] or without [110] intermittent corticosteroid pulses.

Novel therapeutic strategies that are being explored include eculizumab (a monoclonal antibody that inhibits complement protein C5) [111], aquaporumab (a nonpathogenic monoclonal antibody that competitively inhibits NMO-IgG) [112], and tocilizumab (anti-IL-6 receptor monoclonal antibody which prevented NMO relapses and controlled the neurogenic pain of the disease) [113].

Conclusion

NMO is a humoral autoimmune disease characterized by antibody- and complement-mediated astrocytic destruction. Classic manifestations of NMO/NMOSD include severe AON, LETM, and the area postrema syndrome. Serologic testing for NMO-IgG (using the most sensitive and specific methods, i.e., cell-based assays) should always be considered in patients with such symptoms, especially in those without brain MRI lesions that are typical for MS. The vast majority of NMO patients pursue a relapsing course, and as such, immunotherapy to prevent future attacks should be instituted in every NMO patient as soon as possible to avert potentially devastating (or even lethal) relapses.

Disclosures The authors have no relevant financial disclosures.

References

1. Jarius S, Wildemann B. The history of neuromyelitis optica. J Neuroinflammation. 2013;10:8.
2. Lennon VA, Wingerchuk DM, Kryzer TJ, et al. A serum autoantibody marker of neuromyelitis optica: distinction from multiple sclerosis. Lancet. 2004;364:2106–12.
3. Lennon VA, Kryzer TJ, Pittock SJ, Verkman AS, Hinson SR. IgG marker of optic-spinal multiple sclerosis binds to the aquaporin-4 water channel. J Exp Med. 2005;202:473–7.
4. Jarius S, Franciotta D, Bergamaschi R, et al. NMO-IgG in the diagnosis of neuromyelitis optica. Neurology. 2007;68:1076–7.
5. Paul F, Jarius S, Aktas O, et al. Antibody to aquaporin 4 in the diagnosis of neuromyelitis optica. PLoS Med. 2007;4:e133.
6. Takahashi T, Fujihara K, Nakashima I, et al. Anti-aquaporin-4 antibody is involved in the pathogenesis of NMO: a study on antibody titre. Brain. 2007;130:1235–43.
7. Jung JS, Preston GM, Smith BL, Guggino WB, Agre P. Molecular structure of the water channel through aquaporin CHIP. The hourglass model. J Biol Chem. 1994;269:14648–54.
8. Pittock SJ, Weinshenker BG, Lucchinetti CF, et al. Neuromyelitis optica brain lesions localized at sites of high aquaporin 4 expression. Arch Neurol. 2006;63:964–8.
9. Misu T, Fujihara K, Kakita A, et al. Loss of aquaporin 4 in lesions of neuromyelitis optica: distinction from multiple sclerosis. Brain. 2007;130:1224–34.
10. Roemer SF, Parisi JE, Lennon VA, et al. Pattern-specific loss of aquaporin-4 immunoreactivity distinguishes neuromyelitis optica from multiple sclerosis. Brain. 2007;130:1194–205.

11. Lucchinetti CF, Guo Y, Popescu BF, et al. The pathology of an autoimmune astrocytopathy: lessons learned from neuromyelitis optica. Brain Pathol. 2014;24:83–97.
12. Frohman EM, Racke MK, Raine CS. Multiple sclerosis–he plaque and its pathogenesis. N Engl J Med. 2006;354:942–55.
13. Chihara N, Aranami T, Sato W, et al. Interleukin 6 signaling promotes anti-aquaporin 4 auto-antibody production from plasmablasts in neuromyelitis optica. Proc Natl Acad Sci U S A. 2011;108:3701–6.
14. Bennett JL, Lam C, Kalluri SR, et al. Intrathecal pathogenic anti-aquaporin-4 antibodies in early neuromyelitis optica. Ann Neurol. 2009;66:617–29.
15. Bennett JL, O'Connor KC, Bar-Or A, et al. B lymphocytes in neuromyelitis optica. Neurol Neuroimmunol Neuroinflamm. 2015;2:e104.
16. Kinoshita M, Nakatsuji Y. Where do AQP4 antibodies fit in the pathogenesis of NMO? Mult Scler Int. 2012;2012:862169.
17. Bizzoco E, Lolli F, Repice AM, et al. Prevalence of neuromyelitis optica spectrum disorder and phenotype distribution. J Neurol. 2009;256:1891–8.
18. Wingerchuk DM. Neuromyelitis optica: effect of gender. J Neurol Sci. 2009;286:13–8.
19. Cabrera-Gomez JA, Kurtzke JF, Gonzalez-Quevedo A, Lara-Rodriguez R. An epidemiological study of neuromyelitis optica in Cuba. J Neurol. 2009;256:35–44.
20. Sahraian MA, Moinfar Z, Khorramnia S, Ebrahim MM. Relapsing neuromyelitis optica: demographic and clinical features in Iranian patients. Eur J Neurol. 2010;17:794–9.
21. Mealy MA, Wingerchuk DM, Greenberg BM, Levy M. Epidemiology of neuromyelitis optica in the United States: a multicenter analysis. Arch Neurol. 2012;69:1176–80.
22. Cossburn M, Tackley G, Baker K, et al. The prevalence of neuromyelitis optica in South East Wales. Eur J Neurol. 2012;19:655–9.
23. Wingerchuk DM, Weinshenker BG. Neuromyelitis optica (Devic's syndrome). Handb Clin Neurol. 2014;122:581–99.
24. Wingerchuk DM, Lennon VA, Lucchinetti CF, et al. The spectrum of neuromyelitis optica. Lancet Neurol. 2007;6:805–15.
25. Balcer LJ. Optic neuritis. N Engl J Med. 2006;354:1273–80.
26. Toosy AT, Mason DF, Miller DH. Optic neuritis. Lancet Neurol. 2014;13:83–99.
27. Jarius S, Frederikson J, Waters P, et al. Frequency and prognostic impact of antibodies to aquaporin-4 in patients with optic neuritis. J Neurol Sci. 2010;298:158–62.
28. Jarius S, Ruprecht K, Wildemann B, et al. Contrasting disease patterns in seropositive and seronegative neuromyelitis optica: a multicentre study of 175 patients. J Neuroinflammation. 2012;9:14.
29. Jiao Y, Fryer JP, Lennon VA, et al. Updated estimate of AQP4-IgG serostatus and disability outcome in neuromyelitis optica. Neurology. 2013;81:1197–204.
30. Petzold A, Pittock S, Lennon V, et al. Neuromyelitis optica-IgG (aquaporin-4) autoantibodies in immune mediated optic neuritis. J Neurol Neurosurg Psychiatry. 2010;81:109–11.
31. Sotirchos ES, Saidha S, Byraiah G, et al. In vivo identification of morphologic retinal abnormalities in neuromyelitis optica. Neurology. 2013;80:1406–14.
32. Beh SC, Greenberg BM, Frohman T, Frohman EM. Transverse myelitis. Neurol Clin. 2013;31:79–138.
33. Scott TF, Frohman EM, De Seze J, Gronseth GS, Weinshenker BG. Evidence-based guideline: clinical evaluation and treatment of transverse myelitis: report of the Therapeutics and Technology Assessment Subcommittee of the American Academy of Neurology. Neurology. 2011;77:2128–34.
34. Weinshenker BG, O'Brien PC, Petterson TM, et al. A randomized trial of plasma exchange in acute central nervous system inflammatory demyelinating disease. Ann Neurol. 1999;46:878–86.
35. Kanamori Y, Nakashima I, Takai Y, et al. Pain in neuromyelitis optica and its effect on quality of life: a cross-sectional study. Neurology. 2011;77:652–8.
36. Misu T, Fujihara K, Nakashima I, et al. Intractable hiccup and nausea with periaqueductal lesions in neuromyelitis optica. Neurology. 2005;65:1479–82.
37. Apiwattanakul M, Popescu BF, Matiello M, et al. Intractable vomiting as the initial presentation of neuromyelitis optica. Ann Neurol. 2010;68:757–61.

38. Hage Jr R, Merle H, Jeannin S, Cabre P. Ocular oscillations in the neuromyelitis optica spectrum. J Neuroophthalmol. 2011;31:255–9.
39. Jarius S, Lauda F, Wildemann B, Tumani H. Steroid-responsive hearing impairment in NMO-IgG/aquaporin-4-antibody-positive neuromyelitis optica. J Neurol. 2013;260:663–4.
40. Iorio R, Lucchinetti CF, Lennon VA, et al. Syndrome of inappropriate antidiuresis may herald or accompany neuromyelitis optica. Neurology. 2011;77:1644–6.
41. Baba T, Nakashima I, Kanbayashi T, et al. Narcolepsy as an initial manifestation of neuromyelitis optica with anti-aquaporin-4 antibody. J Neurol. 2009;256:287–8.
42. Kanbayashi T, Shimohata T, Nakashima I, et al. Symptomatic narcolepsy in patients with neuromyelitis optica and multiple sclerosis: new neurochemical and immunological implications. Arch Neurol. 2009;66:1563–6.
43. Fung EL-W, Tsung LL-Y, Dale RC. Aquaporin-4 autoantibody: a neurogenic cause of anorexia and weight loss. Dev Med Child Neurol. 2012;54:45–7.
44. Qiu W, Raven S, Wu J-S, et al. Hypothalamic lesions in multiple sclerosis. J Neurol Neurosurg Psychiatry. 2011;82:819–22.
45. Suzuki N, Takahashi T, Aoki M, et al. Neuromyelitis optica preceded by hyperCKemia episode. Neurology. 2010;74:1543–5.
46. Guo Y, Lennon VA, Popescu BF, et al. Autoimmune aquaporin-4 myopathy in neuromyelitis optica spectrum. JAMA Neurol. 2014;71:1025–9.
47. Magana SM, Matiello M, Pittock SJ, et al. Posterior reversible encephalopathy syndrome in neuromyelitis optica spectrum disorders. Neurology. 2009;72:712–7.
48. Bot JCJ, Barkhof F, Polman CH, et al. Spinal cord abnormalities in recently diagnosed MS patients: added value of spinal MRI examination. Neurology. 2004;62:226–33.
49. Nakamura M, Miyazawa I, Fujihara K, et al. Preferential spinal central gray matter involvement in neuromyelitis optica. An MRI study J Neurol. 2008;255:163–70.
50. Takai Y, Misu T, Nakashima I, et al. Two cases of lumbosacral myeloradiculitis with anti-aquaporin-4 antibody. Neurology. 2012;79:1826–8.
51. Matthews L, Marasco R, Jenkinson M, et al. Distinction of seropositive NMO spectrum disorder and MS brain lesion distribution. Neurology. 2013;80:1330–7.
52. Kim W, Park MS, Lee SH, et al. Characteristic brain magnetic resonance imaging abnormalities in central nervous system aquaporin-4 autoimmunity. Mult Scler. 2010;16:1229–36.
53. Khanna S, Sharma HJ, et al. Magnetic resonance imaging of optic neuritis in patients with neuromyelitis optica versus multiple sclerosis. J Neuroophthalmol. 2012;32:216–20.
54. Mealy MA, Whetstone A, Orman G, et al. Longitudinally extensive optic neuritis as an MRI biomarker distinguishes neuromyelitis optica from multiple sclerosis. J Neurol Sci. 2015;355:59–63.
55. Wingerchuk DM, Lennon VA, Pittock SJ, Lucchinetti CF, Weinshenker BG. Revised diagnostic criteria for neuromyelitis optica. Neurology. 2006;66:1485–9.
56. Ketelslegers IA, Modderman PW, Vennegoor A, Killestein J, Hamann D, Hintzen RQ. Antibodies against aquaporin-4 in neuromyelitis optica: distinction between recurrent and monophasic patients. Mult Scler. 2011;17:1527–30.
57. Melamed E, Levy M, Waters PJ, et al. Update on biomarkers in neuromyelitis optica. Neurol Neuroimmunol Neuroinflamm. 2015;2:e134.
58. Mader S, Gredler V, Schanda K, et al. Complement activating antibodies to myelin oligodendrocyte glycoprotein in neuromyelitis optica and related disorders. J Neuroinflammation. 2011;8:184.
59. Rostásy K, Mader S, Schanda K, et al. Anti-myelin oligodendrocyte glycoprotein antibodies in pediatric patients with optic neuritis. Arch Neurol. 2012;69:752–6.
60. Ramanathan S, Reddel SW, Henderson A, et al. Antibodies to myelin oligodendrocyte glycoprotein in bilateral and recurrent optic neuritis. Neurol Neuroimmunol Neuroinflamm. 2014;1:e40.
61. Kitley J, Waters P, Woodhall M, et al. Neuromyelitis optica spectrum disorders with aquaporin-4 and myelin-oligodendrocyte glycoprotein antibodies: a comparative study. JAMA Neurol. 2014;71:276–83.
62. Pittock SJ, Lennon VA, de Seze J, et al. Neuromyelitis optica and non organ-specific autoimmunity. Arch Neurol. 2008;65:78–83.

63. Jarius S, Jacobi C, de Seze J, et al. Frequency and syndrome of specificity of antibodies to aquaporin-4 in neurological patients with rheumatic disorders. Mult Scler. 2011;17:1067–73.

64. Takano R, Misu T, Takahashi T, et al. Astrocytic damage is far more severe than demyelination in NMO: a clinical CSF biomarker study. Neurology. 2010;75:208–16.

65. Uzawa A, Mori M, Ito M, et al. Markedly increased CSF interleukin-6 levels in neuromyelitis optica, but not in multiple sclerosis. J Neurol. 2009;256:2082–4.

66. Matsushita T, Tateishi T, Isobe N, et al. Characteristic cerebrospinal fluid cytokine/chemokine profiles in neuromyelitis optica, relapsing remitting or primary progressive multiple sclerosis. PLoS One. 2013;8:e61835.

67. Wingerchuk DM, Banwell B, Bennett JL, et al. International consensus diagnostic criteria for neuromyelitis optica spectrum disorders. Neurology. 2015;85:177–89.

68. Kleiter I, Gahlen A, Borisow N, et al. Neuromyelitis optica: evaluation of 871 attacks and 1153 treatment courses. Ann Neurol. 2015;79(2):206–16. [Epub ahead of print].

69. Wingerchuk DM, Weinshenker BG. Neuromyelitis optica. Curr Treat Options Neurol. 2008;10:55–66.

70. Keegan M, Pineda AA, McClelland RL, et al. Plasma exchange for severe attacks of CNS demyelination: predictors of response. Neurology. 2002;58:143–6.

71. Watanabe S, Nakashima I, Misu T, et al. Therapeutic efficacy of plasma exchange in NMO-IgG-positive patients with neuromyelitis optica. Mult Scler. 2007;13:128–32.

72. Bonnan M, Valentino R, Olindo S, et al. Plasma exchange in severe spinal attacks associated with neuromyelitis optica spectrum disorder. Mult Scler. 2009;15:487–92.

73. Magana SM, Keegan BM, Weinshenker BG, et al. Beneficial plasma exchange response in central nervous system inflammatory demyelination. Arch Neurol. 2011;68:870–8.

74. Roesner S, Appel R, Gbadamosi J, et al. Treatment of steroid-unresponsive optic neuritis with plasma exchange. Acta Neurol Scand. 2012;126:103–8.

75. Bonnan M, Cabre P. Plasma exchange in severe attacks of neuromyelitis optica. Mult Scler Int. 2012;2012:787630.

76. Merle H, Olindo S, Jeannin S, et al. Treatment of optic neuritis by plasma exchange (add-on) in neuromyelitis optica. Arch Ophthalmol. 2012;130:858–62.

77. Elsone L, Panicker J, Mutch K, et al. Role of intravenous immunoglobulin in the treatment of acute relapses of neuromyelitis optica: experience in 10 patients. Mult Scler. 2014;20:501–4.

78. Papeix C, Vidal JS, de Seze J, et al. Immunosuppressive therapy is more effective than interferon in neuromyelitis optica. Mult Scler. 2007;13:256–9.

79. Shimizu J, Hatanaka Y, Hasagawa M, et al. IFNbeta-1b may severely exacerbate Japanese optic-spinal MS in neuromyelitis optica spectrum. Neurology. 2010;75:1423–7.

80. Kleiter I, Hellwig K, Berthele A, et al. Failure of natalizumab to prevent relapses in neuromyelitis optica. Arch Neurol. 2012;69:239–45.

81. Min JH, Kim BJ, Lee KH, et al. Development of extensive brain lesions following fingolimod (FTY720) treatment in a patient with neuromyelitis optica spectrum disorder. Mult Scler. 2012;18:113–5.

82. Costanzi C, Matiello LCF, et al. Azathioprine: tolerability, efficacy, and predictors of benefit in neuromyelitis optica. Neurology. 2011;77:659–66.

83. Torres J, Pruitt A, Balcer L, et al. Analysis of the treatment of neuromyelitis optica. J Neurol Sci. 2015;351:31–5.

84. Kandiel A, Fraser AG, Korelitz BI, et al. Increased risk of lymphoma among inflammatory bowel disease patients treated with azathioprine and 6-mercaptopurine. Gut. 2005;54:1121–5.

85. Bernatsky S, Clarke AE, Suissa S. Hematologic malignant neoplasms after drug exposure in rheumatoid arthritis. Arch Intern Med. 2008;168:378–81.

86. Lennard L, Van Loon JA, Weinshilboum RM. Pharmacogenetics of acute azathioprine toxicity: relationship to thiopurine methyltransferase genetic polymorphism. Clin Pharmacol Ther. 1989;46:149–54.

87. Jacob A, Matiello M, Weinshenker BG, et al. Treatment of neuromyelitis optica with mycophenolate mofetil: retrospective analysis of 24 patients. Arch Neurol. 2009;66: 1128–33.
88. Cree BA, Lamb S, Morgan K, et al. An open label study of the effects of rituximab in neuromyelitis optica. Neurology. 2005;64:1270–2.
89. Jacob A, Weinshenker BG, Violich I, et al. Treatment of neuromyelitis optica with rituximab: retrospective analysis of 25 patients. Arch Neurol. 2008;65:1443–8.
90. Kim S-H, Kim W, Li XF, et al. Repeated treatment with rituximab based on the assessment of peripheral circulating memory B cells in patients with relapsing neuromyelitis optica over 2 years. Arch Neurol. 2011;68:1412–20.
91. Bedi GS, Brown AD, Delgado SR, et al. Impact of rituximab on relapse rate and disability in neuromyelitis optica. Mult Scler. 2011;17:1225–30.
92. Greenberg BM, Graves D, Remington G, et al. Rituximab dosing and monitoring strategies in neuromyelitis optica patients: creating strategies for therapeutic success. Mult Scler. 2012;18:1022–6.
93. Kim S-H, Huh S-Y, Lee SJ, et al. A 5-year follow-up of rituximab treatment in patients with neuromyelitis optica spectrum disorder. JAMA Neurol. 2013;70:1110–7.
94. Mealy MA, Wingerchuk DM, Palace J, et al. Comparison of relapse and treatment failure rates among patients with neuromyelitis optica: multicenter study of treatment efficacy. JAMA Neurol. 2014;71:324–30.
95. Dervite I, Hober D, Morel P. Acute hepatitis B in a patient with antibodies to hepatitis B surface antigen who was receiving rituximab. N Engl J Med. 2001;344:68–9.
96. Mahale P, Kontoyiannis DP, Chemaly RF, et al. Acute exacerbation and reactivation of chronic hepatitis C virus infection in cancer patients. J Hepatol. 2012;57:1177–85.
97. Tsutsumi Y, Kanamori H, Mori A, et al. Reactivation of hepatitis B virus with rituximab. Expert Opin Drug Saf. 2005;4:599–608.
98. Van Meerten T, Hagenbeek A. CD20-targeted therapy: the next generation of antibodies. Semin Hematol. 2010;47:199–210.
99. Cabre P, Olindo S, Marignier R, et al. Efficacy of mitoxantrone in neuromyelitis optica spectrum: clinical and neuroradiological study. J Neurol Neurosurg Psychiatry. 2013;84: 511–6.
100. Cohen BA, Mikol DD. Mitoxantrone treatment of multiple sclerosis: safety considerations. Neurology. 2004;63:S28–32.
101. Weinstock-Guttman B, Ramanathan M, Lincoff N, et al. Study of mitoxantrone for the treatment of recurrent neuromyelitis optica (Devic disease). Arch Neurol. 2006;63:957–96.
102. Bichuetti DB, Lobato de Oliveira EM, Oliveira DM, et al. Neuromyelitis optica treatment: analysis of 36 patients. Arch Neurol. 2010;67:1131–6.
103. Yaguchi H, Sakushima K, Takahashi I, et al. Efficacy of intravenous cyclophosphamide therapy for neuromyelitis optica spectrum disorder. Intern Med. 2013;52:969–72.
104. Kitley J, Elsone L, George J, et al. Methotrexate is an alternative to azathioprine in neuromyelitis optica spectrum disorders with aquaporin-4 antibodies. J Neurol Neurosurg Psychiatry. 2013;84:918–21.
105. Watanabe S, Misu T, Miyazawa I, et al. Low-dose corticosteroids reduce relapses in neuromyelitis optica: a retrospective analysis. Mult Scler. 2007;13:968–74.
106. Kageyama T, Komori M, Miyamoto K, et al. Combination of cyclosporine A with corticosteroids is effective for the treatment of neuromyelitis optica. J Neurol. 2013;260:627–34.
107. Miyamoto K, Kusunoki S. Intermittent plasmapheresis prevents recurrence in neuromyelitis optica. Ther Apher Dial. 2009;13:505–8.
108. Khatri BO, Kramer J, Dukic M, et al. Maintenance plasma exchange therapy for steroid-refractory neuromyelitis optica. J Clin Apher. 2012;27:183–92.
109. Gartzen K, Limmroth V, Putzki N. Relapsing neuromyelitis optica responsive to glatiramer acetate treatment. Eur J Neurol. 2007;14:e12–3.

110. Bergamaschi R, Uggetti C, Tonietti S, et al. A case of relapsing neuromyelitis optica treated with glatiramer acetate. J Neurol. 2003;250:359–61.
111. Pittock SJ, Lennon VA, McKeon A, et al. Eculizumab in AQP4-IgG-positive relapsing neuromyelitis optica spectrum disorders: an open-label pilot study. Lancet Neurol. 2013;12:554–62.
112. Tradtrantip L, Zhang H, Saadoun S, et al. Anti-aquaporin-4 monoclonal antibody blocker therapy for neuromyelitis optica. Ann Neurol. 2012;71:314–22.
113. Araki M, Matsuoka T, Miyamoto K, et al. Efficacy of the anti-IL 6 receptor antibody tocilizumab in neuromyelitis optica: a pilot study. Neurology. 2014;82:1302–6.

Immunopathogenesis and Treatment of Guillain-Barre Syndrome and Chronic Inflammatory Demyelinating Polyneuropathy

10

Elena Grebenciucova and Kourosh Rezania

Guillain-Barre Syndrome (GBS)

GBS represents a spectrum of polyneuropathies, which arise from immune-mediated attack on different myelin or axonal antigens of peripheral and/or cranial nerves. GBS is the most common cause of flaccid paralysis worldwide after the elimination of poliomyelitis [1]. GBS encompasses a spectrum of diseases (i.e., subtypes) with varied clinical manifestations, reflective of the target antigen of autoimmune attack (myelin vs. axon) as well as the location of immunopathology within the peripheral nervous system (nerve roots, plexi, distal nerves, cranial nerves). Besides the autoimmune etiology, the GBS subtypes share the acute to subacute onset and albuminocytological dissociation in the CSF.

Subtypes of GBS have been defined based on the clinical manifestations, neurophysiological features, and presence of different antibodies to neural glycolipid components. Acute inflammatory demyelinating polyneuropathy (AIDP) constitutes the typical primarily demyelinating form of the disease. AIDP is the most common subtype of GBS in Europe and North America and is typically characterized by acute onset of flaccid, hypo-, or areflexic paralysis [1, 2]. The clinical course consists of progressive weakness within hours to days and maximum weakness and disability within 4 weeks. Muscle weakness (including proximal limb and respiratory) usually dominates the clinical presentation. However, sensory symptoms, usually a distal paresthesia, very often allow distinguishing AIDP from some of its mimics such as myasthenia gravis and botulism. Dysautonomia is prevalent in AIDP and is one of its life-threatening manifestations. A less common, atypical presentation, which is encountered in 8% of the patients, is paraparesis without arm weakness. [3] Patients with paraparetic GBS, however, usually have sensory symptoms and areflexia, as well as abnormal conduction studies in the upper

E. Grebenciucova • K. Rezania, MD (✉)
University of Chicago Medical Center, Department of Neurology, Chicago, IL, USA
e-mail: krezania@neurology.bsd.uchicago.edu

© Springer International Publishing AG 2017
A. Minagar, J.S. Alexander (eds.), *Inflammatory Disorders of the Nervous System*, Current Clinical Neurology, DOI 10.1007/978-3-319-51220-4_10

extremities [3]. Acute motor axonal neuropathy (AMAN) is the second most common form of GBS in North America and Europe, accounting for 6–78% of the cases, and the most common in China and Bangladesh [4]. AMAN patients have a purely motor picture (positive sensory symptoms in only 10% of patients). In contrast to AIDP, dysautonomia and cranial nerve involvement are rare, and deep tendon reflexes are often normal to brisk in AMAN [4]. AMAN is also associated with a more rapid progression early in the course, with earlier peak than AIDP (11.5 vs. 18 days) [5]. Acute motor and sensory axonal neuropathy is the third GBS subtype which has sensory involvement (in contrast to AMAN) and is characterized by less favorable recovery because of axonal degeneration. Miller Fisher syndrome (MFS), the fourth major subtype of GBS, accounts for 5–12% of the GBS cases [6]. MFS typically presents with a triad of ophthalmoparesis, ataxia, and areflexia, and the patients generally do not develop significant weakness or respiratory impairment and have a good prognosis. MFS by itself has different clinical subtypes: acute ataxic neuropathy (without ophthalmoplegia), acute ophthalmoparesis (without ataxia), and a variant with CNS symptoms such as hypersomnolence (Bickerstaff's encephalitis) [1]. Yet another less common, local subtypes of MFS include pharyngeal-cervical-brachial variant, which is characterized by rapidly progressive weakness of oropharyngeal, cervical, and upper extremity muscles accompanied by areflexia of the upper extremities [7].

Examination of cerebrospinal fluid (CSF) demonstrates albuminocytological dissociation in all the variants of GBS. Another useful diagnostic test is nerve conduction study and abnormal nerve conduction study, which demonstrates segmental demyelination in AIDP and axonal neuropathy in AMAN, AMSAN, and MFS and its variants [8]. It should be noted that conduction block, which is characteristic for AMAN, is secondary to functional blockage of axonal salutatory conduction and not secondary to segmental demyelination, leading to the recommendation that at least two sets of nerve conduction studies over time to differentiate AIDP from AMAN [9].

Pathology

AIDP is characterized by lymphocytic (mainly T cell) and macrophage infiltration and associated segmental demyelination, which affect nerve roots, plexi, and proximal portions of the nerves, which are more myelinated [10, 11]. Complement activation has been suggested to play an early role, as deposition of complement activation marker C3d and terminal complement complex C5b-9 on the surface of Schwann cells and myelin degeneration were shown to precede macrophage infiltration in patients who succumbed in early stage of AIDP [12].

On the other hand, postmortem findings in AMAN subtype may show Wallerian degeneration of the motor axons; presence of macrophages within the periaxonal space, which surround or displace the axons; and intact myelin sheath [13]. Some of the AMAN patients with fatal paralysis have had minimal axonal degeneration in the postmortem study consistent with functional impairment of axonal electrical conduction in these cases [13]. Axonal degeneration of the motor and sensory nerves is the hallmark of the neuropathology in AMSAN [13]. Because of the benign clinical course of MFS, the pathological studies are limited. Although segmental demyelination is reported in a patient with MFS [14], the patient more likely had AIDP and associated ophthalmoplegia.

Immunopathogenesis

About two thirds of GBS cases occur after a respiratory or gastrointestinal infection, and the pathogen can be identified in about half of these cases [15]. Some of the more common preceding infections include *C. jejuni* cytomegalovirus, Epstein-Barr virus, *Mycoplasma* pneumonia, *Hemophilus* influenza, influenza A, and hepatitis E virus [2]. The best explanation for the association of GBS and aforementioned infections is molecular mimicry between the components of pathogens and axonal or myelin structures. *C. jejuni* is the most common antecedent infection in GBS, ranging from 26 to 65% of the cases depending on the geographic location [4]. Patients with AMAN after *C. jejuni* infection have high titers of antibodies to GM1 and GD1a, which is the result of cross-reactivity between lipo-oligosaccharides from the bacterial wall of *C. jejuni* and respective gangliosides of the motor nerve axons [16, 17]. On the other hand, lipo-oligosaccharides that mimic the carbohydrate moiety of peripheral nerve gangliosides are expressed in only a subset of *C. jejuni* strains, Penner D: 19 serogroup, as it is different from other serotypes in containing genes for enzymes involved in synthesis of sialic acids which result in molecular mimicry with gangliosides GM1, GD1a ND GD1B [1]. As a result, GBS is a relatively rare outcome of these infections: e.g., only one out of 5000 *C. pylori* gastroenteritis results in GBS [18]. Whether *C. jejuni* infection is a cause of AIDP is a matter of controversy. A previous study showed that only 5 of 22 (23%) of patients with GBS post *C. jejuni* infection had AIDP, but when they were followed by repeated nerve conduction studies, all of those who had prolonged motor distal latencies normalized in less than 2 weeks suggestive for impaired axonal conductivity (seen in AMAN) rather than segmental demyelination seen in AIDP, which is associated with more slowing of the nerve conduction study in the same time period during remyelination [19]. A neuropathy characterized by severe axonal degeneration and seropositivity for IgG or IgM GM1 antibodies has also been reported in patients who received ganglioside injections for chronic pain [20]. IgG antibodies against GQ1b and GD1a are detected in more than 90% of patients with MFS [21–23], as well as patients with AIDP who have ophthalmoplegia. As about half of patients with pharyngeal-cervical-brachial variants are seropositive for IgG anti-GT1a antibodies which cross-reacts with GQ1b, it is considered to be in the broad spectrum of MFS [7].

Differences in anatomical expression of gangliosides explain the diverse phenotypic manifestations of GBS variants. GM1 is suggested to be expressed more in the motor than sensory nerve roots, therefore providing possible explanation for motor involvement of AMAN [23]. On the other hand, GM1/GD1a is also present in the sensory nerves [24]. The predominant or pure motor involvement could be the result of specificity of autoantibodies for epitopes of these gangliosides that are only present in the motor axons. Furthermore, nodes of Ranvier of the distal, intramuscular portion of the motor axons are suggested to be particularly susceptible to complement activation by antibodies to GD1a [25]. The blood-nerve barrier is more permeable in the unmyelinated distal branches of the motor nerves and the nerve roots, making these parts of the peripheral nerves more vulnerable to circulating factors such as autoantibodies and complement [26, 27]. Ophthalmoplegia and areflexia in MFS which is associated with antibodies directed to GQ1b are explained by high expression of GQ1b in the oculomotor nerves and muscle spindles [23].

The autoantigen involved in AIDP is so far unknown, and most of the AIDP patients are not seropositive for antiganglioside antibodies. Some of the putative antigens include proteins which are expressed at the nodes of Ranvier (neurofascin 186, gliomedin, sodium channels, ankyrin, and spectrin) and at the paranode (neurofascin 155, contactin/Caspr 1, and connexins Cx31.3, Cx3232) [23].

A recently identified molecular target is moesin in patients with CMV infection as antibodies against moesin were present in most of AIDP cases after CMV but not with other GBS patients or other neurological disease controls [28]. Moesin is expressed in the microvilli of the Schwann cells and has been proposed to have a critical role in myelination [29].

There is also evidence for involvement of T cells in the pathogenesis of GBS, based on: (1) T cell infiltration is present in experimental allergic neuritis (EAN) which is considered as an animal model of GBS. (2) There is increased frequency of Th1 and Th17 levels in the blood and of T cell-related cytokines (IFN gamma, IL-17, and IL-22) in the cerebrospinal fluid of GBS patients [30–32]. (3) Reduced number and abnormal function of $CD4^+Foxp3^+$ (T_{reg}) cells, which have a critical role in immune homeostasis, have been demonstrated in the blood of GBS patients [32, 33].

Animal Models

Experimental allergic neuritis (EAN) has been considered as an animal model for human GBS. EAN is usually (but not always) a monophasic illness, which is induced by vaccination of rats, mice, rabbits, and guinea pigs with peripheral nerve homogenate or different myelin proteins such as P0, PMP 22, and P2 [34–37]. It presents with weakness and ataxia after a period of about 2 weeks after the vaccination. Perivascular T cell infiltration is noted 2–3 days before the onset of demyelination and paralysis [36, 37]. T cell infiltration results in activation of monocytes to tissue macrophages, which subsequently strip myelin and cause axonal injury by secreting cytokines such as tumor necrosis factor alpha. B cells also play a role in the pathogenesis of EAN, and autoantibodies against the myelin play a synergistic role in causing demyelination, after the blood-nerve barrier has become more permeable because of T cell activation and subsequent infiltration of macrophages [38]. Although the target antigen in EAN remains to be elusive, neurofascin 186 and gliomedin, which are involved in clustering of voltage-gated Na channels at the nodes of

Ranvier, have been suggested as potential antigenic targets [39, 40]. In the EAN model induced by vaccination with peripheral myelin in rat, antibodies to neurofascin and gliomedin cause dismantling of nodal organization and Na channel clusters, therefore leading to conduction block prior to onset of demyelination [39, 40].

B cell immunity, particularly autoantibodies to gangliosides, appears to have a primary role in the pathogenesis of GBS variants. Immunization of Japanese white rabbits with a bovine brain ganglioside mixture or isolated GM1 results in an AMAN phenotype: acute monophasic flaccid paralysis, seropositivity for anti-GM1 antibodies, axonal degeneration, IgG deposits at the nodes of Ranvier and lymphocytic infiltration in the periaxonal space, and lack of segmental demyelination [41, 42]. On the other hand, GQ1b and GD1a antibodies cause conduction block at the motor nerve terminals in a mouse model [25].

Treatment of GBS

Treatment of GBS consists of supportive treatment as well as immunotherapy in more severe cases. Supportive care is better provided in an intensive care unit in the progressive phase of the disease.

Supportive Treatment

1. Respiratory care
   Respiratory failure is one of the most serious short-term complications of GBS. About 25% of patients with GBS who are unable to walk and 30–50% of patients who are admitted to ICU undergo intubation and mechanical ventilation [43]. The need for mechanical ventilation should be anticipated in GBS when there is rapidly progressive course as manifested by time to peak disability less than 7 days, time from the onset of symptoms to hospitalization less than 7 days, and presence of more than 30% reduction of vital capacity, NIF, and PEF during the course of hospitalization [44, 45]. It is essential to anticipate the need for mechanical ventilation (MV) and proceed with elective intubation in selected patients. It is therefore recommended to assess FVC every 2–4 h during the day and every 4–6 h at night in a patient with declining respiratory function. A vital capacity of less than 20 mL/kg, maximal inspiratory pressure less than 30 cm H_2O, maximal expiratory pressure less than 40 cm H_2O, and a reduction of more than 30% in vital capacity, maximal inspiratory pressure, or maximal expiratory pressure anticipate need for oncoming respiratory failure [44]. Elective intubation and MV are recommended in patients with significant respiratory distress, fatigue, sweating, tachycardia, active aspiration, FVC < 15 mL/kg, hypercarbia (PaCO2 48 mm Hg), and hypoxemia (PaO2 on room air <56 mm Hg) [1, 46].

2. Dysautonomia
   Autonomic dysfunction in GBS is more common in the acute stage of the disease, can involve sympathetic or parasympathetic systems, and is a major cause of mortality [2]. In a study on pediatric GBS patients, hypertension and

tachycardia occurred in 70 and 77% of the patients, respectively, and they were more likely with increasing motor weakness [47]. In another study on 156 GBS patients, tachycardia, hypertension, and hypotension were noted in 38, 69, and 11% of the patients, respectively [48]. Less common manifestations include transient ECG changes such as ST segment elevation and diffusely inverted T waves secondary to coronary vasospasm [49]. Careful assessment for fluctuations in blood pressure and pulse rate and appropriate treatment which may involve symptomatic treatment and even insertion of a pacemaker are therefore important aspects of the GBS care, especially during the ICU care, but also during the recovery period [1].

Gastrointestinal dysfunction was noted in 45% of a large cohort of GBS patients [48], while adynamic ileus was reported in 15% of GBS patients admitted to the ICU in another study [50]; however, the authors speculated that some of the cases could have been due to other factors such as abdominal surgery, immobility, and use of medications such as opioids.

About a quarter of GBS patients (39% of AIDP and 19% of the AMAN cases) had urinary symptoms, including urinary retention in about 10% of the cases [51, 52]. Urinary dysfunction in GBS is proposed to be caused by either hypo- or hyper-activity of lumbosacral nerves [52]. Besides incontinence and urinary retention which will require the use of a catheter, patients may develop underactive detrusor, overactive detrusor, and, to a lesser extent, hyperactive sphincter. Urinary symptoms may be persistent and affect the quality of life in the patients who have recovered from the acute phase, i.e., urinary frequency and urgency were present in one third and nocturia in half of the patients who recovered from GBS patients when these patients were followed for 6 years [53].

Immunomodulatory Treatments

GBS was associated with mortality in 10% of patients and severe residual neurological deficit in 20 of cases before the introduction of immunotherapy [54]. As detailed below, immunomodulatory treatments directed at removal (plasma exchange (PLEX)) or modulation of immunoglobulins and probably T cell responses (intravenous immunoglobulins (IVIG)) have been proven to be effective in GBS. In contrast to many other autoimmune neurological diseases, steroids have not shown to hasten recovery nor affect the long-term outcome [55], and their use is not recommended in GBS, neither alone nor combined with PLEX or IVIG [1, 2].

1. Plasma Exchange (PLEX)

   The immunomodulatory action of PLEX is through the removal of autoantibodies and complement components. It is usually administered at five plasma volume exchanges (50 ml/kg each) usually every other day, over a period of up to 2 weeks [56, 57]. PLEX is more effective if done early in the course of the illness, preferentially the first week after the onset of symptoms [58]. However, larger exchanges of 1.5 plasma volumes have also been used. Hughes et al. reviewed four clinical studies involving 585 severely affected GBS patients and concluded that there is significant improvement and less disability in the treated patients after 4 weeks and 1 year after of randomization [56–60]. The treated patients also had a higher chance of full strength recovery (odds ratio 1.24, confidence interval 1.07–1.45), as well as lower disability and higher likelihood for full recovery in 1 year [59]. In milder GBS patients who did not lose the ability to ambulate, patients who received two sessions of PLEX over 3 days had shorter onset of motor recovery (4 vs. 8 days) and better improvement after 1 month compared to those who did not receive PLEX [57]. On the other hand, in GBS patients who could not stand unaided, there was a higher likelihood of regaining full motor strength in 1 year after four sessions of PLEX (x1.5 plasma volume each) than after two sessions (64% vs. 48%) [57]. Six exchanges were similar in efficacy to four in the severe GBS cases in the latter study.

2. Intravenous Immunoglobulin (IVIG)
IVIG has become the preferred treatment for GBS because of the availability and convenience of use [1]. The therapeutic effect of IVIG in GBS may arise from blocking pathogenic autoantibodies and antibody-mediated complement activation [8]. On the other hand, IVIG has shown to result in reduced number of Th1 and Th17 and expansion of the population of T_{reg} cells in GBS patients [31, 32]. IVIG, when started within 2 weeks of onset of weakness, has been shown to be effective in AIDP patients with more severe disease manifested as inability to walk 10 m unaided (GBS disability scale score $\geq$3) [59]. IVIG treatment has been demonstrated to be as effective as PLEX if given within 2 weeks in patients who lose the ability to walk [61, 62]. The dosage of IVIG used in the GBS clinical trials has been 2 g/kg divided over 5 days [59]. The same dose can be divided over 2–4 days in selected cases, although a study suggested more posttreatment relapses in children who received the dose in 2 days [63]. It has been suggested that some patients may have a better response with a higher dose than 2 g/kg total or a second course of treatment, for the following reasons: (1) about 10% of the IVIG-treated GBS patients have a relapse, which usually responds to further treatment with IVIG [64], and (2) a subgroup of GBS have poor initial response and slower recovery, which has been correlated with lower levels of serum immunoglobulin concentrations due to different pharmacokinetics [65]. The latter subgroup may benefit from a higher dose or a second course of treatment [65].

Although the optimal immunomodulatory treatment for AMAN is still unclear, PLEX has been suggested to be more efficient and cost-effective than IVIG [2, 66]. The prognosis of MFS is generally good without treatment. Although the recovery started earlier in the MFS patients who received IVIG, the final outcome was not changed by the use of PLEX or IVIG in a study [67].

3. Oncoming Treatments
Considering the role of anti-ganglioside antibodies and complement activation in the pathogenesis of GBS variants, modulation of complement activation through

monoclonal antibodies and synthetic serine protease inhibitors is emerging as a new treatment for GBS [8]. Eculizumab is a humanized monoclonal antibody, which binds plasma C5 and blocks its cleavage to C5b, therefore preventing the formation of membrane attack complex [68]. Eculizumab prevented the occurrence of anti-GQ1b-mediated neuropathy in a murine model [69]. Nafamostat, a synthetic serine protease inhibitor which is used as a short-acting anticoagulant during hemodialysis, has been shown to ameliorate the phenotype of anti-GM1 antibody-mediated neuropathy in a rabbit model due to its anticomplement activity [70].

Chronic Inflammatory Demyelinating Polyneuropathy (CIDP)

The term CIDP refers to a chronic form of an acquired inflammatory polyneuropathy that is clinically differentiated from AIDP by its time course. CIDP encompasses a spectrum of phenotypic variants with common features of chronicity, demyelination evident on the nerve conduction studies, and albuminocytological dissociation in the CSF.

Clinical Manifestations

Classical CIDP is characterized by symmetrical proximal and distal muscle weakness, sensory loss, and hyporeflexia or areflexia, with either a relapsing or progressive course [71]. Proximal weakness and upper extremity involvement are common in classical CIDP, which is in contrast to most other types of polyneuropathy which are generally characterized by a more distal pattern of involvement [72]. Sensory changes may include numbness, paresthesias, and difficulty with proprioception and balance. Neuropathic pain is a rather infrequent feature in CIDP [73], but rarely pain is the presenting feature [74]. Respiratory compromise and dysautonomia are uncommon in CIDP (in contrast to GBS) and occur in less than 10% of patients [75]. Facial, ocular, and oropharyngeal involvement is infrequent as well and is estimated to occur in about 15% of patients [76]. CIDP is differentiated from GBS by its time course: the time to nadir in CIDP is more than 8 weeks (it is usually <2 weeks and maximally 4 weeks in GBS) [2]. In two thirds of those affected, the disease has a progressive course, with the remainder experiencing relapses.

CIDP Variants

Only 50% of patients with CIDP present with classic features described above [77]. Other variants of CIDP include sensory-predominant, motor-predominant, ataxic, chronic inflammatory sensory polyradiculopathy (CISP), and multifocal acquired demyelinating sensory and motor (MADSAM) neuropathy.

Five to thirty-five percent of CIDP patients present with sensory symptoms in their lower extremities [78]. Despite this purely sensory presentation from the clinical standpoint, motor nerve conduction abnormalities consistent with demyelination can be found in many of these patients, and a pure sensory variant of CIDP has only been reported rarely [79, 80]. On the other hand, many of the patients with purely sensory variant will develop motor involvement years later [81]. Sensory CIDP may mimic sensory ganglionopathy if the sensory action potentials are absent and motor conduction studies are entirely normal. In these instances, nerve biopsy may be required for the diagnosis [79, 82]. A rare (~5%) predominantly sensory ataxic form of CIDP (chronic immune sensory polyradiculopathy (CISP)) is a distinct clinical entity that involves large fibers of the dorsal roots rather than distal sensory nerves [83, 84]. In these cases peripheral nerve conduction studies may be unrevealing, and somatosensory conduction potentials may need to confirm demyelination of the sensory nerve roots [85]. The motor-predominant variant of CIDP presents with relatively symmetric proximal and distal muscle weakness, demyelination on the nerve conduction study, and minimal or absent sensory involvement, which occurs in about 7–10% of patients with CIDP, more commonly in young adults <20 years of age [78, 86, 87]. The main differential diagnosis for motor variant of CIDP is multifocal motor neuropathy. Multifocal acquired demyelinating sensory and motor (MADSAM, aka Lewis-Sumner syndrome) neuropathy is a focal variant which occurs in about 6–15% of CIDP patients [78]. MADSAM presents with an asymmetrical muscle weakness and sensory changes, usually starting in one or both upper extremities. Later in its clinical course, MADSAM may become more diffuse and involve both lower extremities as well.

It is differentiated from axonal mononeuritis multiplex by the presence of segmental demyelination in the nerve conduction study, involving both motor and sensory nerves.

Pathology

Postmortem studies as well as MRI and ultrasonography have demonstrated involvement of nerve roots, plexi, and proximal nerve trunks, as well as focal involvement of more distal portion of peripheral nerves in CIDP patients [88, 89]. The classic histopathological findings include demyelination, remyelination (thick myelin sheath and onion bulb formation), endoneurial edema, and presence of inflammatory infiltrates (CD4, CD8 lymphocytes) in the perineurium and endoneurium [73]. Macrophages intercalate between the layers of Schwann cell membranes, including outer mesaxon, extending their elongated processes into the myelin lamellae and breaking them down [90]. Due to the focal distribution of lesions, up to 20% of biopsies may show no inflammatory changes. Only 10–50% of nerve biopsies show inflammatory cell infiltrates, due to the focal nature of the disease [90]; on the other hand, 20–40% only show features of axonal degeneration [73, 91, 92].

Immunopathogenesis

CIDP is an autoimmune disease as proven by its response to immunomodulatory treatments, presence of inflammatory infiltrates in the peripheral nerves, and development of a chronic relapsing EAN in animal models, similar to CIDP from the pathological and electrophysiological standpoint [93, 94].

Immunopathogenesis of CIDP is complex and involves both cellular and humoral arms of the immune system, affecting peripheral myelin. Breakdown in the blood-nerve-barrier (BNB), which protects the microenvironment of the nerve from exogenous proteins such as potentially pathogenic immunoglobulins, plays a key role in the pathogenesis of CIDP. Abnormal permeability of BNB can be detected via contrast enhancement seen in the MRI of the inflamed nerve trunks and plexi of patients with CIDP [95, 96].

Similar to AIDP, the target antigen remains unknown in CIDP, but unlike GBS, CIDP is characteristically not preceded by an antecedent infection. Although about a third of cases were preceded by an infection in a previous study [97], other studies have challenged that data by finding that the antecedent infections were present in only 10% of patients with CIDP, which does not differ from the prevalence of in the general population [98]. On the other hand, the onset has not been consistently linked to any one specific antecedent infection, with the exception of rare association of CIDP and HIV infection [99, 100]. CIDP has been rarely reported in association with malignant melanoma, which is explained by presence of shared antigens, such as myelin-associated glycoprotein and different gangliosides, between melanocytes and Schwann cells, as they both are derived from neuroectodermal origin [101–104].

Cellular Immunity

Aberrant T cell activation plays an important role in the pathogenesis of CIDP as suggested by several lines of evidence: (i) sural nerve biopsies of CIDP patients frequently demonstrate endoneurial infiltration by CD4+, CD8+ T cells, and macrophages [105]; (ii) changes in T cell subsets, function, and interleukin profiles have been reported in the blood and CSF of patients with CIDP [106]; and (iii) gamma delta T cells, which are capable of recognizing nonprotein antigens such as gangliosides, were observed in 14 of 20 CIDP nerve biopsy specimens [107].

It is yet unclear whether the initial activation of T cells occurs in lymphoid organs or within the peripheral nerve. Upon the activation of peripheral CD4+ T cells, they release multiple inflammatory cytokines (interleukin (IL)-2, interferon-γ (IFNγ), and IL-17 as well as the chemokines (interferon gamma-induced protein (IP)-10 and macrophage inflammatory protein 3 β (MIP3β) and stimulate the increase in the expression of the endothelial adhesion molecules (VCAM, ICAM, ELAM) that mediate the adherence and transmigration of T cells through BNB and into the nerve compartment. When in the endoneurium, T cells release pro-inflammatory cytokines and metalloproteinases (MMP), further breaking down the BNB. Both MMP-2 and MMP-9 were found to be upregulated in nerves of CIDP patients [108]. As T cells transmigrate BNB, they become locally activated due to the upregulation of MHC II and co-stimulatory molecules B7-1 and B7-2 by infiltrating macrophages as well as Schwann cells. An antigen-driven, major histocompatibility complex class I-restricted CD8+ T cell-mediated immune attack has also been suggested to play a role in the pathogenesis of CIDP [109, 110]. An oligoclonal or polyclonal repertoire of CD8+ T cells is found in peripheral nerves of patients with CIDP which correlates with the same expansion in their blood [109]. On the other hand, IVIG corrects this prominent oligoclonal repertoire of CD8+ T cells [110].

Another important checkpoint that controls the extent of inflammatory reaction and autoimmunity is T_{reg} cells. In patients with CIDP, T_{reg} cells are reduced in number and have been found to be less functional than in healthy controls [111, 112]. The B7-1/B7-2 CD28/CTLA4 signaling pathways are important in the lymphocyte activation and homeostasis of T_{reg} cells, with CD28 signaling promoting and CTLA4 signaling downregulate T cell activation [36, 113]. The importance of the aforementioned pathways in the pathogenesis of CIDP is demonstrated by occurrence of a spontaneous autoimmune neuropathy in B7-2 knockout nonobese diabetic mice (see below).

Endoneurial macrophages and Schwann cells may function as antigen-presenting cells particularly in regard with nonprotein antigens, as indicated by overexpression of MHC-like molecules CD1a and CD1b in these cells in the nerve biopsies of CIDP patients [114, 115]. Moreover, Schwann cells may participate as accessory cells in T cell activation as they express CD58 molecule (LFA-3) [115]. Macrophages recruited into the site of inflammation represent one of the dominant effector cells in CIDP [116]. They form clusters around the endoneurial vessels and participate in antigen presentation, in the release of pro-inflammatory cytokines, and at the end stage in stripping away the damaged myelin and phagocytizing it.

Humoral Immunity

Different lines of evidence suggest that humoral immunity has an important role in the pathogenesis of CIDP. Firstly, sural nerve biopsies of some patients with CIDP have shown complement and immunoglobulin deposition on the surface of Schwann cells and compact myelin [117, 118]; secondly, serum proteins from CIDP patients bind to the segments of healthy nerves, which results in demyelination and conduction blocks, when injected interneurally [119]; thirdly, the efficacy of plasma exchange in the treatment of CIDP implicates the important role of humoral factors in its pathogenesis.

It is therefore plausible that after the BNB is first damaged by the action of T cells and macrophages detailed above, autoantibodies mediate demyelination by complement fixation and by directing macrophages to the antigenic targets via Fc receptors, leading to opsonization and phagocytosis.

Although the target antigen in CIDP remains elusive, antibodies to a number of myelin and axonal antigens such as glycolipids GM1, LM1, and LM1-containing ganglioside complex, beta tubulin, galactocerebroside, chondroitin sulfate, and proteins P0, P2, and P0-related glycoprotein have been reported in sera from CIDP patients [120, 121]. On the other hand, these antibodies have not been detected in most patients with CIDP, and only antibodies against PO were shown to be pathogenic in vivo with passive transfer or intraneural injection [122]. The presence of these autoantibodies may represent an epiphenomenon of the ongoing inflammation rather than denote causality.

Proteins in the non-compact myelin in the nodal, paranodal, and juxtanodal regions have an important role for the maintenance of structural integrity of the nodes of Ranvier and therefore saltatory conduction. As the search for a target anti-gen among major compact myelin proteins has been so far unsuccessful, the atten-tion has shifted toward non-compact myelin proteins such as gliomedin, neurofascin, contactin, and Caspr 1 [40, 123, 124]. The complex of contactin/Caspr/neurofas-cin-155 has a critical function in the integrity of paranodal junctions [125]. In a study by Deveaux et al., 30% of patients with CIDP had IgG antibodies that bound to the nodes of Ranvier and paranodes of the rodent nerves, and the binding was specific to gliomedin, neurofascin 186, and contactin [123]. Another study showed that 13 of 533 Japanese patients with CIDP had an IgG4 antibody to contactin 1; seropositivity was associated with sensory ataxia and poor responsiveness to IVIG treatment [126]. In another study and using the same group of patients, antibodies to neurofascin-155 were identified in 7% of the patients [127]; those who were seropositive were more likely to have sensory ataxia (42%), tremors (13%), and demyelinating CNS lesions (8%) and also were poorly responsive to IVIG [127]. Poor response to IVIG in patients positive to neurofascin-155 and contactin 1 has been suggested to be due to the fact that antibodies are of IgG4 type, which do not result in complement fixation and have low affinity to Fc receptors, two postulated immunomodulatory mechanisms of IVIG [127].

Antibodies to contactin/Caspr/neurofascin-155 complex are pathogenic as serum of anti-contactin-positive CIDP patients prevents adhesive interaction between con-tactin. Caspr and neurofascin-155 therefore alter the structure of paranodal junc-tions in myelinated neuronal culture [125].

Animal Models

Immunization of rabbits with a high dose of bovine myelin results in a relapsing or progressive form of EAN [93]. Chronic EAN has been created in the Lewis rats by immunization with myelin after treatment with low-dose cyclosporine A (CsA), which is explained by inhibition of T cell apoptosis and therefore perpetuation of inflammatory response by low-dose CsA [128]. Higher doses of CsA actually resulted in attenuation of the disease severity, attributed to suppression of overall T cell responses, which leads to prevention of the occurrence of EAN [128].

Spontaneous autoimmune polyneuropathy (SAP) in nonobese diabetic (NOD) mice is another model of inflammatory neuropathy 36. The NOD mouse strain is a model of type 1 diabetes, but it also has the propensity to develop other autoimmune diseases. When B7-2 was knocked out in these mice, they did not develop insulitis and diabetes, but on the other hand, all female and one third of male mice developed a chronic demyelinating neuropathy beginning at 20 weeks of age with pathological (heavy infiltration by CD4+, CD8+ T cells and dendritic cells in peripheral nerves and dorsal root ganglia) and electrophysiological (demyelination, conduction block-ing) characteristics of CIDP 129. There was overexpression of B7-1 by the antigen presenting cells in that model. The disease was reproduced by treatment of NOD mice with antibody against B7-2, and by transfer of CD4+ T cells but not by sera from SAP animals [129]. Interferon gamma secreting Th1 cells that are reactive against certain episodes of myelin protein zero (P0) are shown to have a critical role in SAP in B7-2 deficient mouse model [130].

Treatment

CIDP is considered a treatable form of autoimmune neuropathy, and therefore a variety of immunomodulatory and immunosuppressive agents have been studied for its treatment.

Several controlled and retrospective studies as well as a few randomized trials have confirmed the efficacy of current first-line treatments: corticosteroids, IVIG, and PLEX [131–133]. Approximately, 50–70% of patients with CIDP respond to one of these treatments, with another 50% of the remainder responding to one of the other therapies [78, 134].

Corticosteroids

Steroids are the oldest treatment used for CIDP. The mechanism of action of steroids is multimodal and includes decrease in circulating lymphocytes, inflammatory cytokines, macrophage activation, and lymphocyte transmigration. A 3-month, randomized, placebo-controlled trial showed the efficacy of high-dose prednisone (120 mg) on alternate days in 28 CIDP patients [135]. A clinical response to steroid treatment occurs between 2 weeks and several months with an average of about 8 weeks [91, 121]. Although oral steroids are effective, daily dosing is commonly poorly tolerated due to multiple side effects (osteoporosis, weight gain, glycemic control, stomach irritation). As a result, pulse treatments with intravenous methylprednisolone or oral dexamethasone have been investigated as an alternative approach. When the efficacy of dexamethasone 40 mg daily for 4 days a month was compared to prednisolone at 60 mg in a double-blind, randomized, controlled trial, remission occurred in about 40% of patients at both arms at 12 months [136]. The median time to remission was however shorter in the dexamethasone (20 weeks) versus prednisone group (39 weeks). Another retrospective study evaluated intravenous methylprednisolone, loading dose of 1 g/day for 3–5 days followed 1 g/week for 4–8 weeks, and then a slow taper over a period of 2 months to 2 years [137]. There was favorable response as assessed by remission rate and improved disability score, in 13 out of 16 patients at 6-month follow-up, and IV methylprednisolone regimen was equal in efficacy to IVIG and oral prednisolone arms in that study. There were fewer steroid-related side effects in the IV methylprednisolone than the prednisone arm.

Intravenous Immunoglobulins (IVIG)

IVIG has been used as a preferred treatment for CIDP for almost two decades.

Axonal loss, as demonstrated by muscle atrophy clinically or low or absent motor potentials on EMG, is an important predictor of lack of response to IVIG [138].

The mechanism of action of IVIG in CIDP is multimodal and includes blocking or decreased production of pathogenic antibodies and decreased complement deposition [139]. IVIG also modulates cellular immune system and decreases the concentration of adhesion molecules and cytokine secretion by the endothelial cells [139]. Wong et al. showed significantly reduced ratio of sialylated/agalactosylated IgG-Fc in CIDP patients, and decrease in that ratio was associated with more severe disease [140]. Treatment with IVIG resulted in increased levels of sialylated IgG-Fc which correlated with clinical improvement [140]. The effect of IVIG on the T cell profile and T_{reg} cells is described above [32].

IVIG is administered at 2 g/kg divided over 3–5 days and followed by maintenance infusions of 0.5–1 g/kg every 2–4 weeks. The frequency and dose of the maintenance therapy are adjusted based on the clinical response of the patient. IVIG is overall well tolerated by most patients. Infusion reactions include chills, rash, nausea, headache, and myalgias. These can be prevented or improved by premedicating patients with acetaminophen and diphenhydramine and slowing the infusion rate [141]. Other serious but not common side effects include renal failure (typically in patient with underlying renal insufficiency), congestive heart failure (in patients with pre-existing heart disease), anaphylactic reactions (more common in IgA-deficient patients), and thromboembolic events such as deep venous thrombosis and ischemic stroke. Other rare side effects include aseptic meningitis, neutropenia, and uveitis [141]. The efficacy of IVIG was proven in the CIDP Efficacy (ICE) trial, which is thus far the largest and longest (up to 48 weeks) randomized, double-blind, placebo-controlled, crossover trial in this disease. The trial used a loading dose of 2 g/kg administered over 2 to 5 days, followed by maintenance infusions of 1 g/kg administered every 3 weeks for 6 months, and demonstrated improvement in adjusted INCAT disability score and grip strength and lower rate of relapse compared to the placebo arm [142].

Subcutaneous IG (SCIg) is being investigated as an alternative to IVIG in those patients who cannot tolerate IVIG infusions. These have been used for two decades for other autoimmune disorders and require more frequent administration but at lower doses. Recent randomized trials showed efficacy of SCIg in improving the muscle strength in CIDP patients who were previously responsive to IVIG [143, 144].

Two IVIG formulations (Gammagard 5% IVIG and Kiovig 10% IVIG) were compared for their efficacy and side effect profile in a study, which demonstrated similar efficacy and side effect profile [145]. No randomized trials of IVIG versus SCIg have thus far been conducted. The effectiveness of IVIG versus pulsed IV methylprednisolone (500 mg IV daily for 4 days, followed by a monthly administration for 6 months) was compared in a randomized controlled trial, which showed that IVIG was less frequently discontinued because of inefficacy or side effects at 6 months (87.5% vs. 47.6%, respectively); however, the relapse rate after discontinuation was higher in the IVIG group, while in the patients who remained in the methylprednisolone group, no patients relapsed at 6 months of treatment [146].

Plasma Exchange (PLEX)

PLEX has been demonstrated to be effective in CIDP in multiple studies, including the two short-term randomized placebo-controlled trials [147, 148]. In the study by

Hahn et al., PLEX was effective in 80% of the patients as indicated by improvement in grip strength, clinical disability grade, and the mean neurologic disability score, as well as summated motor potential amplitudes and conduction velocities [148]. Of those patients who responded to the plasma exchange, most improved within 4 weeks of receiving therapy with no significant difference in responsiveness between those with progressive and relapsing disease, i.e., five of seven patients with progressive course and seven of eight patients with relapsing course improved in that study. Despite good response initially, after discontinuation of therapy, about two thirds of patients will experience deterioration within several weeks [133, 148]. There are no specific guidelines for the use of PLEX in CIDP beyond 4 weeks; clinical response, timing, and degree of deterioration should be used to guide decision-making regarding frequency of subsequent PLEX sessions. Usually, a maintenance therapy with one PLEX session at least every 8 weeks may be needed, sometimes in addition to other immunomodulatory medications [121].

Plasma exchange administration requires a central catheter placement and about three to five sessions per treatment. Adverse effects include bleeding, infection at the site of the catheter, hypotension, anemia, and hypocalcemia due to citrate toxicity [133]. Pre-existing coagulation abnormalities, thrombocytopenia, and hemodynamic instability warrant the use of another treatment modality.

Other Treatments

A large number of immunosuppressants (azathioprine, cyclophosphamide, methotrexate, cyclosporine A, mycophenolate mofetil, rituximab) and immunomodulatory drugs (alpha and beta interferon) have been tried for CIDP. Although some of the aforementioned medications are commonly used in CIDP patients as steroid-sparing drugs, none have been shown to be effective in CIDP in randomized, controlled trials [149]. When azathioprine was added to a regimen of alternate-day steroid treatment, the outcome was not different [150]; on the other hand, azathioprine has been used in the treatment of CIDP patients who also had diabetes in small case series [151, 152]. A double-blinded randomized study did not show efficacy of a weekly dose of oral methotrexate in patients in CIDP who were also on IVIG and prednisone [153]. Interferon B1a was shown not to be effective in a cohort of ten patients with treatment-resistant CIDP in a randomized, double-blind, placebo-controlled study [154]. High-dose cyclophosphamide (200 mg/kg over 4 days) infusion was reported to be effective in a cohort of four CIDP patients who had failed other treatments, with remissions that could last more than 3 years [155]. Cyclosporine has been reported to be effective to sustain remission in a child with CIDP and to reduce the required dose of prednisolone in another [156]. In a retrospective study on eight CIDP patients, neuropathy disability score improved in all eight, and in six of eight, the concomitant medications could be stopped or dose reduced by >50% [157]. On the other hand, another study on 21 CIDP patients suggested efficacy of mycophenolate in only one third of patients [158]. Autologous hematopoietic stem cell transplantation (AHSCT) has been successfully used for treatment-resistant CIDP [159]. In a prospective study, 11 patients with therapy-refractory CIDP underwent AHSCT with a median follow-up time of 28 months. Eight had a drug-free remission at their last follow-up [159].

Other treatment modalities are being investigated, including agents affecting B cells, T cells, transmigration molecules, and signal transduction pathways.

Rituximab, which is a monoclonal antibody against CD20 and acts by depleting the precursors of antibody-producing B cells, was used in 13 patients with refractory CIDP, eight of whom had concurrent hematological disease (B cell lymphoma, Waldenstrom macroglobulinemia, and IgM monoclonal gammopathy of unknown significance) [160]. Nine of 13 (7 of 8 with hematological disease) showed improved in that study, with median duration of 2 months from rituximab infusion to a response and mean duration of response of 1 year. In another study, rituximab was used in four patients with anti-CNTN1/NF155-positive, IVIG-resistant, CIDP patients [161]. The autoantibody titer diminished in all the patients and three of the four improved clinically.

Alemtuzumab is a monoclonal antibody directed against the CD52, therefore resulting in lymphocytic depletion via apoptosis. In a cohort of seven patients with treatment-resistant CIDP who underwent treatment with alemtuzumab, two had remissions and another two needed a lower dose of IVIG [162]. Fingolimod, a sphingosine-1-phosphate receptor modulator approved for relapsing-remitting multiple sclerosis, is currently under investigation for the treatment of CIDP in a randomized, double-blind, placebo-controlled trial.

Supportive Therapies

Physical therapy and supportive equipment such as canes, walking sticks, walkers, braces, and ankle-foot orthotics may be helpful in assisting CIDP patients in walking and other activities of daily living. Physical therapy may help maintain range of motion and prevent joint contractures. Neuropathic pain, anxiety, depression, and fatigue may need to be treated with symptomatic medications. Exercise can be helpful in combatting fatigue and encouraging endurance.

References

1. Yuki N, Hartung HP. Guillain-Barre syndrome. N Engl J Med. 2012;366:2294–304.
2. van den Berg B, Walgaard C, Drenthen J, Fokke C, Jacobs BC, van Doorn PA. Guillain-Barre syndrome: pathogenesis, diagnosis, treatment and prognosis. Nat Rev Neurol. 2014;10:469–82.
3. van den Berg B, Fokke C, Drenthen J, van Doorn PA, Jacobs BC. Paraparetic Guillain-Barre syndrome. Neurology. 2014;82:1984–9.
4. Kuwabara S, Yuki N. Axonal Guillain-Barre syndrome: concepts and controversies. Lancet Neurol. 2013;12:1180–8.
5. Hiraga A, Kuwabara S, Ogawara K, et al. Patterns and serial changes in electrodiagnostic abnormalities of axonal Guillain-Barre syndrome. Neurology. 2005;64:856–60.
6. Aranyi Z, Kovacs T, Sipos I, Bereczki D. Miller Fisher syndrome: brief overview and update with a focus on electrophysiological findings. Eur J Neurol. 2012;19:15–20. e11–13

7. Wakerley BR, Yuki N. Pharyngeal-cervical-brachial variant of Guillain-Barre syndrome. J Neurol Neurosurg Psychiatry. 2014;85:339–44.
8. Wakerley BR, Yuki N. Guillain-Barre syndrome. Expert Rev Neurother. 2015;15:847–9.
9. Uncini A, Manzoli C, Notturno F, Capasso M. Pitfalls in electrodiagnosis of Guillain-Barre syndrome subtypes. J Neurol Neurosurg Psychiatry. 2010;81:1157–63.
10. Asbury AK, Arnason BG, Adams RD. The inflammatory lesion in idiopathic polyneuritis. Its role in pathogenesis. Medicine. 1969;48:173–215.
11. Prineas JW. Pathology of the Guillain-Barre syndrome. Ann Neurol. 1981;9(Suppl):6–19.
12. Hafer-Macko CE, Sheikh KA, Li CY, et al. Immune attack on the Schwann cell surface in acute inflammatory demyelinating polyneuropathy. Ann Neurol. 1996;39:625–35.
13. Griffin JW, Li CY, Ho TW, et al. Guillain-Barre syndrome in northern China. The spectrum of neuropathological changes in clinically defined cases. Brain (A Journal of Neurology). 1995;118(Pt 3):577–95.
14. Phillips MS, Stewart S, Anderson JR. Neuropathological findings in Miller Fisher syndrome. J Neurol Neurosurg Psychiatry. 1984;47:492–5.
15. Jacobs BC, Rothbarth PH, van der Meche FG, et al. The spectrum of antecedent infections in Guillain-Barre syndrome: a case-control study. Neurology. 1998;51:1110–5.
16. Yuki N, Taki T, Inagaki F, et al. A bacterium lipopolysaccharide that elicits Guillain-Barre syndrome has a GM1 ganglioside-like structure. J Exp Med. 1993;178:1771–5.
17. Koga M, Takahashi M, Masuda M, Hirata K, Yuki N. Campylobacter gene polymorphism as a determinant of clinical features of Guillain-Barre syndrome. Neurology. 2005;65:1376–81.
18. Tam CC, Rodrigues LC, Petersen I, Islam A, Hayward A, O'Brien SJ. Incidence of Guillain-Barre syndrome among patients with Campylobacter infection: a general practice research database study. J Infect Dis. 2006;194:95–7.
19. Kuwabara S, Ogawara K, Misawa S, et al. Does Campylobacter jejuni infection elicit "demyelinating" Guillain-Barre syndrome? Neurology. 2004;63:529–33.
20. Illa I, Ortiz N, Gallard E, Juarez C, Grau JM, Dalakas MC. Acute axonal Guillain-Barre syndrome with IgG antibodies against motor axons following parenteral gangliosides. Ann Neurol. 1995;38:218–24.
21. Willison HJ, Yuki N. Peripheral neuropathies and anti-glycolipid antibodies. Brain (A Journal of Neurology). 2002;125:2591–625.
22. Kusunoki S, Kaida K. Antibodies against ganglioside complexes in Guillain-Barre syndrome and related disorders. J Neurochem. 2011;116:828–32.
23. Dalakas MC. Pathogenesis of immune-mediated neuropathies. Biochim Biophys Acta. 1852;2015:658–66.
24. Gong Y, Tagawa Y, Lunn MP, et al. Localization of major gangliosides in the PNS: implications for immune neuropathies. Brain (A Journal of Neurology). 2002;125:2491–506.
25. McGonigal R, Rowan EG, Greenshields KN, et al. Anti-GD1a antibodies activate complement and calpain to injure distal motor nodes of Ranvier in mice. Brain (A Journal of Neurology). 2010;133:1944–60.
26. Burkel WE. The histological fine structure of perineurium. Anat Rec. 1967;158:177–89.
27. Olsson Y. Microenvironment of the peripheral nervous system under normal and pathological conditions. Crit Rev Neurobiol. 1990;5:265–311.
28. Sawai S, Satoh M, Mori M, et al. Moesin is a possible target molecule for cytomegalovirus-related Guillain-Barre syndrome. Neurology. 2014;83:113–7.
29. Gatto CL, Walker BJ, Lambert S. Local ERM activation and dynamic growth cones at Schwann cell tips implicated in efficient formation of nodes of Ranvier. J Cell Biol. 2003;162:489–98.
30. Li S, Yu M, Li H, Zhang H, Jiang Y. IL-17 and IL-22 in cerebrospinal fluid and plasma are elevated in Guillain-Barre syndrome. Mediators Inflamm. 2012;2012:260473.
31. Li S, Jin T, Zhang HL, et al. Circulating Th17, Th22, and Th1 cells are elevated in the Guillain-Barre syndrome and downregulated by IVIg treatments. Mediators Inflamm. 2014;2014:740947.

32. Maddur MS, Rabin M, Hegde P, et al. Intravenous immunoglobulin exerts reciprocal regulation of Th1/Th17 cells and regulatory T cells in Guillain-Barre syndrome patients. Immunol Res. 2014;60:320–9.

33. Sakaguchi S, Yamaguchi T, Nomura T, Ono M. Regulatory T cells and immune tolerance. Cell. 2008;133:775–87.

34. Waksman BH, Adams RD. Allergic neuritis: an experimental disease of rabbits induced by the injection of peripheral nervous tissue and adjuvants. J Exp Med. 1955;102:213–36.

35. Rostami A, Gregorian SK, Brown MJ, Pleasure DE. Induction of severe experimental autoimmune neuritis with a synthetic peptide corresponding to the 53-78 amino acid sequence of the myelin P2 protein. J Neuroimmunol. 1990;30:145–51.

36. Soliven B. Animal models of autoimmune neuropathy. ILAR (Journal/National Research Council, Institute of Laboratory Animal Resources). 2014;54:282–90.

37. Astrom KE, Webster HD, Arnason BG. The initial lesion in experimental allergic neuritis. A phase and electron microscopic study. J Exp Med. 1968;128:469–95.

38. Taylor JM, Pollard JD. Dominance of autoreactive T cell-mediated delayed-type hypersensitivity or antibody-mediated demyelination results in distinct forms of experimental autoimmune neuritis in the Lewis rat. J Neuropathol Exp Neurol. 2001;60:637–46.

39. Lonigro A, Devaux JJ. Disruption of neurofascin and gliomedin at nodes of Ranvier precedes demyelination in experimental allergic neuritis. Brain (A Journal of neurology). 2009;132:260–73.

40. Devaux JJ. Antibodies to gliomedin cause peripheral demyelinating neuropathy and the dismantling of the nodes of Ranvier. Am J Pathol. 2012;181:1402–13.

41. Yuki N, Yamada M, Koga M, et al. Animal model of axonal Guillain-Barre syndrome induced by sensitization with GM1 ganglioside. Ann Neurol. 2001;49:712–20.

42. Susuki K, Yuki N, Schafer DP, et al. Dysfunction of nodes of Ranvier: a mechanism for anti-ganglioside antibody-mediated neuropathies. Exp Neurol. 2012;233:534–42.

43. van Doorn PA, Ruts L, Jacobs BC. Clinical features, pathogenesis, and treatment of Guillain-Barre syndrome. Lancet Neurol. 2008;7:939–50.

44. Lawn ND, Fletcher DD, Henderson RD, Wolter TD, Wijdicks EF. Anticipating mechanical ventilation in Guillain-Barre syndrome. Arch Neurol. 2001;58:893–8.

45. Sharshar T, Chevret S, Bourdain F, Raphael JC. French Cooperative Group on Plasma Exchange in Guillain-Barre S. Early predictors of mechanical ventilation in Guillain-Barre syndrome. Crit Care Med. 2003;31:278–83.

46. Ropper AH, Kehne SM. Guillain-Barre syndrome: management of respiratory failure. Neurology. 1985;35:1662–5.

47. Dimario Jr FJ, Edwards C. Autonomic dysfunction in childhood Guillain-Barre syndrome. J Child Neurol. 2012;27:581–6.

48. Ruts L, Drenthen J, Jongen JL, et al. Pain in Guillain-Barre syndrome: a long-term follow-up study. Neurology. 2010;75:1439–47.

49. Hiraga A, Nagumo K, Suzuki K, Sakakibara Y, Kojima S. [A patient with Guillain-Barre syndrome and recurrent episodes of ST elevation and left ventricular hypokinesis in the anterior wall]. No to shinkei =. Brain Nerve. 2003;55:517–20.

50. Burns TM, Lawn ND, Low PA, Camilleri M, Wijdicks EF. Adynamic ileus in severe Guillain-Barre syndrome. Muscle Nerve. 2001;24:963–5.

51. Sakakibara R, Hattori T, Kuwabara S, Yamanishi T, Yasuda K. Micturitional disturbance in patients with Guillain-Barre syndrome. J Neurol Neurosurg Psychiatry. 1997;63:649–53.

52. Sakakibara R, Uchiyama T, Kuwabara S, et al. Prevalence and mechanism of bladder dysfunction in Guillain-Barre Syndrome. NeurourolUrodyn. 2009;28:432–7.

53. Amatya B, Khan F, Whishaw M, Pallant JF. Guillain-Barre syndrome: prevalence and long-term factors impacting bladder function in an Australian community cohort. J Clin Neurol. 2013;9:144–50.

54. Winer JB, Hughes RA, Osmond C. A prospective study of acute idiopathic neuropathy. I. Clinical features and their prognostic value. J Neurol Neurosurg Psychiatry. 1988;51:605–12.

55. Hughes RA, van Doorn PA. Corticosteroids for Guillain-Barre syndrome. Cochrane Database Syst Rev. 2012;8:CD001446.
56. Efficiency of plasma exchange in Guillain-Barre syndrome: role of replacement fluids. French Cooperative Group on Plasma Exchange in Guillain-Barre syndrome. Ann Neurol. 1987;22:753–61.
57. Appropriate number of plasma exchanges in Guillain-Barre syndrome. The French Cooperative Group on Plasma Exchange in Guillain-Barre Syndrome. Ann Neurol. 1997;41:298–306.
58. Plasmapheresis and acute Guillain-Barre syndrome. The Guillain-Barre syndrome Study Group. Neurology. 1985;35:1096–1104.
59. Hughes RA, Swan AV, Raphael JC, Annane D, van Koningsveld R, van Doorn PA. Immunotherapy for Guillain-Barre syndrome: a systematic review. Brain (A Journal of Neurology). 2007;130:2245–57.
60. Greenwood RJ, Newsom-Davis J, Hughes RA, et al. Controlled trial of plasma exchange in acute inflammatory polyradiculoneuropathy. Lancet. 1984;1:877–9.
61. van der Meche FG, Schmitz PI. A randomized trial comparing intravenous immune globulin and plasma exchange in Guillain-Barre syndrome. Dutch Guillain-Barre Study Group. N Engl J Med. 1992;326:1123–9.
62. Randomised trial of plasma exchange, intravenous immunoglobulin, and combined treatments in Guillain-Barre syndrome. Plasma Exchange/Sandoglobulin Guillain-Barre Syndrome Trial Group. Lancet. 1997;349:225–30.
63. Korinthenberg R, Schessl J, Kirschner J, Monting JS. Intravenously administered immunoglobulin in the treatment of childhood Guillain-Barre syndrome: a randomized trial. Pediatrics. 2005;116:8–14.
64. Kleyweg RP, van der Meche FG. Treatment related fluctuations in Guillain-Barre syndrome after high-dose immunoglobulins or plasma-exchange. J Neurol Neurosurg Psychiatry. 1991;54:957–60.
65. Kuitwaard K, de Gelder J, Tio-Gillen AP, et al. Pharmacokinetics of intravenous immunoglobulin and outcome in Guillain-Barre syndrome. Ann Neurol. 2009;66:597–603.
66. Dada MA, Kaplan AA. Plasmapheresis treatment in Guillain-Barre syndrome: potential benefit over IVIg in patients with axonal involvement. Ther Apher Dial (Official Peer-Reviewed Journal of the International Society for Apheresis, the Japanese Society for Apheresis, the Japanese Society for Dialysis Therapy). 2004;8:409–12.
67. Mori M, Kuwabara S, Fukutake T, Hattori T. Intravenous immunoglobulin therapy for Miller Fisher syndrome. Neurology. 2007;68:1144–6.
68. Hillmen P, Hall C, Marsh JC, et al. Effect of eculizumab on hemolysis and transfusion requirements in patients with paroxysmal nocturnal hemoglobinuria. N Engl J Med. 2004;350:552–9.
69. Halstead SK, Zitman FM, Humphreys PD, et al. Eculizumab prevents anti-ganglioside antibody-mediated neuropathy in a murine model. Brain (A Journal of Neurology). 2008;131:1197–208.
70. Phongsisay V, Susuki K, Matsuno K, et al. Complement inhibitor prevents disruption of sodium channel clusters in a rabbit model of Guillain-Barre syndrome. J Neuroimmunol. 2008;205:101–4.
71. Van den Bergh PY, Hadden RD, Bouche P, et al. European Federation of Neurological Societies/Peripheral Nerve Society guideline on management of chronic inflammatory demyelinating polyradiculoneuropathy: report of a joint task force of the European Federation of Neurological Societies and the Peripheral Nerve Society – first revision. Eur J Neurol. 2010;17:356–63.
72. Gorson KC, Katz J. Chronic inflammatory demyelinating polyneuropathy. Neurol Clin. 2013;31:511–32.
73. Saperstein DS, Katz JS, Amato AA, Barohn RJ. Clinical spectrum of chronic acquired demyelinating polyneuropathies. Muscle Nerve. 2001;24:311–24.
74. Boukhris S, Magy L, Khalil M, Sindou P, Vallat JM. Pain as the presenting symptom of chronic inflammatory demyelinating polyradiculoneuropathy (CIDP). J Neurol Sci. 2007;254:33–8.

75. Henderson RD, Sandroni P, Wijdicks EF. Chronic inflammatory demyelinating polyneuropathy and respiratory failure. J Neurol. 2005;252:1235–7.
76. Dyck PJ, Lais AC, Ohta M, Bastron JA, Okazaki H, Groover RV. Chronic inflammatory polyradiculoneuropathy. Mayo Clin Proc. 1975;50:621–37.
77. Mathey EK, Park SB, Hughes RA, et al. Chronic inflammatory demyelinating polyradiculoneuropathy: from pathology to phenotype. J Neurol Neurosurg Psychiatry. 2015;86:973–85.
78. Viala K, Maisonobe T, Stojkovic T, et al. A current view of the diagnosis, clinical variants, response to treatment and prognosis of chronic inflammatory demyelinating polyradiculoneuropathy. J Peripher Nerv Syst. 2010;15:50–6.
79. Oh SJ, Joy JL, Kuruoglu R. "Chronic sensory demyelinating neuropathy": chronic inflammatory demyelinating polyneuropathy presenting as a pure sensory neuropathy. J Neurol Neurosurg Psychiatry. 1992;55:677–80.
80. Rajabally YA, Wong SL. Chronic inflammatory pure sensory polyradiculoneuropathy: a rare CIDP variant with unusual electrophysiology. J Clin Neuromuscul Dis. 2012;13:149–52.
81. van Dijk GW, Notermans NC, Franssen H, Wokke JH. Development of weakness in patients with chronic inflammatory demyelinating polyneuropathy and only sensory symptoms at presentation: a long-term follow-up study. J Neurol. 1999;246:1134–9.
82. Simmons Z, Tivakaran S. Acquired demyelinating polyneuropathy presenting as a pure clinical sensory syndrome. Muscle Nerve. 1996;19:1174–6.
83. Yato M, Ohkoshi N, Sato A, Shoji S, Kusunoki S. Ataxic form of chronic inflammatory demyelinating polyradiculoneuropathy (CIDP). Eur J Neurol. 2000;7:227–30.
84. Sinnreich M, Klein CJ, Daube JR, Engelstad J, Spinner RJ, Dyck PJ. Chronic immune sensory polyradiculopathy: a possibly treatable sensory ataxia. Neurology. 2004;63:1662–9.
85. Yiannikas C, Vucic S. Utility of somatosensory evoked potentials in chronic acquired demyelinating neuropathy. Muscle Nerve. 2008;38:1447–54.
86. Sabatelli M, Madia F, Mignogna T, Lippi G, Quaranta L, Tonali P. Pure motor chronic inflammatory demyelinating polyneuropathy. J Neurol. 2001;248:772–7.
87. Hattori N, Misu K, Koike H, et al. Age of onset influences clinical features of chronic inflammatory demyelinating polyneuropathy. J Neurol Sci. 2001;184:57–63.
88. Pitarokoili K, Schlamann M, Kerasnoudis A, Gold R, Yoon MS. Comparison of clinical, electrophysiological, sonographic and MRI features in CIDP. J Neurol Sci. 2015;357:198–203.
89. Matsuda M, Ikeda S, Sakurai S, Nezu A, Yanagisawa N, Inuzuka T. Hypertrophic neuritis due to chronic inflammatory demyelinating polyradiculoneuropathy (CIDP): a postmortem pathological study. Muscle Nerve. 1996;19:163–9.
90. Vital C, Vital A, Lagueny A, et al. Chronic inflammatory demyelinating polyneuropathy: immunopathological and ultrastructural study of peripheral nerve biopsy in 42 cases. Ultrastruct Pathol. 2000;24:363–9.
91. Barohn RJ, Kissel JT, Warmolts JR, Mendell JR. Chronic inflammatory demyelinating polyradiculoneuropathy. Clinical characteristics, course, and recommendations for diagnostic criteria. Arch Neurol. 1989;46:878–84.
92. Gorson KC, Allam G, Ropper AH. Chronic inflammatory demyelinating polyneuropathy: clinical features and response to treatment in 67 consecutive patients with and without a monoclonal gammopathy. Neurology. 1997;48:321–8.
93. Harvey GK, Pollard JD, Schindhelm K, Antony J. Chronic experimental allergic neuritis. An electrophysiological and histological study in the rabbit. J Neurol Sci. 1987;81:215–25.
94. Adam AM, Atkinson PF, Hall SM, Hughes RA, Taylor WA. Chronic experimental allergic neuritis in Lewis rats. Neuropathol Appl Neurobiol. 1989;15:249–64.
95. Crino PB, Grossman RI, Rostami A. Magnetic resonance imaging of the cauda equina in chronic inflammatory demyelinating polyneuropathy. Ann Neurol. 1993;33:311–3.
96. Morgan GW, Barohn RJ, Bazan 3rd C, King RB, Klucznik RP. Nerve root enhancement with MRI in inflammatory demyelinating polyradiculoneuropathy. Neurology. 1993;43:618–20.
97. McCombe PA, Pollard JD, McLeod JG. Chronic inflammatory demyelinating polyradiculoneuropathy. A clinical and electrophysiological study of 92 cases. Brain (A Journal of Neurology). 1987;110(Pt 6):1617–30.

98. Chio A, Cocito D, Bottacchi E, et al. Idiopathic chronic inflammatory demyelinating polyneuropathy: an epidemiological study in Italy. J Neurol Neurosurg Psychiatry. 2007;78:1349–53.

99. Gibbels E, Diederich N. Human immunodeficiency virus (HIV)-related chronic relapsing inflammatory demyelinating polyneuropathy with multifocal unusual onion bulbs in sural nerve biopsy. A clinicomorphological study with qualitative and quantitative light and electron microscopy. Acta Neuropathol. 1988;75:529–34.

100. Chimowitz MI, Audet AM, Hallet A, Kelly Jr JJ. HIV-associated CIDP. Muscle Nerve. 1989;12:695–6.

101. Bird SJ, Brown MJ, Shy ME, Scherer SS. Chronic inflammatory demyelinating polyneuropathy associated with malignant melanoma. Neurology. 1996;46:822–4.

102. Weiss MD, Luciano CA, Semino-Mora C, Dalakas MC, Quarles RH. Molecular mimicry in chronic inflammatory demyelinating polyneuropathy and melanoma. Neurology. 1998;51:1738–41.

103. Rousseau A, Salachas F, Baccard M, Delattre JY, Sanson M. Chronic inflammatory polyneuropathy revealing malignant melanoma. J Neurooncol. 2005;71:335–6.

104. Noronha AB, Harper JR, Ilyas AA, Reisfeld RA, Quarles RH. Myelin-associated glycoprotein shares an antigenic determinant with a glycoprotein of human melanoma cells. J Neurochem. 1986;47:1558–65.

105. Schmidt B, Toyka KV, Kiefer R, Full J, Hartung HP, Pollard J. Inflammatory infiltrates in sural nerve biopsies in Guillain-Barre syndrome and chronic inflammatory demyelinating neuropathy. Muscle Nerve. 1996;19:474–87.

106. Chi LJ, Xu WH, Zhang ZW, Huang HT, Zhang LM, Zhou J. Distribution of Th17 cells and Th1 cells in peripheral blood and cerebrospinal fluid in chronic inflammatory demyelinating polyradiculoneuropathy. J Peripher Nerv Syst. 2010;15:345–56.

107. Winer J, Hughes S, Cooper J, Ben-Smith A, Savage C. gamma delta T cells infiltrating sensory nerve biopsies from patients with inflammatory neuropathy. J Neurol. 2002;249:616–21.

108. Renaud S, Erne B, Fuhr P, et al. Matrix metalloproteinases-9 and -2 in secondary vasculitic neuropathies. Acta Neuropathol. 2003;105:37–42.

109. Schneider-Hohendorf T, Schwab N, Uceyler N, Gobel K, Sommer C, Wiendl H. CD8+ T-cell immunity in chronic inflammatory demyelinating polyradiculoneuropathy. Neurology. 2012;78:402–8.

110. Mausberg AK, Dorok M, Stettner M, et al. Recovery of the T-cell repertoire in CIDP by IV immunoglobulins. Neurology. 2013;80:296–303.

111. Chi LJ, Wang HB, Wang WZ. Impairment of circulating CD4+CD25+ regulatory T cells in patients with chronic inflammatory demyelinating polyradiculoneuropathy. J Peripher Nerv Syst. 2008;13:54–63.

112. Sanvito L, Makowska A, Gregson N, Nemni R, Hughes RA. Circulating subsets and CD4(+)CD25(+) regulatory T cell function in chronic inflammatory demyelinating polyradiculoneuropathy. Autoimmunity. 2009;42:667–77.

113. Ledbetter JA, Imboden JB, Schieven GL, et al. CD28 ligation in T-cell activation: evidence for two signal transduction pathways. Blood. 1990;75:1531–9.

114. Khalili-Shirazi A, Gregson NA, Londei M, Summers L, Hughes RA. The distribution of CD1 molecules in inflammatory neuropathy. J Neurol Sci. 1998;158:154–63.

115. Van Rhijn I, Van den Berg LH, Bosboom WM, Otten HG, Logtenberg T. Expression of accessory molecules for T-cell activation in peripheral nerve of patients with CIDP and vasculitic neuropathy. Brain (A Journal of Neurology). 2000;123(Pt 10):2020–9.

116. Sommer C, Koch S, Lammens M, Gabreels-Festen A, Stoll G, Toyka KV. Macrophage clustering as a diagnostic marker in sural nerve biopsies of patients with CIDP. Neurology. 2005;65:1924–9.

117. Dalakas MC, Engel WK. Immunoglobulin and complement deposits in nerves of patients with chronic relapsing polyneuropathy. Arch Neurol. 1980;37:637–40.

118. Hays AP, Lee SS, Latov N. Immune reactive C3d on the surface of myelin sheaths in neuropathy. J Neuroimmunol. 1988;18:231–44.

119. Yan WX, Taylor J, Andrias-Kauba S, Pollard JD. Passive transfer of demyelination by serum or IgG from chronic inflammatory demyelinating polyneuropathy patients. Ann Neurol. 2000;47:765–75.
120. Koller H, Kieseier BC, Jander S, Hartung HP. Chronic inflammatory demyelinating polyneuropathy. N Engl J Med. 2005;352:1343–56.
121. Dalakas MC, Medscape. Advances in the diagnosis, pathogenesis and treatment of CIDP. Nat Rev Neurol. 2011;7:507–17.
122. Yan WX, Archelos JJ, Hartung HP, Pollard JD. P0 protein is a target antigen in chronic inflammatory demyelinating polyradiculoneuropathy. Ann Neurol. 2001;50:286–92.
123. Devaux JJ, Odaka M, Yuki N. Nodal proteins are target antigens in Guillain-Barre syndrome. J Peripher Nerv Syst. 2012;17:62–71.
124. Querol L, Nogales-Gadea G, Rojas-Garcia R, et al. Antibodies to contactin-1 in chronic inflammatory demyelinating polyneuropathy. Ann Neurol. 2013;73:370–80.
125. Labasque M, Hivert B, Nogales-Gadea G, Querol L, Illa I, Faivre-Sarrailh C. Specific contactin N-glycans are implicated in neurofascin binding and autoimmune targeting in peripheral neuropathies. J Biol Chem. 2014;289:7907–18.
126. Miura Y, Devaux JJ, Fukami Y, et al. Contactin 1 IgG4 associates to chronic inflammatory demyelinating polyneuropathy with sensory ataxia. Brain (A Journal of Neurology). 2015;138:1484–91.
127. Devaux JJ, Miura Y, Fukami Y, et al. Neurofascin-155 IgG4 in chronic inflammatory demyelinating polyneuropathy. Neurology. 2016;86:800–7.
128. McCombe PA, van der Kreek SA, Pender MP. The effects of prophylactic cyclosporin A on experimental allergic neuritis (EAN) in the Lewis rat. Induction of relapsing EAN using low dose cyclosporin A. J Neuroimmunol. 1990;28:131–40.
129. Salomon B, Rhee L, Bour-Jordan H, et al. Development of spontaneous autoimmune peripheral polyneuropathy in B7-2-deficient NOD mice. J Exp Med. 2001;194:677–84.
130. Kim HJ, Jung CG, Jensen MA, Dukala D, Soliven B. Targeting of myelin protein zero in a spontaneous autoimmune polyneuropathy. J Immunol. 2008;181:8753–60.
131. Hughes RA, Mehndiratta MM. Corticosteroids for chronic inflammatory demyelinating polyradiculoneuropathy. Cochrane Database Syst Rev. 2012;8:CD002062.
132. Eftimov F, Winer JB, Vermeulen M, de Haan R, van Schaik IN. Intravenous immunoglobulin for chronic inflammatory demyelinating polyradiculoneuropathy. Cochrane Database Syst Rev. 2013;12:CD001797.
133. Mehndiratta MM, Hughes RA. Plasma exchange for chronic inflammatory demyelinating polyradiculoneuropathy. Cochrane Database Syst Rev. 2012;9:CD003906.
134. Cocito D, Paolasso I, Antonini G, et al. A nationwide retrospective analysis on the effect of immune therapies in patients with chronic inflammatory demyelinating polyradiculoneuropathy. Eur J Neurol. 2010;17:289–94.
135. Dyck PJ, O'Brien PC, Oviatt KF, et al. Prednisone improves chronic inflammatory demyelinating polyradiculoneuropathy more than no treatment. Ann Neurol. 1982;11:136–41.
136. van Schaik IN, Eftimov F, van Doorn PA, et al. Pulsed high-dose dexamethasone versus standard prednisolone treatment for chronic inflammatory demyelinating polyradiculoneuropathy (PREDICT study): a double-blind, randomised, controlled trial. Lancet Neurol. 2010;9:245–53.
137. Lopate G, Pestronk A, Al-Lozi M. Treatment of chronic inflammatory demyelinating polyneuropathy with high-dose intermittent intravenous methylprednisolone. Arch Neurol. 2005;62:249–54.
138. Iijima M, Yamamoto M, Hirayama M, et al. Clinical and electrophysiologic correlates of IVIg responsiveness in CIDP. Neurology. 2005;64:1471–5.
139. Buttmann M, Kaveri S, Hartung HP. Polyclonal immunoglobulin G for autoimmune demyelinating nervous system disorders. Trends Pharmacol Sci. 2013;34:445–57.
140. Wong AH, Fukami Y, Sudo M, Kokubun N, Hamada S, Yuki N. Sialylated IgG-Fc: a novel biomarker of chronic inflammatory demyelinating polyneuropathy. J Neurol Neurosurg Psychiatry. 2016;87:275–9.

141. Brannagan 3rd TH. Intravenous gamma globulin (IVIg) for treatment of CIDP and related immune-mediated neuropathies. Neurology. 2002;59:S33–40.
142. Hughes RA, Donofrio P, Bril V, et al. Intravenous immune globulin (10% caprylate-chromatography purified) for the treatment of chronic inflammatory demyelinating polyradiculoneuropathy (ICE study): a randomised placebo-controlled trial. Lancet Neurol. 2008;7:136–44.
143. Markvardsen LH, Debost JC, Harbo T, et al. Subcutaneous immunoglobulin in responders to intravenous therapy with chronic inflammatory demyelinating polyradiculoneuropathy. Eur J Neurol. 2013;20:836–42.
144. Markvardsen LH, Harbo T, Sindrup SH, et al. Subcutaneous immunoglobulin preserves muscle strength in chronic inflammatory demyelinating polyneuropathy. Eur J Neurol. 2014;21:1465–70.
145. Kuitwaard K, van den Berg LH, Vermeulen M, et al. Randomised controlled trial comparing two different intravenous immunoglobulins in chronic inflammatory demyelinating polyradiculoneuropathy. J Neurol Neurosurg Psychiatry. 2010;81:1374–9.
146. Nobile-Orazio E, Cocito D, Jann S, et al. Intravenous immunoglobulin versus intravenous methylprednisolone for chronic inflammatory demyelinating polyradiculoneuropathy: a randomised controlled trial. Lancet Neurol. 2012;11:493–502.
147. Dyck PJ, Daube J, O'Brien P, et al. Plasma exchange in chronic inflammatory demyelinating polyradiculoneuropathy. N Engl J Med. 1986;314:461–5.
148. Hahn AF, Bolton CF, Pillay N, et al. Plasma-exchange therapy in chronic inflammatory demyelinating polyneuropathy. A double-blind, sham-controlled, cross-over study. Brain (A Journal of Neurology). 1996;119(Pt 4):1055–66.
149. Hughes RA, Swan AV, van Doorn PA. Cytotoxic drugs and interferons for chronic inflammatory demyelinating polyradiculoneuropathy. Cochrane Database Syst Rev. 2004:CD003280.
150. Dyck PJ, O'Brien P, Swanson C, Low P, Daube J. Combined azathioprine and prednisone in chronic inflammatory-demyelinating polyneuropathy. Neurology. 1985;35:1173–6.
151. Stewart JD, McKelvey R, Durcan L, Carpenter S, Karpati G. Chronic inflammatory demyelinating polyneuropathy (CIDP) in diabetics. J Neurol Sci. 1996;142:59–64.
152. Haq RU, Pendlebury WW, Fries TJ, Tandan R. Chronic inflammatory demyelinating polyradiculoneuropathy in diabetic patients. Muscle Nerve. 2003;27:465–70.
153. Group RMCT. Randomised controlled trial of methotrexate for chronic inflammatory demyelinating polyradiculoneuropathy (RMC trial): a pilot, multicentre study. Lancet Neurol. 2009;8:158–64.
154. Hadden RD, Sharrack B, Bensa S, Soudain SE, Hughes RA. Randomized trial of interferon beta-1a in chronic inflammatory demyelinating polyradiculoneuropathy. Neurology. 1999;53:57–61.
155. Brannagan 3rd TH, Pradhan A, Heiman-Patterson T, et al. High-dose cyclophosphamide without stem-cell rescue for refractory CIDP. Neurology. 2002;58:1856–8.
156. Visudtibhan A, Chiemchanya S, Visudhiphan P. Cyclosporine in chronic inflammatory demyelinating polyradiculoneuropathy. Pediatr Neurol. 2005;33:368–72.
157. Bedi G, Brown A, Tong T, Sharma KR. Chronic inflammatory demyelinating polyneuropathy responsive to mycophenolate mofetil therapy. J Neurol Neurosurg Psychiatry. 2010;81:634–6.
158. Gorson KC, Amato AA, Ropper AH. Efficacy of mycophenolate mofetil in patients with chronic immune demyelinating polyneuropathy. Neurology. 2004;63:715–7.
159. Press R, Askmark H, Svenningsson A, et al. Autologous haematopoietic stem cell transplantation: a viable treatment option for CIDP. J Neurol Neurosurg Psychiatry. 2014;85:618–24.
160. Benedetti L, Briani C, Franciotta D, et al. Rituximab in patients with chronic inflammatory demyelinating polyradiculoneuropathy: a report of 13 cases and review of the literature. J Neurol Neurosurg Psychiatry. 2011;82:306–8.
161. Querol L, Rojas-Garcia R, Diaz-Manera J, et al. Rituximab in treatment-resistant CIDP with antibodies against paranodal proteins. Neurol Neuroimmunol Neuroinflamm. 2015;2:e149.
162. Marsh EA, Hirst CL, Llewelyn JG, et al. Alemtuzumab in the treatment of IVIG-dependent chronic inflammatory demyelinating polyneuropathy. J Neurol. 2010;257:913–9.

Myasthenia Gravis: Clinical Features, Immunology, and Therapies

11

Wael Richeh, John D. Engand, and Richard M. Paddison

Introduction

Myasthenia gravis (MG) is a disorder of the neuromuscular junction. Most cases of MG are autoimmune in origin although rarely there are cases of congenital genetic origin. The autoimmune disease is characterized by fluctuating muscle weakness which worsens with exertion and improves with rest. The disease usually involves the extraocular muscle initially and may progress to involve bulbar and limb musculature, resulting in generalized MG {1,2}. The disorder is of unknown etiology; however, the role of antibodies directed against the nicotinic acetylcholine receptor is well established in the pathogenesis. Since MG is eminently treatable, recognition of the signs and symptoms of MG is crucial. Recent progress in treatment options has led to a significant reduction in morbidity and mortality [1, 2].

Epidemiology

Acquired MG prevalence is approximately 20 per 100,000 in the US population. Gender and age both appear to influence the occurrence of MG. Below the age of 40 years, the female/male ratio is about 3:1. Between 40 and 50 years, it is roughly equal, but over the age of 50, MG occurs more commonly in men. Childhood MG is uncommon in Europe and North America, comprising 10 to 15% of cases.

W. Richeh, MD (✉)
LSUHSC School of Medicine, Department of Neurology,
433 Bolivar St, New Orleans, LA, USA

Shannon Clinic, Brain and Spine Institute, San Angelo, Texas, USA
e-mail: wael.richeh@yahoo.com

J.D. Engand, MD • R.M. Paddison
LSUHSC School of Medicine, Department of Neurology,
433 Bolivar St, New Orleans, LA, USA

© Springer International Publishing AG 2017
A. Minagar, J.S. Alexander (eds.), *Inflammatory Disorders of the Nervous System*, Current Clinical Neurology, DOI 10.1007/978-3-319-51220-4_11

In Asian countries, up to 50% of patients have onset before 15 years, and these patients present mainly with purely ocular manifestations [4, 5].

Pathogenesis

The nerve terminals innervating the neuromuscular junctions (NMJ) of skeletal muscles arise from the terminal arborization of α-motor neurons of the ventral horns of the spinal cord and brain stem. The NMJ itself consists of a synaptic cleft and a 20 nm thick space which contains acetylcholinesterase (AChE) along with other supporting proteins/proteoglycans. The NMJ postsynaptic membrane has deep folds with acetylcholine receptors (AChRs) tightly packed on the top of these folds.

When the nerve action potential reaches the synaptic bouton, depolarization opens voltage-gated calcium channels on the presynaptic membrane, triggering release of acetylcholine (ACh) into the synaptic cleft. The ACh diffuses into the synaptic cleft to reach postsynaptic membrane receptors where it triggers the end plate potential (EPP). ACh is then hydrolyzed by AChE within the synaptic cleft.

Muscle-specific receptor tyrosine kinase (MuSK), a postsynaptic transmembrane protein, forms part of the receptor for agrin, a protein present on synaptic basal lamina. Agrin/MuSK interaction triggers and maintains rapsyn-dependent clustering of AChR and other postsynaptic proteins [13]. Rapsyn, a peripheral membrane protein on the postsynaptic membrane, is necessary for the clustering of AChR. Mice lacking agrin or MuSK fail to form NMJs and die at birth due to profound muscle weakness [2, 24].

NMJ physiology influences susceptibility to MG muscle weakness. EPP generated in normal NMJ is several times larger than the threshold needed to generate the postsynaptic action potential. This neuromuscular transmission "safety factor" is reduced in MG patients. Reduction in number or activity of the AChR molecules at the NMJ decreases the EPP. The EPP may be adequate at rest to generate an action potential, but when the quantal release of ACh is reduced after repetitive activity, the EPP may fall below the threshold needed to trigger the action potential [22]. This results in blocking of muscle fiber contraction and muscle weakness. If the EPP at rest is consistently below the action potential threshold, persistent weakness occurs.

Effector Mechanisms of Anti-AChR Antibodies (Anti-AChR Abs)

Anti-AChR Abs affect NMT by at least three mechanisms [2]: (i) complement binding and activation at the NMJ, (ii) antigenic modulation (accelerated AChR endocytosis of molecules cross-linked by antibodies), (iii) and functional AChR block—preventing normal ACh from attaching and acting on the AChR.

Role of CD4+ T Cells in MG

Pathogenic anti-AChR Abs are high-affinity IgGs, and their synthesis requires activated CD4+ T cells to interact with and stimulate B cells. Thymectomy is believed to benefit patients with MG by removal of these AChR-specific CD4+ T cells [20]. Treatment with anti-CD4+ antibodies has also been shown to have a positive therapeutic impact. AIDS patients with reduction in CD4+ T cells notice myasthenic symptom improvement.

Role of CD4+ T-Cell Subtypes and Cytokines in MG and EAMG (Experimental Autoimmune MG)

CD4+ T cells are classified into two main subtypes: Th1 and Th2 cells. Th1 cells secrete pro-inflammatory cytokines, such as IL-2, IFN-γ, and TNF-α, which are important in cell-mediated immune responses. Th2 cells secrete anti-inflammatory cytokines, like IL-4, IL-6, and IL-10, which are important inducers of humoral immune responses. IL-4 further stimulates differentiation of Th3 cells that secrete TGF-β, which is involved in immunosuppressive mechanisms [17].

MG patients have abundant anti-AChR Th1 cells in the blood that recognize many AChR epitopes and are capable of inducing B cells to produce high-affinity anti-AChR antibodies. Th1 cells are indispensible in the development of EAMG as proven in animal models. Therapies against Th1 cytokines (TNF-α and IFN-γ) have been proven in animal models to improve EAMG symptoms [22, 23].

Anti-AChR Th2 cells have a complex role in EAMG pathogenesis. They can be protective, but their cytokines IL-5, IL-6, and IL-10 may also facilitate EAMG development [2]. CD4+ T cells that express CD25 marker and transcription factor Foxp3 are called "Tregs" and are important in maintaining self-tolerance. Tregs in MG patients may be functionally impaired and have been shown to increase after thymectomy with concomitant symptom improvement. Natural killer (NK) and natural killer T (NKT) cells also have important roles in MG and EAMG. Natural killer T (NKT) cells with Tregs help in regulating anti-AChR response. Mouse models have shown inhibition of EAMG development after stimulation of NKT cells [23]. IL-18, secreted by antigen-presenting cells (APCs), stimulates NK cells to produce IFN-γ, which permits and enhances Th1 cells to induce EAMG. IL-18-deficient mice are resistant to EAMG, and pharmacologic block of IL-18 suppresses EAMG. MG patients have been shown to have increased serum level of IL-18, which tends to decrease with clinical improvement [15].

Other Autoantigens in MG

Seronegative MG patients are those patients who have clinical MG but do not demonstrate anti-AChR antibodies in blood. Some of these patients have anti-MuSK antibodies (up to 40% of this subgroup). Other ethnic groups or locations (e.g., Chinese and Norwegians) have lower frequencies of anti-MuSK antibodies in seronegative MG patients. MG patients with anti-MuSK antibodies do not have anti-AChR Abs, except as reported in a group of Japanese patients [16].

Agrin/MuSK signaling pathway maintains the structural and functional integrity of the postsynaptic NMJ apparatus in the adult muscle cell. Anti-MuSK antibodies affect the agrin-dependent AChR cluster maintenance at the NMJ, leading to reduced AChR numbers. Complement-mediated damage may also be responsible for decreasing the AChR numbers at the NMJ when targeted by anti-MuSK Abs. Some human muscle cell culture studies have shown cell cycle arrest, downregulation of AChR subunit with rapsyn, and other muscle protein expression, on exposure to sera from anti-MuSK-positive MG patients [2]. Other antimuscle cell protein antibodies (e.g., antititin and antiryanodine receptor antibodies) are also postulated to have pathogenic roles in autoimmune MG.

Immunological Test

The most commonly used immunological test for the diagnosis of MG measures the serum concentrations of anti-AChR antibodies and is highly specific for myasthenia gravis [46]. False positives are rare and may occur with low titers in LEMS (5%), motor neuron disease (3–5%), and polymyositis (<1%).

The sensitivity of this test is approximately 85% for gMG and 50% for oMG [47, 48]. Anti-AChR antibody concentrations cannot be used to predict the severity of disease in individual patients since the concentration of the antibodies does not correlate with the clinical picture. Seronegativity may occur with immunosuppression or if the test is done too early in the disease [49, 50]. As indicated above, striated muscle antibodies against muscle cytoplasmic proteins (titin, myosin, actin, and ryanodine receptors) are detected mainly in patients with thymomatous MG and also in some thymoma patients without MG [24, 51]. The presence of these antibodies in early-onset MG raises the suspicion of a thymoma. Titin antibodies and other striated muscle antibodies are also found in up to 50% of patients with late-onset and nonthymomatous MG and are less helpful as predictors of thymoma in patients over 50 years [51]. Anti-KCNA4 antibodies might be a useful marker to identify patients with thymoma but can be also seen in myocarditis/myositis [52]. Patients with gMG who are anti-AChR antibody negative should be tested for anti-MuSK antibodies which are found in approximately 40% of patients in this group. As noted, low-affinity anti-AChR antibodies binding to clustered AChRs have been found in 66% of sera from patients with seronegative gMG [53]. Whether low-affinity antibodies are present in oMG remains to be determined, but this cell-based assay might eventually provide a more sensitive diagnostic test in this subgroup. Chest CT or MRI is done in all patients with confirmed MG to exclude the presence of a thymoma. Iodinated contrast agents should be used with caution because they might exacerbate myasthenic weakness [54, 55]. MG often coexists with thyroid disease, so baseline testing of thyroid function should be obtained at the time of diagnosis.

Clinical Feature

The cardinal feature of MG is fluctuating weakness that is fatigable, worsening with repetitive activities and improving with rest. Weakness is worsened by exposure to heat, infection, and stress [3]. The fluctuating nature of weakness distinguishes MG from other disorders which present with weakness. Typically, the weakness involves specific skeletal muscle groups. The distribution of the weakness is generally ocular, bulbar, proximal extremities, and neck, and in a few patients, it involves the respiratory muscles. In patients with MG, the weakness is mild in 26%, moderate in 36%, and severe in 39%, associated with dysphagia, depressed cough, and reduced vital capacity [27]. Extraocular muscle (EOM) weakness is by far the most common initial symptom of MG, occurring in approximately 85% of patients. Generalized progression will develop in 50% of these patients within 2 years [27]. Early MG usually presents with fluctuating ptosis and diplopia. Diplopia can be elicited by having the patient look laterally for 20–30 s resulting in eye muscle fatigue. The ptosis can be unilateral or bilateral, and sustained up-gaze for 30 or more seconds will usually induce it. The ptosis can be severe enough to totally occlude vision. The most commonly involved EOM is the medial rectus. But, on clinical examination, usually more than one extraocular muscle is weak with pupillary sparing. The weakness does not follow any pattern of specific nerve or muscle involvement, distinguishing it from other disorders such as vertical gaze paresis, distinct cranial nerve palsy, or internuclear ophthalmoplegia (INO).

Bulbar muscle involvement during the course of MG can be seen in approximately 60% of patients. It may present as fatigable chewing, particularly on chewing solid food with jaw closure more involved than jaw opening [38, 39]. Painless dysphagia and dysarthria may be the initial presentation in approximately 15% of patients [39]. The lack of ocular involvement in these patients may result in misdiagnosis as motor neuron disease or primary myopathy. Weakness involving respiratory muscles is rarely the presenting feature of MG, but respiratory insufficiency certainly may occur later as the disease progresses [35]. Respiratory muscle weakness can lead to myasthenic crisis which can be life threatening, requiring mechanical ventilation. It can be precipitated by infections and certain medications such as aminoglycosides, telithromycin, neuromuscular blocking agents, magnesium sulfate, beta-blockers, and fluoroquinolone antibiotics.

Involvement of the limbs in MG produces predominantly proximal muscle weakness. The upper extremities tend to be more often affected than the lower extremities. Occasionally predominant distal muscle weakness occurs [40]. Facial muscles are frequently involved and can make the patient appear expressionless. Neck extensor and flexor muscles are commonly affected. The weight of the head may overcome the extensors, producing a "dropped head syndrome." Although it has become evident that the natural course of MG with adequate treatment is general improvement in 57% and remission in 13% after the first 2 years, severe weakness can be accompanied by high mortality. Only 20% of patients remain unchanged, and mortality from the disease is 5–9%. Only 4% of the patients who survive the first 2 years become worse. Of those who will develop generalized myasthenia, virtually, all do so by 2–3 years [3].

Clinical Classification

The Myasthenia Gravis Foundation of America (MGFA) clinical classification divides MG into five main classes and several subclasses [26]. It is designed to identify subgroups of patients with MG who share distinct clinical features or severity of disease that may indicate different prognoses or responses to therapy. It should not be used to measure outcome and is as follows:

Class I MG is characterized by the following:

1. Any ocular muscle weakness.
2. May have weakness of eye closure.
3. All other muscle strengths are normal.

Class II MG is characterized by the following:

1. Mild weakness affecting muscles other than ocular muscles
2. May also have ocular muscle weakness of any severity

Class IIa MG is characterized by the following:

1. Predominantly affecting limb muscles, axial muscles, or both
2. May also have lesser involvement of oropharyngeal muscles

Class IIb MG is characterized by the following:

1. Predominantly affecting oropharyngeal muscles, respiratory muscles, or both
2. May also have lesser or equal involvement of limb muscles, axial muscles, or both

Class III MG is characterized by the following:

1. Moderate weakness affecting muscles other than ocular muscles
2. May also have ocular muscle weakness of any severity

Class IIIa MG is characterized by the following:

1. Predominantly affecting limb muscles, axial muscles, or both
2. May also have lesser involvement of oropharyngeal muscles

Class IIIb MG is characterized by the following:

1. Predominantly affecting oropharyngeal muscles, respiratory muscles, or both
2. May also have lesser or equal involvement of limb muscles, axial muscles, or both

Class IV MG is characterized by the following:

1. Severe weakness affecting muscles other than ocular muscles
2. May also have ocular muscle weakness of any severity

Class IVa MG is characterized by the following:

1. Predominantly affecting limb muscles, axial muscles, or both
2. May also have lesser involvement of oropharyngeal muscles

Class IVb MG is characterized by the following:

1. Predominantly affecting oropharyngeal muscles, respiratory muscles, or both
2. May also have lesser or equal involvement of limb muscles, axial muscles, or both

Class V MG is characterized by the following:

1. Intubation with or without mechanical ventilation, except when employed during routine postoperative management.
2. The use of feeding tube without intubation places the patient in class IVb [2, 13].

Diagnosis

Serological Testing

MG is a condition which fulfills all the major criteria for a disorder mediated by autoantibodies against the acetylcholine receptor (AChR-Ab) or against a receptor-associated protein, muscle-specific tyrosine kinase (MuSK-Ab).

Patients with positive AChR-Ab or MuSK-Ab assays have seropositive myasthenia gravis (SPMG). Demonstration of these antibodies is possible in approximately 90% of patients with generalized MG and provides the laboratory confirmation of the disease [1, 2]. In those patients with purely ocular MG, the sensitivity of AChR-Ab testing is considerably lower, detectable in about half of patients. There are rare cases of ocular myasthenia that are MuSK-Ab positive, but most large case series of ocular myasthenia gravis have not found patients who are MuSK-Ab positive.

Acetylcholine receptor antibodies Immunologic assay to detect the presence of circulating AChR-Ab is the first step in the laboratory confirmation of MG. There are three AChR-Ab assays: binding, blocking, and modulating. Most authors use the term AChR-Ab as synonymous with the binding antibodies, and these are what are referenced in most studies that report the diagnostic sensitivity of these tests in MG for the reasons discussed below. These antibodies are polyclonal and are present in approximately 85% of patients with generalized disease. Essentially all patients (98 to 100%) with myasthenia gravis and thymoma are seropositive for these antibodies [7, 8]. The negative predictive value of thymoma in the absence of acetylcholine antibodies (binding) is high at 99.7% [8].

The assay for the binding antibody is the most sensitive. One study found these antibodies in 93, 88, and 71% of individuals with moderate to severe generalized myasthenia gravis, mild generalized myasthenia, and ocular myasthenia, respectively [9]. Others have found binding AChR-Ab in 80 to 90% of those with generalized disease [2, 10, 11] and in 40 to 55% of those with ocular myasthenia. Binding AChR antibodies are measured by standard radioimmunoassay and are highly specific for MG. There are virtually no false-positive results in healthy or disease-matched populations [12–14]. There are rare false positives in low titers in Lambert-Eaton myasthenic syndrome (5%), motor neuron disease (3–5%), and polymyositis (<1%) [9, 14, 15]. They are also rarely seen in some disorders that are not usually confused with myasthenia: primary biliary cholangitis, systemic lupus erythematosus, thymoma without myasthenia, and in first-degree relatives of patients with myasthenia gravis [16, 17].

Blocking AChR-Ab are present in about half of patients with generalized disease. They are present in fewer than 1% of patients with negative binding antibodies, but they have no significant false positives.

Assays for modulating AChR-Ab increase the sensitivity by ≤5% when added to the binding studies [11], and false-positive results are more of a problem [17].

Binding antibody studies are sufficient in most circumstances. The blocking and modulating antibody assays add relatively little to the diagnostic sensitivity [14]. However, the demonstration of blocking antibodies may be helpful if a possible false-positive binding antibody result is suspected.

AChR-Ab titers correlated poorly with disease severity between patients. A low-titer or even antibody-negative patient may have much more severe clinical disease than a patient with high titers. However, in an individual patient, the titers tend to fall with successful immunotherapy, and they parallel clinical improvement.

Ideally, serologic testing for AChR-Ab should be performed prior to initiating immunomodulating therapy for myasthenia gravis, as such therapy can sometimes lead to apparent seronegativity [11]. In one cohort of 143 seropositive patients, 9% became seronegative after treatment when retested in clinical remission. In addition, repeat serologic testing 6–12 months after initial testing has been reported to detect positive seroconversion in approximately 15% of patients with myasthenia gravis who were initially seronegative [11, 18].

MuSK antibodies Antibodies to the muscle-specific receptor tyrosine kinase (MuSK) are present in 38–50% of those with generalized myasthenia gravis who are AChR-Ab negative [11, 19–25]. MuSK is a receptor tyrosine kinase that mediates agrin-dependent AChR clustering and neuromuscular junction formation during development. MuSK antibody-positive MG may have a different cause and pathologic mechanism than AChR-Ab-positive disease [19, 26].

MuSK antibodies are generally not present in those with well-established ocular MG, but they have been detected in a few cases [27, 28]. Although nearly half of patients with AChR-Ab-negative myasthenia gravis will have MuSK antibodies, those with AChR-Ab-positive myasthenia do not have antibodies to MuSK in most studies to date [19–24]. However, one group found that 11% of patients with AChR-Ab-positive myasthenia did have antibodies to MuSK as well [29]. MuSK antibodies appear to be much less common in some AChR-Ab-negative myasthenia populations, being found in only 1 of 27 Taiwanese patients [30] and 0 of 17 Scandinavian patients [31].

One consistent finding is that patients with AChR-Ab-negative MG and MuSK antibodies have a much lower frequency of thymic pathology than patients with AChR-Ab-positive MG [32–35]. Thymic hyperplasia is frequent in AChR-Ab-positive myasthenia, but this pathology is much less frequent in the MuSK-Ab-positive group.

In the appropriate clinical setting (i.e., a patient with the typical clinical features of myasthenia gravis (see "Clinical features" below) who is AChR-Ab negative), MuSK antibody testing can clarify the diagnosis and perhaps direct treatment [20]. However, the initial management of clinically apparent MG should be the same for patients with or without AChR antibodies. This would change only if future studies find additional therapeutic differences related to MuSK antibody status.

Seronegative myasthenia The term seronegative MG, also called antibody-negative MG, refers to the 6–12% of patients with myasthenia who have negative standard assays for both AChR antibodies and MuSK antibodies. The term was previously used only for those who were AChR antibody negative, regardless of MuSK antibody status.

Patients with seronegative MG are more likely to have purely ocular disease than those who are seropositive. There is also a trend for those with generalized seronegative MG to have a better outcome after treatment [25].

Seronegative MG is an autoimmune disorder with most of the same features as seropositive myasthenia gravis [18, 25]. The electrophysiologic findings are identical. Patients with seronegative MG respond in a similar fashion to pyridostigmine, plasma exchange, glucocorticoids, and immunosuppressive therapies, as well as thymectomy.

Newer diagnostic antibody assays may further reduce the percentage of patients that are considered seronegative. As an example, approximately 50% of patients with seronegative MG have low-affinity AChR antibodies (also called clustered AChR antibodies) when tested by a specialized cell-based immunofluorescence assay. Other studies have demonstrated antibodies against LRP4, an agrin receptor required for agrin-induced activation of MuSK and AChR clustering and neuromuscular junction formation. These antibodies have been found in 2–50% of patients with seronegative MG. These assays are not commercially available and are not yet in widespread clinical use.

Electrophysiological Tests

The two principal electrophysiologic tests for the diagnosis of MG are repetitive nerve stimulation (RNS) study and single-fiber electromyography (SFEMG). RNS tests neuromuscular transmission. It is performed by stimulating the nerve supramaximally at 2–3 Hz. A 10% decrement between the first and the fifth evoked muscle action potential is consistent with a diagnosis of MG. In the absence of the decrement, exercise can be used to induce exhaustion of muscles and document decrement. The test is abnormal in approximately 75% of patients with gMG and 50% of patients with oMG [44, 45].

SFEMG is the most sensitive diagnostic test for MG. It is done by using a special needle electrode that allows identification of action potentials from individual muscle fibers. It allows simultaneous recording of the action potentials of two muscle fibers innervated by the same motor axon. The variability in time of the second action potential relative to the first is called "jitter." In MG, the jitter will increase because the safety factor of transmission at the neuromuscular junction is reduced. SFEMG reveals abnormal jitter in 95–99% of patients with MG if appropriate muscles are examined [44, 45]. Although highly sensitive, increased jitter is not specific for primary NMJ disease. It may be abnormal in motor neuron disease, polymyositis, peripheral neuropathy, Lambert-Eaton myasthenic syndrome (LEMS), and other neuromuscular disorders. However, it is specific for a disorder of neuromuscular transmission when no other abnormalities are seen on standard needle EMG examination [42].

Management

Management of MG should be individualized according to patient characteristics and the severity of the disease. There are two approaches for management of MG based on the pathophysiology of the disease. The first is by increasing the amount of ACh that is available to bind with the postsynaptic receptor using an acetylcholinesterase inhibitor agent, and the second is by using immunosuppressive medications that decrease the binding of acetylcholine receptors by antibodies.

There are four basic therapies used to treat MG:

1. Symptomatic treatment with acetylcholinesterase inhibitors
2. Rapid short-term immunomodulating treatment with plasma exchange (PE) and intravenous immunoglobulin (IVIg)
3. Chronic long-term immunomodulating treatment with glucocorticoids and other immunosuppressive drugs
4. Surgical treatment

Acetylcholinesterase Inhibitors

Acetylcholinesterase inhibitors are the first-line treatment in patients with MG. Response to treatment varies from marked improvement in some patients to little or no improvement in others. Acetylcholinesterase inhibitors are used as a symptomatic therapy and act by increasing the amount of available acetylcholine at the NMJ [46]. They do not alter disease progression or outcome. Pyridostigmine is the most commonly used drug. It has a rapid onset of action within 15 to 30 min, reaching peak activity in about 2 h. The effect lasts for about 3–4 h. The initial oral dose is 15–30 mg every 4–6 h and is titrated upwards depending on the patient's response. Adverse side effects of pyridostigmine are mostly due to the cholinergic properties of the drug such as abdominal cramping, diarrhea, increased salivation and bronchial secretions, nausea, sweating, and bradycardia. Nicotinic side effects are also frequent and include muscle fasciculation and cramping. High doses of pyridostigmine exceeding 450 mg daily, administered to patients with renal failure, have been reported to cause worsening of muscle weakness [47].

Short-Term Immunomodulating Therapies

Plasma exchange (PE) and intravenous immunoglobulin (IVIg) have rapid onset of action with improvement within days, but this is a transient effect. They are used in certain situations such as myasthenic crisis and preoperatively before thymectomy or other surgical procedures. They can be used intermittently to maintain remission in patients with MG who are not well controlled despite the use of chronic immuno-modulating drugs.

Plasma Exchange (PE)

PE improves strength in most patients with MG by directly removing AChR from the circulation [48]. Typically one exchange is done every other day for a total of four to six times. Adverse effects of PE include hypotension, paresthesias, infections, thrombotic complications related to venous access, and bleeding tendencies due to decreased coagulation factors [50].

Intravenous Immunoglobulin Therapy (IVIg)

IVIg are preparations of immunoglobulins isolated from pooled human plasma by ethanol cryoprecipitation. IVIg is usually administered for 5 days at a dose of 0.4 g/kg/day. Different doses and schedules involving fewer infusions at higher doses are also used. The mechanism of action of IVIg is complex. Therapeutic mechanisms include inhibition of cytokines, competition with autoantibodies, and inhibition of complement deposition. Interference with the binding of Fc receptor on macrophages, Ig receptor on B cells, and interference with antigen recognition by sensitized T cells are other mechanisms [50]. More specific techniques to remove pathogenic anti-AChR antibodies utilizing immunoadsorption have been developed recently and offer a more targeted approach to MG treatment. Clinical trials showed significant reduction of blocking antibodies with concomitant clinical improvement in patients treated with immunoadsorption techniques [41].

IVIg is considered to be relatively safe, but rare cases of severe complications such as thrombosis, renal insufficiency, volume overload, and hemolytic anemia are reported [42].

Compared to plasma exchange, IVIg is similar in terms of efficacy and complication rates [43]. However, plasma exchange (PE) has considerable cost advantages over IVIg with a cost-benefit ratio of 2:1 for treatment of myasthenia gravis [44].

Long-Term Immunotherapies

The goal of immune-directed therapy of MG is to induce a remission or near remission of the disease.

Corticosteroids

Corticosteroids were the first and most commonly used immunosuppressant medications in MG. Prednisone is generally used when symptoms of MG are not adequately controlled by cholinesterase inhibitors alone. Good response can be achieved with initial high doses which are then tapered to the lowest dose to maintain the response. Temporary exacerbation can occur after starting high doses of prednisone within the first 7–10 days and can last for several days [35, 36]. In mild cases, cholinesterase inhibitors are usually used to manage this worsening. In cases of severe exacerbation, PE or IVIg can be given before or with corticosteroid therapy to prevent or reduce the severity of corticosteroid-induced weakness and to induce a more rapid response. Oral prednisone might be more effective than anticholinesterase drugs in oMG and should therefore at least be considered in all patients with oMG [37, 38].

Nonsteroidal Immunosuppressive Agents

Azathioprine, a purine analog, reduces nucleic acid synthesis, thereby interfering with T- and B-cell proliferation. It has been utilized as an immunosuppressant agent in MG since the 1970s and is effective in 70–90% of patients with MG [45]. It usually takes up to 15 months to detect clinical response. When used in combination with prednisone, it might be more effective and better tolerated than prednisone alone [49]. Adverse side effects include hepatotoxicity and leukopenia [50]. The patients being considered for treatment with azathioprine should be screened for thiopurine methyltransferase (TPMT) deficiency either by plasma levels or genetic testing. Those people who have low levels of TPMT are at higher risk of adverse effects from azathioprine and should not receive the drug.

Mycophenolate mofetil selectively blocks purine synthesis, thereby suppressing both T-cell and B-cell proliferation. Widely used in the treatment of MG, its efficacy in MG was actually suggested by a few nonrandomized clinical trials [31, 32].

The standard dose used in MG is 1000 mg twice daily, but doses up to 3000 mg daily can be used. Higher doses are associated with myelosuppression, and complete blood counts should be monitored at least once monthly. The drug is contraindicated in pregnancy and should be used with caution in renal diseases, GI diseases, bone marrow suppression, and elderly patients [33].

Cyclophosphamide administered intravenously and orally is an effective treatment for MG [34]. More than half of the patients become asymptomatic within

1 year of treatment. Undesirable side effects include hair loss, nausea, vomiting, anorexia, and skin discoloration, which limit its use to the management of patients who do not respond to other immunosuppressive treatments [2].

Cyclosporine blocks the synthesis of IL-2 cytokine receptors and other proteins critical to the function of CD4+ T cells. Cyclosporine is used mainly in patients who do not tolerate or respond to azathioprine. Large retrospective studies have supported its use as a steroid-sparing agent [45].

Tacrolimus has been used successfully to treat MG at low doses. It has the theoretical advantage of less nephrotoxicity than cyclosporine. However, there are more controlled trial data supporting the use of cyclosporine. Like other immunosuppressive agents, tacrolimus also has the potential for severe side effects [2].

MG patients resistant to therapy have been successfully treated with cyclophosphamide in combination with bone marrow transplant or with rituximab, a monoclonal antibody against the B-cell surface marker CD20 [26].

Etanercept, a soluble and a recombinant tumor necrosis factor (TNF) receptor blocker, has also been shown to have steroid-sparing effects in studies on small groups of patients [2, 27].

Surgical Management

Thymectomy Surgical treatment is strongly recommended for patients with thymoma. The clinical efficacy of thymectomy for patients with autoimmune MG without thymoma has been questioned because the evidence supporting its use has not been demonstrated in randomized controlled trials. However, many case reports and series suggest that thymectomy is also of benefit in generalized autoimmune MG, especially when performed in younger patients. The benefit of thymectomy evolves over several years. Thymectomy is advised as soon as the patient's degree of weakness is sufficiently controlled to permit surgery. Patients undergoing surgery are usually pretreated with low-dose glucocorticoids and IVIg or PE. Thymectomy may not be a viable therapeutic approach for anti-MuSK antibody-positive patients because their thymus glands lack the germinal centers and infiltrates of lymphocytes that characterize thymi in patients who have anti-AChR antibodies. This supports a different pathologic mechanism in anti-MuSK-Ab-positive and anti-AChR-Ab-positive MG [78, 79]. Most experts still consider thymectomy to be a therapeutic option in anti-AChR-Ab-positive generalized MG with disease onset before the age of 50 years [2].

Prognosis

Given current treatment, which combines cholinesterase inhibitors, immunosuppressive drugs, PE, IVIg, immunosuppressive therapy, and supportive care in an intensive care unit (ICU) setting (when appropriate), most patients with MG have a near-normal life span. Mortality is now 3–4%, with principal risk factors being age older than 40 years, short history of progressive disease, and thymoma. Prior to modern therapies, the mortality from MG was as high as 30–40%. Fortunately, in most cases the term "gravis" is no longer applicable to most patients.

Morbidity results from intermittent impairment of muscle strength, which may cause aspiration, increased incidence of pneumonia, falls, and even respiratory failure if not treated [14]. In addition, the medications used to control the disease may produce adverse effects.

Today, the only terribly feared condition arises when the weakness involves the respiratory muscles. Weakness might become so severe as to require ventilatory assistance. Those patients are said to be in myasthenic crisis.

The disease frequently presents (40%) with only ocular symptoms. However, the EOMs are almost always involved within the first year. Of patients who show only ocular involvement at the onset of MG, only 16% still have exclusively ocular disease at the end of 2 years.

In patients with generalized weakness, the nadir of maximal weakness usually is reached within the first 3 years of the disease. As a result, half of the disease-related mortality also occurs during this period. Those who survive the first 3 years of disease usually achieve a steady state or improve. Worsening of disease is uncommon after 3 years.

Thymectomy results in complete remission of the disease in a number of patients. However, the prognosis is highly variable.

A retrospective study of 38 patients with MG indicated that the disease, particularly late-onset MG, is associated with a high risk for cancers outside of the thymus, whether or not the patient also has thymoma [16]. Extrathymic neoplasms occurred in 12 of the study patients. All of these tumors were solid and heterogeneous to their organ of origin. Some of the tumors were diagnosed before and some after the patients were diagnosed with MG.

Altogether the tumors represented nine different types of neoplasm, as follows:

- Two each of squamous cell carcinoma of the mouth, invasive bladder cancer, and prostate adenocarcinoma
- One each of basal cell skin cancer; lung, gastric, breast, and colon adenocarcinoma; and renal cell cancer

The only statistically significant variable among the patients was age, with the extrathymic tumors being found only in patients over 50 years. None of the patients with these neoplasms had thyroid disease or an autoimmune disease other than MG.

Congenital Myasthenic Syndromes

Congenital myasthenic syndromes (CMS) are characterized by fatigable weakness of skeletal muscle (e.g., ocular, bulbar, limb muscles) with onset at or shortly after birth or in early childhood. Rarely symptoms may not manifest until later in childhood. Cardiac and smooth muscles are not involved. Severity and course of disease are highly variable, ranging from minor symptoms to progressive disabling weakness. In some subtypes of CMS, myasthenic symptoms may be mild, but sudden severe exacerbations of weakness or even sudden episodes of respiratory insufficiency may be precipitated by fever, infections, or stress. Major findings of the neonatal onset subtype include feeding difficulties; poor suck and cry; choking spells; eyelid ptosis; and facial, bulbar, and generalized weakness. In addition arthrogryposis multiplex congenita may be present, and respiratory insufficiency with sudden apnea and cyanosis may occur. Later childhood onset subtypes show abnormal muscle fatigability with difficulty in activities such as running or climbing stairs; motor milestones may be delayed; fluctuating eyelid ptosis and fixed or fluctuating extraocular muscle weakness are common presentations.

Diagnosis/Testing

The diagnosis of CMS is based on clinical findings, a decremental EMG response of the compound muscle action potential (CMAP) on low-frequency (2–3 Hz) stimulation, absence of anti-acetylcholine receptor (AChR) and anti-MuSK antibodies in the serum, and lack of improvement of clinical symptoms with immunosuppressive therapy. Mutations in one of multiple genes encoding proteins expressed at the NMJ are currently known to be associated with subtypes of CMS, including the genes encoding different subunits of the acetylcholine receptor:

- CHRNE (εAChR subunit)
- CHRNA1 (αAChR subunit)
- CHRNB1 (βAChR subunit)
- CHRND (δAChR subunit)
- AGRN encoding agrin
- CHAT encoding choline O-acetyltransferase
- COLQ encoding acetylcholinesterase collagenic tail peptide
- DOK7 encoding protein Dok-7
- GFPT1 encoding glucosamine-fructose-6-phosphate aminotransferase 1
- MUSK encoding muscle, skeletal receptor tyrosine protein kinase
- RAPSN encoding rapsyn (43-kd receptor-associated protein of the synapse)
- SCN4A encoding the sodium channel protein type 4 subunit alpha

Management

Treatment of manifestations: Most individuals with CMS benefit from acetylcholinesterase (AChE) inhibitors and/or the potassium channel blocker 3,4-diaminopyridine (3,4-DAP); however, caution must be used in giving 3,4-DAP to young children and individuals with fast-channel CMS (FCCMS). Individuals with COLQ and DOK7 mutations usually do not respond to long-term treatment with AChE inhibitors. Some individuals with slow-channel CMS (SCCMS) are treated with quinidine, which has some major side effects and may be detrimental in individuals with acetylcholine receptor (AChR) deficiency. Fluoxetine is reported to be beneficial for SCCMS. Ephedrine and albuterol have been beneficial in a few individuals, especially as a therapeutic option for those with DOK7 or COLQ mutations.

Prevention of primary manifestations: Prophylactic anticholinesterase therapy to prevent sudden respiratory insufficiency or apneic attacks provoked by fever or infections in those with mutations in CHAT or RAPSN. Parents of infants are advised to use apnea monitors and be trained in CPR.

Agents/circumstances to avoid: Drugs known to affect neuromuscular transmission and exacerbate symptoms of myasthenia gravis (e.g., ciprofloxacin, chloroquine, procaine, lithium, phenytoin, beta-blockers, procainamide, quinidine).

Evaluation of relatives at risk: If the disease-causing mutations in the family are known, molecular genetic testing can be used to clarify the genetic status of at-risk asymptomatic family members, especially newborns or young children, who could benefit from early treatment to prevent sudden respiratory failure.

Genetic Counseling

Congenital myasthenic syndromes are inherited in an autosomal recessive or, less frequently, autosomal dominant manner.

In autosomal recessive CMS (AR-CMS), the parents of an affected child are obligate heterozygotes and therefore carry one mutant allele. Heterozygotes (carriers) are asymptomatic. At conception, each sibling of an affected individual has a 25% chance of being affected, a 50% chance of being an asymptomatic carrier, and a 25% chance of being unaffected and not a carrier.

In autosomal dominant CMS (AD-CMS), some individuals have an affected parent, while others have a de novo mutation. The proportion of cases caused by de novo mutations is unknown. Each child of an individual with AD-CMS has a 50% chance of inheriting the mutation.

Prenatal testing for pregnancies at increased risk is possible through laboratories offering either testing for the gene of interest or custom testing.

The Future and Myasthenia

Complement inhibition is an attractive therapeutic approach for MG because it is effective in RODENT EAMG (e.g., ref. 24).

Moreover, anti-C5 inhibitors show short-term safety and are effective in a variety of human disorders, including myocardial infarction [10], coronary artery bypass graft surgery [11], and lung transplantation [12]. Thus, therapeutic approaches based on inhibition of complement activation will likely be tried for MG in the future.

However, the ultimate goal for MG treatment is to eradicate the rogue anti-AChR autoimmune response specifically and reestablish tolerance to the AChR without affecting the other functions of the immune system or causing other adverse effects.

Such targeted immunosuppressive approaches are still far from clinical use. However, their success in EAMG suggests that approaches for specific modulation of the autoimmune anti-AChR response may become part of MG patient care in the next decade. We will summarize here the different approaches that have proven successful for the prevention and treatment of EAMG induced by immunization with AChR. We will also analyze the possible technical and biological limitations to their application for the treatment of human MG.

Approaches that have proven successful in rodent EAMG include the following: (a) administration of AChR or parts of its sequence in a manner known to induce tolerance; (b) depletion of AChR-specific B cells or T cells; and (c) interference with formation of the complex between MHC class II molecules, epitope peptide, T-cell receptor, and CD4 molecule.

Antigen presentation under special circumstances may lead to antigen-specific tolerance in adult animals rather than activated CD4$^+$ T cells. Earlier studies showed that in rats, presentation of AChR epitopes by unsuitable APCs (fixed B cells that had been incubated with AChR under conditions favoring AChR uptake and processing) caused unresponsiveness of the AChR-specific CD4$^+$ T cells to further stimulation with AChR [13]. More recently, several studies have demonstrated that DCs, especially after treatment with TGF-β, IFN-γ, or IL-10, when injected into rats with developing or ongoing EAMG, suppressed or ameliorated the myasthenic symptoms [14–16]. The effect was correlated with a reduced production of anti-AChR Abs without a reduced proliferative response of T cells to the AChR. Approaches based on the use of tolerance-inducing APCs, which should present all AChR epitopes and therefore influence all AChR-specific T cells, might be useful for the treatment of MG. Should pulsing of the APCs with human AChR be needed, biosynthetic human AChR subunits could be used as antigens.

Mucosal or subcutaneous administration of AChR or synthetic or biosynthetic AChR peptides to rodents—approaches known to induce antigen-specific tolerance in adult animals—prevented or delayed EAMG development [19]. Depending on the dose of the antigen administered, anergy/deletion of antigen-specific T cells (at high doses) and/or expansion of cells producing immunosuppressive cytokines (TGF-β, IL-4, IL-10) (at low doses) are major mechanisms in mucosal tolerance induction. The use of mucosal toleration procedures in human MG, however, is problematic because those procedures can be a double-edged sword [20]; they reduce AChR-specific CD4$^+$ T-cell responses but may also stimulate AChR-specific B cells to produce Abs, thereby worsening the disease. Also, a large amount of human AChRs would be required, which may be difficult to obtain.

Conjugates of a toxin with AChR or synthetic AChR sequences, when administered to animals with EAMG, eliminated B cells producing anti-AChR Abs [21]. This is probably because the AChR moiety of the conjugate docks onto the membrane-bound Abs of AChR-specific B cells, which can then be killed by the toxic domain. This approach has two caveats. First, the toxin may damage other cells. Second, anti-AChR CD4$^+$ T cells can recruit new B cells to synthesize more anti-AChR Abs.

AChR-specific CD4$^+$ T cells can be specifically eliminated in vitro by APCs genetically engineered to express relevant portions of the AChR, Fas ligand (to eliminate the activated AChR-specific T cells with which they interact), and a portion of Fas-associated death domain, which prevents self-destruction by the Fas ligand [22]. It is not known yet whether this strategy can be safely used to modulate EAMG in vivo.

Activation of CD4⁺ T cells requires interaction and stable binding of several proteins on the surfaces of the CD4⁺ T cell and of the APC. In experimental systems, interfering with formation of this complex usually reduced the activity of autoimmune CD4⁺ T cells. This may be obtained by administering or inducing Abs that recognize the binding site for the antigen of the T-cell receptor (known as T-cell vaccination) [23]. T-cell vaccination is already used in clinical trials for the treatment of multiple sclerosis, rheumatoid arthritis, and psoriasis [24]. It is effective in EAMG, and it is a promising future strategy for the treatment of MG [24]. The mechanisms of action of T-cell vaccination are complex, and they likely include the induction of modulatory CD4⁺ and CD8⁺ T cells [24]. Another approach used synthetic peptide analogs of an epitope recognized by autoimmune CD4⁺ T cells that bind the MHC class II molecules but cannot stimulate the specific CD4⁺ cells. These are known as altered peptide ligands (APLs). APLs compete with peptide epitopes derived from the autoantigen, thereby turning off the autoimmune response. APLs might also stimulate modulatory anti-inflammatory CD4⁺ T cells or anergize the pathogenic CD4⁺ T cells [25]. The rich epitope repertoire of anti-AChR CD4⁺ T cells in MG patients reduces the therapeutic potential of approaches that interfere with activation of specific CD4⁺ T cells; targeting only a few epitopes may not significantly reduce the anti-AChR response. Moreover, these treatments are likely to produce only transient improvement that ceases when administration of the anti-T-cell Ab is discontinued.

MG and EAMG have offered unique opportunities to investigate the molecular mechanisms of an Ab-mediated autoimmune disease. Many factors have contributed to making MG the best understood human autoimmune disease. These include the simplicity of the pathogenic mechanism in MG, where NMJ failure explains all symptoms; the deeper understanding of the structure and the function of the NMJ and its molecular components, most notably, the AChR; and the increasing understanding of the mechanisms that modulate immune responses and maintain tolerance. Hopefully increasing knowledge of the immunobiology of MG will form a foundation for designing new and specific therapeutic approaches aimed at curbing the rogue autoimmune response and reestablishing immunological tolerance without interfering with the other immune functions.

If this expectation is fulfilled, MG, which has been a benchmark to understanding autoimmunity in humans, will become a reference point for the design of specific immunosuppressive treatments of other autoimmune Ab-mediated diseases.

References

1. Robertson N. Enumerating neurology. Brain. 2000;123(4):663–4.
2. Conti-Fine BM, Milani M, Kaminski HJ. Myasthenia gravis: past, present, and future. J Clin Investig. 2006;116(11):2843–54.

3. Grob D, Brunner N, Namba T, Pagala M. Lifetime course of myasthenia gravis. Muscle Nerve. 2008;37(2):141–9.
4. Zhang X, Yang M, Xu J, et al. Clinical and serological study of myasthenia gravis in hu bei province, China. J Neurol Neurosurg Psychiatry. 2007;78(4):386–90.
5. Kurukumbi M, Weir RL, Kalyanam J, Nasim M, Jayam-Trouth A. Rare association of thymoma, myasthenia gravis and sarcoidosis: a case report. J Med Case Reports. 2008;2:245.
6. Marsteller HB. The first American case of myasthenia gravis. Arch Neurol. 1988;45(2):185–7.
7. Wilks, Sir Samuel, Bart. In: Roll Munk's, editor. Reprinted by RCPs, 1955, P.86.
8. Willis T. Pathologiae cerebri et nervosi generis specimen. Oxford, UK: Ja Allestry; 1667.
9. Jolly F. Ueber myasthenia gravis pseudoparalytica, vol. 32. Berlin: Klin Wochenschr; 1895.
10. Hughes T. The early history of myasthenia gravis. Neuromuscul Disord. 2005;15(12):878–86.
11. Walker MB. Case showing the effect of prostigmin on myasthenia gravis. J R Soc Med. 1935;28:759–61.
12. Pascuzzi RM. The history of myasthenia gravis. Neurol Clin. 1994;12(2):231–42.
13. Nastuk WL, Strauss AJL, Osserman KE. Search for a neuromuscular blocking agent in the blood of patients with myasthenia gravis. Am J Med. 1959;26(3):394–409.
14. Simpson JA. Myasthenia gravis, a new hypothesis. Scott Med. 1960;5:419–36.
15. Patrick J, Lindstrom J. Autoimmune response to acetylcholine receptor. Science. 1973;180(4088):871–2.
16. Sathasivam S. Steroids and immunosuppressant drugs in myasthenia gravis. Nat Clin Pract Neurol. 2008;4(6):317–27.
17. Gilhus NE, Owe JF, Hoff JM, Romi F, Skele GO, Aarli JA. Myasthenia gravis: a review of available treatment approaches. Autoimmune Diseases. 2011;10:1–6.
18. Leite MI, Waters P, Vincent A. Diagnostic use of autoantibodies in myasthenia gravis. Autoimmunity. 2010;43(5–6):371–9.
19. Meriggioli MN, Sanders DB. Autoimmune myasthenia gravis: emerging clinical and biological heterogeneity. Lancet Neurol. 2009;8(5):475–90.
20. Vernino S, Lennon VA. Autoantibody profiles and neurological correlations of thymoma. Clin Cancer Res. 2004;10(21):7270–5.
21. Leite MI, Schröbel P, Jones M, et al. Fewer thymic changes in MuSK antibody-positive than in MuSK antibody-negative MG. Ann Neurol. 2005;57(3):444–8.
22. Vincent A, McConville J, Farrugia ME, Newsom-Davis J. Seronegative myasthenia gravis. Semin Neurol. 2004;24(1):125–33.
23. Morgenthaler TI, Brown LR, Colby TV, Harper CM, Coles DT. Thymoma. Mayo Clin Proc. 1993;68(11):1110–23.
24. Romi F, Skeie GO, Gilhus NE, Aarli JA. Striational antibodies in myasthenia gravis: reactivity and possible clinical significance. Arch Neurol. 2005;62(3):442–6.
25. Romi F, Skeie GO, Aarli JA, Gilhus NE. The severity of myasthenia gravis correlates with the serum concentration of titin and ryanodine receptor antibodies. Arch Neurol. 2000;57(11):1596–600.
26. Jaretzki A, Barohn RJ, Ernstoff RM, et al. Myasthenia gravis: recommendations for clinical research standards. Ann Thorac Surg. 2000;70(1):327–34.
27. Hughes BW, Kusner LL, Kaminski HJ. Molecular architecture of the neuromuscular junction. Muscle Nerve. 2006;33(4):445–61.
28. Glass DJ, Bowen DC, Stitt TN, et al. Agrin acts via a MuSK receptor complex. Cell. 1996;85(4):513–23.
29. Morgutti M, Conti-Tronconi BM, Sghirlanzoni A, Clementi F. Cellular immune response to acetylcholine receptor in myasthenia gravis: II. Thymectomy and corticosteroids. Neurology. 1979;29(5):734–8.
30. Weiner HL. Induction and mechanism of action of transforming growth factor-β-secreting Th3 regulatory cells. Immunol Rev. 2001;182:207–14.

31. Christadoss P, Goluszko E. Treatment of experimental autoimmune myasthenia gravis with recombinant human tumor necrosis factor receptor Fc protein. J Neuroimmunol. 2002;122(1–2):186–90.
32. Feferman T, Maiti PK, Berrih-Aknin S, et al. Overexpression of IFN-induced protein 10 and its receptor CXCR3 in myasthenia gravis. J Immunol. 2005;174(9):5324–31.
33. Shi FD, Wang HB, Li H, et al. Natural killer cells determine the outcome of B cell-mediated autoimmunity. Nat Immunol. 2000;1(3):245–51.
34. Jander S, Stoll G. Increased serum levels of the interferon-γ-inducing cytokine interleukin-18 in myasthenia gravis. Neurology. 2002;59(2):287–9.
35. Keesey JC. Clinical evaluation and management of myasthenia gravis. Muscle Nerve. 2004;29(4):484–505.
36. Vincent A, Leite MI. Neuromuscular junction autoimmune disease: muscle specific kinase antibodies and treatments for myasthenia gravis. Curr Opin Neurol. 2005;18(5):519–25.
37. Grob D, Arsura L, Brunner NG, Namba T. The course of myasthenia gravis and therapies affecting outcome. Ann N Y Acad Sci. 1987;505:472–99.
38. Pal S, Sanyal D. Jaw muscle weakness: a differential indicator of neuromuscular weakness-preliminary observations. Muscle Nerve. 2011;43(6):807–11.
39. Grob D. Course and management of myasthenia gravis. JAMA. 1953;153(6):529–32.
40. Werner P, Kiechl S, Löscher W, Poewe W, Willeit J. Distal myasthenia gravis—frequency and clinical course in a large prospective series. Acta Neurol Scand. 2003;108(3):209–10.
41. Pascuzzi RM. The edrophonium test. Semin Neurol. 2003;23(1):83–8.
42. Meriggioli MN, Sanders DB. Advances in the diagnosis of neuromuscular junction disorders. Am J Phys Med Rehabil. 2005;84(8):627–38.
43. Sethi KD, Rivner MH, Swift TR. Ice pack test for myasthenia gravis. Neurology. 1987;37(8):1383–5.
44. Sanders DB, Howard JF, Johns TR. Single-fiber electromyography in myasthenia gravis. Neurology. 1979;29(1):68–76.
45. Oh SJ, Kim DE, Kuruoglu R, Bradley RJ, Dwyer D. Diagnostic sensitivity of the laboratory tests in myasthenia gravis. Muscle Nerve. 1992;15(6):720–4.
46. Lindstrom JM, Seybold ME, Lennon VA. Antibody to acetylcholine receptor in myasthenia gravis. Prevalence, clinical correlates, and diagnostic value. Neurology. 1976;26(11):1054–9.
47. Lennon VA. Serologic profile of myasthenia gravis and distinction from the Lambert-Eaton myasthenic syndrome. Neurology. 1997;48(4):S23–7.
48. Vincent A, Newsom-Davis J. Acetylcholine receptor antibody as a diagnostic test for myasthenia gravis: results in 153 validated cases and 2967 diagnostic assays. J Neurol Neurosurg Psychiatry. 1985;48(12):1246–52.
49. Mittag TW, Caroscio J. False-positive immunoassay for acetylcholine-receptor antibody in amyotrophic lateral sclerosis. N Engl J Med. 1980;302(15):868.
50. Koon HC, Lachance DH, Harper CM, Lennon VA. Frequency of seronegativity in adult-acquired generalized myasthenia gravis. Muscle Nerve. 2007;36(5):651–8.
51. Cikes N, Momoi MY, Williams CL, et al. Striational autoantibodies: quantitative detection by enzyme immunoassay in myasthenia gravis, thymoma, and recipients of D-penicillamine or allogeneic bone marrow. Mayo Clin Proc. 1988;63(5):474–81.
52. Suzuki S, Satoh T, Yasuoka H, et al. Novel autoantibodies to a voltage-gated potassium channel KV1.4 in a severe form of myasthenia gravis. J Neuroimmunol. 2005;170(1–2):141–9.
53. Leite MI, Jacob S, Viegas S, et al. IgG1 antibodies to acetylcholine receptors in "seronegative" myasthenia gravis. Brain. 2008;131(7):1940–52.
54. Chagnac Y, Hadani M, Goldhammer Y. Myasthenic crisis after intravenous administration of iodinated contrast agent. Neurology. 1985;35(8):1219–20.
55. Eliashiv S, Wirguin I, Brenner T, Argov Z. Aggravation of human and experimental myasthenia gravis by contrast media. Neurology. 1990;40(10):1623–5.
56. Drachman DB. Medical progress: myasthenia gravis. N Engl J Med. 1994;330(25): 1797–810.

57. Bosch EP, Subbiah B, Ross MA. Cholinergic crisis after conventional doses of anticholinesterase medications in chronic renal failure. Muscle Nerve. 1991;14(10):1036–7.
58. Batocchi AP, Evoli A, Schino CD, Tonali P. Therapeutic apheresis in myasthenia gravis. Ther Apher. 2000;4(4):275–9.
59. Gold R, Schneider-Gold C. Current and future standards in treatment of myasthenia gravis. Neurotherapeutics. 2008;5(4):535–41.
60. Samuelsson A, Towers TL, Ravetch JV. Anti-inflammatory activity of IVIG mediated through the inhibitory Fc receptor. Science. 2001;291(5503):484–6.
61. Psaridi-Linardaki L, Trakas N, Mamalaki A, Tzartos SJ. Specific immunoadsorption of the autoantibodies from myasthenic patients using the extracellular domain of the human muscle acetylcholine receptor α-subunit. Development of an antigen-specific therapeutic strategy. J Neuroimmunol. 2005;159(1–2):183–91.
62. Brannagan TH, Nagle KJ, Lange DJ, Rowland LP. Complications of intravenous immune globulin treatment in neurologic disease. Neurology. 1996;47(3):674–7.
63. Barth D, Nabavi Nouri M, Ng E, Nwe P, Bril V. Comparison of IVIg and PLEX in patients with myasthenia gravis. Neurology. 2011;76(23):2017–23.
64. Robinson J, Eccher M, Bengier A, Liberman J. Costs and charges for plasma exchange (PLEX) versus intravenous immunoglobulin (IVIg) in the treatment of neuromuscular disease. Neurology. 2012;78:PD6.008.
65. Pascuzzi RM, Branch Coslett H, Johns TR. Long-term corticosteroid treatment of myasthenia gravis: report of 116 patients. Ann Neurol. 1984;15(3):291–8.
66. Evoli A, Batocchi AP, Palmisani MT, Lo Monaco M, Tonali P. Long-term results of corticosteroid therapy in patients with myasthenia gravis. Eur Neurol. 1992;32(1):37–43.
67. Kupersmith MJ, Moster M, Bhiiiyan S, Warren F, Weinberg H. Beneficial effects of corticosteroids on ocular myasthenia gravis. Arch Neurol. 1996;53(8):802–4.
68. Bhanushali MJ, Wuu J, Benatar M. Treatment of ocular symptoms in myasthenia gravis. Neurology. 2008;71(17):1335–41.
69. Palace J, Newsom-Davis J, Lecky B. A randomized double-blind trial of prednisolone alone or with azathioprine in myasthenia gravis. Neurology. 1998;50(6):1778–83.
70. Kissel JT, Levy RJ, Mendell JR, Griggs RC. Azathioprine toxicity in neuromuscular disease. Neurology. 1986;36(1):35–9.
71. Chaudhry V, Cornblath DR, Griffin JW, O'Brien R, Drachman DB. Mycophenolate mofetil: a safe and promising immunosuppressant in neuromuscular diseases. Neurology. 2001;56(1):94–6.
72. Ciafaloni E, Massey JM, Tucker-Lipscomb B, Sanders DB. Mycophenolate mofetil for myasthenia gravis: an open-label pilot study. Neurology. 2001;56(1):97–9.
73. Meriggioli MN, Ciafaloni E, Al-Hayk KA, et al. Mycophenolate mofetil for myasthenia gravis: an analysis of efficacy, safety, and tolerability. Neurology. 2003;61(10):1438–40.
74. Spring PJ, Spies JM. Myasthenia gravis: options and timing of immunomodulatory treatment. BioDrugs. 2001;15(3):173–83.
75. Tindall RSA, Phillips JT, Rollins JA, Wells L, Hall K. A clinical therapeutic trial of cyclosporine in Myasthenia gravis. Ann N Y Acad Sci. 1993;681:539–51.

Idiopathic Inflammatory Myopathies

12

Robert N. Schwendimann

Introduction

In 1975, Bohan and Peter described clinical features of polymyositis and dermatomyositis. They stated: "polymyositis is an inflammatory myopathy of unknown cause to which the term dermatomyositis is applied in the presence of the characteristic skin rash" [4]. Today we know that DM is not simply PM with a rash. While they share certain characteristics clinically, they differ greatly in their pathophysiology, histology, and immunology. More recently, sporadic inclusion body myopathy (IBM) and auto-immune necrotizing myopathy (NM) have been added to this group of idiopathic inflammatory myopathies (IIM). IBM and NM also share common characteristics with DM and PM but differ somewhat in their clinical presentations. IBM also differs greatly from the other IIMs in treatment. DM, PM, and NM are extremely important because they are potentially treatable. This review will recount the clinical features of these myopathies along with an approach to diagnosis and treatment. It will also amplify what is known about IBM and autoimmune necrotizing myopathy as far as clinical presentation, diagnostic features, immunological features, treatment, and prognosis.

The clinical feature common to all of these disorders includes weakness, primarily of proximal muscles. Patients with DM, PM, and NM typically complain of difficulty arising from a chair, going up or down stairs, or working with their arms above their heads. Neck weakness and difficulty in swallowing are quite common as well. Usually the extraocular muscles are spared, and respiratory difficulties are uncommon except in severe and/or acute cases. The pattern of weakness is somewhat different in IBM where distal finger and wrist weakness occurs along with proximal weakness in the quadriceps muscles. Early atrophy in these muscles often occurs with IBM. Myalgias may occur in all of these, but pain is more common in NM [2, 5, 6, 8].

R.N. Schwendimann, MD
Department of Neurology, LSU Health Sciences Center,
1501 King Highway, Shreveport, LA 71130, USA
e-mail: RSchwe@lsuhsc.edu

© Springer International Publishing AG 2017
A. Minagar, J.S. Alexander (eds.), *Inflammatory Disorders of the Nervous System*, Current Clinical Neurology, DOI 10.1007/978-3-319-51220-4_12

Dermatomyositis

The onset of weakness in DM is usually acute to subacute, worsening over several weeks. It is more common in females than males. The weakness is proximal and typically symmetrical. Difficulty with swallowing and with speech may occur along with neck weakness sometimes leading to head drop. A characteristic purplish-colored (heliotrope) skin rash occurs over the eyelids and upper chest (in a V-pattern if anterior and in a shawl pattern if posterior), the dorsal metacarpal and interphalangeal joints, and the extensor surface of the elbows, knuckles (Gottron papules), knees, and ankles. The nails may be involved and show dilated capillary loops at the base of the nails [2, 5, 6, 8]. In children, the rash may be more severe and there can sometimes be subcutaneous calcifications. About 6% of patients have no skin abnormalities. There is also a small group of patients that have skin manifestations of DM with no evidence of muscular involvement [5]. Other systemic manifestations include interstitial lung disease, cardiac abnormalities, and malignancies. Malignancies include lung, ovarian, and various GI cancers (pancreas, stomach, colon/rectal). Juvenile DM is associated with a high incidence of leukemia and lymphoma [13].

Evaluation after neuromuscular examination includes screening laboratory studies considering other causes of muscle weakness, including the muscular dystrophies, metabolic myopathies (Pompe's disease, McArdle's disease), mitochondrial myopathies, and thyroid-related myopathies. An acute or subacute onset is much more typical of inflammatory myopathy [10]. The creatine kinase (CK) and aldolase levels are typically elevated, up to 50 times the upper limit of normal, though normal values can also occur. Electrodiagnostic studies reveal normal nerve conduction velocities. The needle electrode exam acutely shows evidence of "myopathic" motor units with brief duration, low amplitude, polyphasic units. EMG also shows evidence of increased insertional activity with spontaneous positive waves and fibrillations seen prominently. There is early recruitment of motor units. Complex repetitive discharges may be identified. This activity may occur in any muscle, including paraspinous groups. The EMG may be helpful in identifying muscle suitable for biopsy [2, 5, 6, 8]. Magnetic resonance imaging of the muscle may show changes suggesting active inflammation, edema, and fatty infiltration. It can also help in identifying muscles suitable for biopsy [11]. Muscle biopsy shows evidence of perivascular, perimysial, and perifascicular inflammation. There is deposition of membrane attack complex (MAC) around small blood vessels that is seen early. Inflammatory infiltrates consist of macrophages, B cells, and CD4+ plasmacytoid dendritic cells. There is evidence of perifascicular atrophy (which is the classic pathological finding in DM) and decrease in capillary density at the periphery of the fascicle. Invasion of non-necrotic muscle fibers is not prominent in DM. Electron microscopy has shown tubuloreticular inclusions in the intramuscular arterioles and capillaries (Fig. 12.1a–e) [2, 5, 6, 8].

A number of myositis-specific antibodies may be associated with both DM and, in some cases, PM. Anti-Mi-2 autoantibody is associated with classical DM associated with typical skin lesions. Its presence is associated with a good response to treatment and a lower incidence of underlying cancer. The anti-TIF-1 gamma (transcriptional intermediary factor 1) antibody is predictive of malignancy. NXP-2 (nuclear matrix protein 2) may be positive in younger patients with subcutaneous calcinosis but also suggests a high incidence of malignancy. The anti-Jo antibody (anti-histidyl-transfer RNA synthetase) occurs in both PM and DM. Patients with this antibody may develop an anti-synthetase syndrome consisting of fever, arthralgia, Raynaud's phenomena, interstitial lung disease, seronegative arthritis, mechanics hands (roughening and cracking of skin), and a rash that differs from the typical rash of DM. Interstitial lung disease is common, seen in 75–90% of cases [3].

The cause of DM is not known, but there appears to be an autoimmune pathogenesis. Membrane attack complex is activated and is deposited on endothelial cells. This leads to necrosis and reduction of endomysial capillaries and ischemia. There is muscle fiber destruction that resembles microinfarcts. The hypoperfusion related to these changes leads to the perifascicular atrophy seen in tissue biopsies. Release of proinflammatory cytokines upregulates adhesion molecules on endothelial cells. This facilitates migration of B cells, CD+4 T cells, and plasmacytoid dendritic cells to perimysial and endomysial spaces. There are also molecular biomarkers of type 1 interferon in both muscle and skin of patients with DM [5, 8].

Polymyositis

The clinical symptoms of polymyositis (PM) are very much the same as those seen in DM. PM usually affects a slightly older age group and is unlikely to occur in children. Like DM, it is more common in females. There is no rash. PM has become a term to describe inflammatory myopathies that are not DM or sporadic inclusion body myopathy or some other myopathic disorder such as a muscular dystrophy. Patients suspected of PM also have proximal muscle weakness as seen in other inflammatory myopathies. There are elevations in CK values and electrodiagnostic studies are consistent with those seen in a myopathic process. Patients with PM may also have evidence of anti-synthetase syndrome with positive anti-Jo antibodies. Associated malignancies also occur in association with PM. Muscle biopsy shows variability of fiber size and evidence of endomysial inflammation with cellular infiltrates that are primarily CD8+ cytotoxic T cells and macrophages. These cells may be seen invading non-necrotic muscle fibers that express major histocompatibility complex (MHC) class 1 antigen. Normal muscle fibers do not express this antigen. There are no vacuoles. MHC expression is probably induced by cytokines secreted by active T cells. These include IL1, IL-6, and IL-15. The triggering mechanism of these changes is unknown though viral infections have been suspected as a cause [2, 5, 6, 8].

Inclusion Body Myositis

Sporadic inclusion body myositis (sIBM) is much more common in males and typically affects an older age group. The age-adjusted prevalence in people over 50 years of age is 3.5/100,00 making it the most common inflammatory myopathy in this age group. IBM is characterized by slowly progressive weakness in the distal upper extremities and in the proximal lower extremities. There is often early weakness and atrophy in the quadriceps group that makes stair climbing and arising from a seated position difficult. This is followed by distal weakness in the arms that usually involves finger and wrist flexors more than finger and wrist extensor muscles. This pattern of weakness is considered by most to be pathognomonic for diagnosis of IBM. Difficulty in swallowing occurs in up to 70% of patients [7].

Diagnosis of IBM involves a clinical performance of the usual testing done in myopathic diseases. The level of CK may be elevated, but may also be normal. Electrodiagnostic studies usually show normal nerve conduction tests though there may be evidence of a mild axonal sensory polyneuropathy. Needle electrode exams show changes suggesting myopathy, though there can also be evidence of motor unit potentials that appear neurogenic (higher amplitude, longer duration, polyphasia). This finding is due to reinnervation of denervated fibers and split muscle fibers. The MRI in IBM shows more pronounced muscle atrophy than inflammation or edema. The anterior muscle groups of the arms and the legs are affected. Another distinctive feature is severe fatty atrophy of the medial gastrocnemius and relative sparing of the rectus femoris. Muscle biopsy shows changes that are similar to those seen in polymyositis: evidence of endomysial inflammation. The inflammatory cells involved are CD8+ T cells that invade non-necrotic muscle fibers. These cells express MHC class I antigen as well. In addition to these changes, there are chronic

---

Fig. 12.1 Dermatomyositis: A complement-mediated microangiopathy. Panel **a** shows a cross section of a hematoxylin and eosin-stained muscle biopsy sample with classic dermatomyositis perifascicular atrophy (layers of atrophic fibers at the periphery of the fascicle [*arrows*]) and some inflammatory infiltrates. Panel **b** shows the deposition of complement (membranolytic attack complex, in *green*) on the endothelial cell wall of endomysial vessels (stained in *red* with *Ulex europaeus* lectin), which leads to destruction of endothelial cells (shown in orange, indicating the superimposition of *red* and *green*). Consequently, in the muscles of patients with dermatomyositis (shown in Panel **c**), as compared with a myopathic control (Panel **d**), the density of the endomysial capillaries (in *yellow-red*) is reduced, especially at the periphery of the fascicle, with the lumen of the remaining capillaries dilated in an effort to compensate for the ischemic process. 1,2 Panel **e** shows a schematic diagram of a proposed immunopathogenesis of dermatomyositis. Activation of complement component 3 (C3) (probably triggered by antibodies against endothelial cells) is an early event leading to the formation of C3b, C3bNEO, and membrane attack complexes (MACs), which are deposited on the endothelial cell wall of the endomysial capillaries; this results in the destruction of capillaries, ischemia, or microinfarcts, which are most prominent in the periphery of the fascicles, as well as in perifascicular atrophy. Cytokines released by activated complement lead to the activation of CD4+ T cells, macrophages, B cells, and CD123+ plasmacytoid dendritic cells; enhance the expression of vascular-cell adhesion molecules (VCAMs) and intercellular adhesion molecule (ICAM) on the endothelial cell wall; and facilitate lymphoid cell transmigration to endomysial tissue through the action of their integrins, late activation antigen (VLA)-4, and lymphocyte function-associated antigen (LFA)-1, which bind VCAM-1 and ICAM-1. The perifascicular regions contain fibers that are in a state of remodeling and regeneration (expressing TGF-β, NCAM, and Mi-2), cell stress (expressing heat shock protein 70 [HSP70] and HSP90), and immune activation (expressing major histocompatibility complex [MHC] class I antigen, chemokines, and STAT1), as well as molecules associated with innate immunity (such as MxA, ISG15, and retinoic acid-inducible gene 1 [RIG-1]) (The figure and legend obtained from Dalakas [6] Copyright permission obtained)

changes with increased connective tissue and varied fiber size. Muscle fibers with rimmed vacuoles that are lined with granular material that stains bluish-red on hematoxylin and eosin (H&E) stain and modified Gomori trichrome stain are a hallmark of IBM. "Ragged red" or cytochrome oxidase negative fibers represent abnormal mitochondria. Congophilic amyloid deposits are best visualized with crystal violet or fluorescent optics. Some of these features may be absent on biopsy material and may falsely lead to a diagnosis of polymyositis. A poor response to treatment for polymyositis may lead to repeat biopsies in order to look more diligently for the pathological features of IBM (Fig. 12.2a–e) [2, 5–8].

IBM has features of both an autoimmune disease and a degenerative disease highlighted by the congophilic amyloid deposits seen in some muscle fibers. These

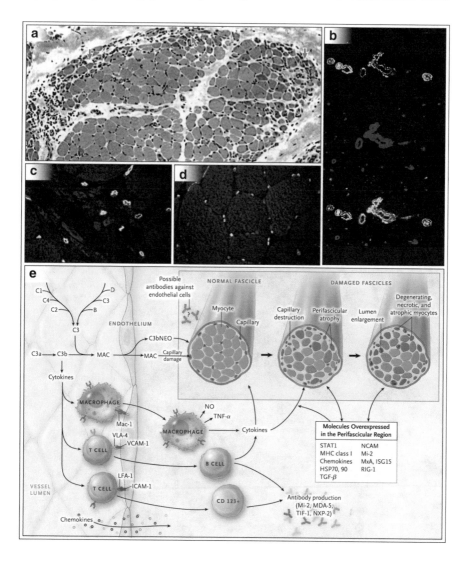

deposits react immunologically against amyloid pr-42 precursor protein, amyloid beta-42, apolipoprotein E, alpha-synuclein, presenilin, ubiquitin, and phosphorylated tau, similar to what is seen in Alzheimer's disease [5, 6, 8].

Immune-Mediated Necrotizing Myopathy

This type of myopathy has recently been added to the previously discussed inflammatory myopathies. It is felt to be a distinct myopathy that is immune mediated. It represents up to 20% of all inflammatory myopathies and occurs more frequently than polymyositis. It can affect any age group but usually occurs in adults. Clinically, the onset is similar to DM and PM with symptoms of proximal muscle weakness that progresses over days to weeks. Muscle pain may be more prominent than in other myopathies. Necrotizing myopathy often occurs in association with other

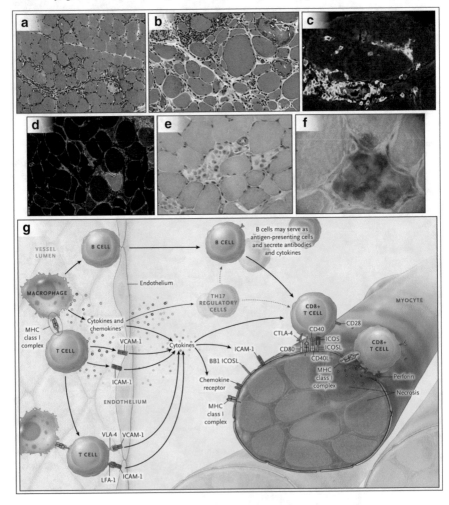

connective tissue diseases such as scleroderma or mixed-connective tissue disease. It may occur following viral infections or in association with cancer (GI tract adeno-carcinomas, small cell carcinoma of the lung). Onset may coincide with use of statin drugs to lower cholesterol. The myopathy may persist following withdrawal of the statin [2, 5, 6]. These cases are often associated with antibodies against signal rec-ognition particle (SRP) or 3-hydroxy-3-methylglutaryl-coenzyme A reductase (HMGCR) [11].

Diagnostic findings are similar to other myopathies. The creatine kinase is often very high, up to 50 times the upper limit of normal in acute stage. EMG shows typi-cal changes associated with myopathy and is not significantly different from changes in DM and PM. It is important to screen for other autoimmune disorders with appro-priate testing and to also carefully screen for underlying cancers. Presence of anti-signal recognition particle (anti-SRP) antibody may be associated with a dilated cardiomyopathy that may not respond to usual treatment with immunosuppressants. Positive HMGCR antibodies may be found in patients who have taken statin drugs [11]. These antibodies are not present in patients whose muscle symptoms have improved after cessation of the statin. MRI of muscles may reveal evidence of inflammation and edema. MRI of muscles, particularly the vastus lateralis, vastus medialis, and medial head of the gastrocnemius, soleus, and anterior tibial muscles, shows hyperintensity of short tau inversion recovery images (STIR) that is associ-ated with fatty infiltration [9].

Fig. 12.2 Main inflammatory features of polymyositis, inclusion body myositis, and necrotizing autoimmune myositis and a proposed immunopathogenic scheme for polymyositis and inclusion body myositis. Panels **a** and **b** show cross sections of hematoxylin and eosin-stained muscle biopsy samples from a patient with polymyositis (Panel **a**) and a patient with inclusion body myositis (Panel **b**), in which scattered inflammatory foci with lymphocytes invading or surrounding healthy-appearing muscle fibers are visible. In inclusion body myositis, there are also chronic myopathic features (increases in connective tissue and atrophic and hypertrophic fibers) and autophagic vacu-oles with bluish-red material, most prominent in fibers not invaded by T cells (*arrow*). In both polymyositis and inclusion body myositis, the cells surrounding or invading healthy fibers are CD8+ T cells, stained in green with an anti-CD8+ monoclonal antibody (Panel **c**); also visible is widespread expression of MHC class I, shown in green in Panel **d**, even in fibers not invaded by T cells. In contrast, in necrotizing autoimmune myositis (a cross section stained with trichrome is shown in Panel **e**), there are scattered necrotic fibers invaded by macrophages (Panel **f**), which are best visualized with an acid phosphatase reaction (in *red*). Panel **g** shows a proposed mechanism of T cell-mediated muscle damage in polymyositis and inclusion body myositis. Antigen-specific CD8+ cells, expanded in the periphery and subsequently in the endomysium, cross the endothelial cell wall and bind directly to aberrantly expressed MHC class I on the surface of muscle fibers through their T cell receptors, forming the MHC-CD8 complex. Upregulation of costimulatory molecules (BB1 and ICOSL) and their ligands (CD28, CTLA-4, and ICOS), as well as ICAM-1 or LFA-1, stabilizes the synaptic interaction between CD8+ cells and MHC class I on muscle fibers. Regulatory Th17 cells play a fundamental role in T cell activation. Perforin granules released by the autoaggressive T cells mediate muscle fiber necrosis. Cytokines, such as interferon-γ, interleu-kin-1, and tumor necrosis factor (TNF) released by the activated T cells, may enhance MHC class I upregulation and T cell cytotoxicity. Activated B cells or plasmacytoid dendritic cells are clonally expanded in the endomysium and may participate in the process in a still-undefined role, either as antigen-presenting cells or through the release of cytokines and antibody production (The figure and legend obtained from Dalakas [6] Copyright permission obtained)

Muscle biopsy shows evidence of muscle necrosis with macrophages surrounding the necrotic fibers. Unlike PM and IBM, no CD8+ cells or vacuoles are seen. Non-necrotic fibers may express MHC-1 and membrane attack complex deposition [2, 5, 6].

Treatment of Inflammatory Myopathies

The treatment of DM, PM, and necrotizing myopathy is quite similar and can be considered together. Inclusion body myopathy does not respond to these treatments. Corticosteroids are considered first-line treatment. While there are different ways to begin therapy, usually high-dose therapy at 0.75–1.5 mg/kg per day orally is started [2, 5, 6, 8, 12].

Dermatomyositis, polymyositis, and necrotizing myopathy usually respond to treatment with immunosuppressants. There are no recognized effective treatments for IBM at the present time. Treatment with high-dose oral corticosteroids is usually the first-line treatment for DM, PM, and necrotizing myopathy. In severe cases, high-dose IV steroids can be administered (methylprednisolone 1000 mg/day for 3 days). Treatment with steroids and other immunosuppressants is based on experience rather than controlled trials. Typical treatment begins with oral prednisone at 1 mg/kg up to 100 mg a day for 4–6 weeks or until muscle strength improves and the CK values have normalized. It is best to judge the results of treatment on improvement in strength rather than the CK values however. Each treating physician may have his/her protocol as to how the prednisone should be tapered, but a reduction in dose by 10 mg every 4 weeks until the patient is taking 20 mg daily is one way to taper the drug. Once the 20 mg dose is reached, dose should be further reduced by 5 mg daily every 4 weeks until a dose of 10 mg per day is reached. Further reduction by 2.5 mg/day every 4 weeks is then initiated though most patients will require a small maintenance dose long term. An alternate day regimen may be helpful in lessening some of the side effects of the prednisone. It is good practice to obtain a bone density scan prior to initiating corticosteroid therapy. Repeat scans should be performed on a yearly basis. Other recommendations include calcium and vitamin D supplements or treatment with a bisphosphonate. Patients should be instructed to eat a low sodium, high protein, low carbohydrate diet. Blood sugar and potassium levels should be monitored.

Other first-line therapies include physical and occupation therapy and speech and swallowing evaluations [2, 5, 6, 8, 12].

There are numerous second-line therapies for these myopathies as well. Methotrexate in doses ranging from 7.5 to 25 mg per week is often the first of these to be considered. Renal function, liver enzymes, and complete blood counts should be monitored. Patients should receive supplemental folate therapy along with the methotrexate. Since methotrexate can cause pulmonary fibrosis, it should be avoided in patients with interstitial lung disease or who demonstrate presence of anti-Jo antibodies [5].

Other second-line drugs include azathioprine, mycophenolate mofetil, cyclosporine, tacrolimus, and rituximab. All have been reported to be useful treatments. In refractory patients, intravenous immunoglobulin (IVIg) at 2 mg/kg/day over 3–5 days has been reported to be beneficial. There are various approaches to the use of these drugs that will not be discussed [12].

Treatment of Inclusion Body Myositis

At the present time, there are no effective drug treatments for IBM. The usual treatments for other inflammatory have all been tried, but none have been of any therapeutic benefit. These treatments have included prednisone, azathioprine, IVIg, methotrexate, lithium, beta-interferon, and many others. There are current trials with the monoclonal antibody bimagrumab (BYM338) that inhibits activin type II receptors that have the effect of inhibiting muscle atrophy. This treatment has been shown to cause an increase in thigh muscle mass measured with MRI in a small group of patients. Follistatin is a myostatin inhibitor that has the potential to increase muscle mass. Other trials with arimoclomol, etanercept, and alemtuzumab have been completed though results of the trials are not published [1, 7, 12]. Further information about drug trials can be obtained through the website, Clinicaltrials.gov.

Current therapy of IBM is supportive. There is evidence that exercise can be facilitated by physical and occupation therapists. The major goal is to maintain strength and prevent falls. The use of assistive devices and orthoses may help in achieving these same goals [5].

Summary

What was generally felt to be one inflammatory myopathy 40 years ago are now recognized to be four distinct diseases today. While there are common features from a clinical standpoint, they are different in their histology and pathology. There are also differences in the response to therapy. The use of magnetic imaging and the recognition of muscle-specific antibodies are useful in separating these conditions from one another. There is active clinical research in finding new treatments for IBM and improving treatments for the other inflammatory myopathies.

References

1. Alfano LN, Lowes LP. Emerging therapeutic options for sporadic inclusion body myositis. Ther Clin Risk Manag. 2015;11:1459–67.
2. Amato AA, Greenberg SA. Inflammatory myopathies. Continuum (Minneap Minn). 2013;19:119–30.
3. Betteridge Z, McHugh N. Myositis-specific autoantibodies: an important tool to support diagnosis of myositis. J Intern Med. 2015; doi:10.1111/joim.12451.
4. Bohan A, Peter JB. Polymyositis and dermatomyositis. N Engl J Med. 1975;292:344–7.

5. Chhibber S, Amato AA. Clinical evaluation and management of inflammatory myopathies. Semin Neurol. 2015;35:347–59.
6. Dalakas MC. Inflammatory muscle disease. N Engl J Med. 2015;372:1734–47.
7. Dimachkie MM, Barohn RJ. Inclusion body myositis. Curr Neurol Neurosci Rep. 2013;13:321. doi:10.1007/s11910-012-0321-4.
8. Findlay AR, Goyal NA, Mozaffar T. An overview of polymyositis and dermatomyositis. Muscle Nerve. 2015;51:638–56.
9. Maurer B, Walker UA. Role of MRI in diagnosis and management of idiopathic inflammatory myopathies. Curr Rheumatol Rep. 2015;17:67. doi:10.1007/s11926-015-0544-x.
10. Michelle EH, Mammen AL. Myositis mimics. Curr Rheumatol Rep. 2015;17:63. doi:10.1007s11926-015-054-0.
11. Mohassel P, Mammen AL. Statin-associated autoimmune myopathy and anti-HMGCR auto-antibodies. Muscle Nerve. 2013;48:477–83.
12. Needham M, Mastaglia FL. Immunotherapies for immune-mediated myopathies: a current perspective. Neurotherapeutics. 2016;13:132–46.
13. Tiniakou E, Mammen AL. Idiopathic myopathies and malignancy: a comprehensive review. Clin Rev Allergy Immunol. 2015; doi:10.1007/s12016-015-8511.x.

The Venous Connection: The Role of Veins in Neurodegenerative Disease

13

Clive Beggs

Context

The cerebral venous drainage system has often been viewed simply as a series of collecting vessels passively channelling blood from the brain back to the heart. However, recent studies suggest that this system may be far from passive and that in fact it plays an important role in regulating intracranial pressure (ICP) [1], the stiffness of the brain parenchyma [2] and the dynamics of the cerebrospinal fluid (CSF) in the cranium [3]. Anomalies of the cervical veins have also been reportedly linked with several neurologic conditions, including multiple sclerosis (MS) [4–6], Parkinson's disease [7], Meniere's disease [8, 9] and Alzheimer's disease [10, 11]. As such, this raises intriguing questions as to whether or not changes in the cerebral venous drainage system can alter the biomechanics of the intracranial space, resulting in neurodegeneration. In this review we investigate this issue and explore the connection between veins and neurologic disease.

Veins and Neurodegeneration

Since the earliest years of research into MS, there has been suspicion that the venous system might be involved in its aetiology, with Dawson [12], Putnam [13, 14] and others [15–19] all implicating veins in the pathophysiology of the disease. MS plaques are often venocentric and frequently form in the periventricular white matter (WM) [6]. The formation of fingerlike plaques at the junction of the

C. Beggs, PhD
Buffalo Neuroimaging Analysis Center, Department of Neurology, School of Medicine and Biomedical Sciences, University at Buffalo, 100 High St, Buffalo 14203, NY, USA

Institute for Sport, Physical Activity and Leisure, Carnegie Faculty, Leeds Beckett University, Leeds LS1 3HE, UK
e-mail: c.beggs@leedsbeckett.ac.uk

© Springer International Publishing AG 2017
A. Minagar, J.S. Alexander (eds.), *Inflammatory Disorders of the Nervous System*, Current Clinical Neurology, DOI 10.1007/978-3-319-51220-4_13

subependymal and medullary veins was first reported by Dawson [12] in the early twentieth century. Later, Putnam and Adler [14], commenting on the appearance of these 'Dawson fingers', observed that the medullary veins were enclosed in a sleeve of plaque and that, adjacent to these plaques, the veins were grossly distorted and distended. Others [19–22] have also shown that inflammatory lesions tend to form axially around veins in the WM, with Tallantyre et al. [23] finding 80% of MS lesions to be perivenous in nature. MS lesions in the grey matter have also been associated with veins, with Kidd et al. [21] finding the majority of cortical lesions arising within the territory of the principal vein, V5, whose course begins in the WM [24], and the remaining cortical lesions forming in the region drained by its branches or those of the superficial veins. Others have confirmed these observations, finding intracortical [25–27], leucocortical [25] and subcortical [20] lesions all to be perivenous in nature.

It is thought that the infiltration of leukocytes across the blood-brain barrier (BBB) into the central nervous system (CNS) is an essential step in the pathophysiology of MS. Chemokines on the endothelial lumen bind to receptors on the leukocytes, and it is thought that this initiates a cascade of events that culminates in breaching of the BBB [28]. The ease with which the leukocytes are able to enter the brain parenchyma depends on the chemokines present and the characteristics of the endothelia. While the BBB has traditionally been considered a uniform element, there is evidence of heterogeneity within the BBB [28], which varies depending on its location within the cerebral vascular bed. In particular, there is considerable heterogeneity in the tight junctions between the endothelial cells [29, 30], which appear weaker and more leaky in the cerebral collecting veins [31]. Furthermore, the expression of the chemokine CXCL12 (which regulates leukocyte access to the CNS parenchyma) at the abluminal endothelial membrane appears altered in the postcapillary venules in MS [28], something that correlates with the perivascular infiltration of T-cells [32, 33]. It has also been shown that the blood flow characteristics of the venules tend to promote margination [28, 34], with the result that the leukocytes are displaced to the periphery of the vessels [34], where they come into contact with the endothelial cells [35], something that may enhance intercellular interactions, leading to the attachment of leukocytes to the endothelial wall.

Perivenous WM changes have also been associated with ageing. In a series of related studies, Chung and co-workers [36–38] investigated jugular venous reflux (JVR) in elderly individuals. They found JVR to be associated with severe age-related WM changes, similar to those associated with leukoaraiosis [38]. Leukoaraiosis is characterised by WM morphological changes around the periventricular veins [39–42] that are thought to be associated with chronic cerebral ischemia [43]. In cases of ischemic injury, histological changes of the WM can range from coagulative necrosis and cavitation to non-specific tissue changes such as sponginess, patchy demyelination and astrocytic proliferation [43]. Such changes are consistent with the lesions seen in patients with leukoaraiosis [44], suggesting that the condition is linked with ischemia [43]. In particular, leukoaraiosis is characterised by noninflammatory collagenosis of the periventricular veins [39, 41], resulting in thickening of the vessel walls and narrowing, or even occlusion, of the lumen [39]. Moody et al. [39] found a strong association between the probability of severe leukoaraiosis and periventricular venous collagenosis.

A strong epidemiological link exists between leukoaraiosis and cerebrovascular disease [45–47]. Arterial hypertension and cardiac disease are also frequently associated with leukoaraiosis [43], and these are thought to induce arteriolosclerotic changes in the arteries and arterioles of the WM, replacing the smooth muscle cells by fibro-hyaline material, causing thickening of the vessel walls and narrowing of the vascular lumen [48]. Indeed, arteriolosclerosis is frequently found within areas of leukoaraiosis [49, 50]. Furthermore, the arterioles supplying the deep WM, which are some of the longest in the brain, frequently become tortuous with ageing [42, 51–53], with the result that there is a trend towards increased tortuosity in individuals with leukoaraiosis [42]. This tortuosity usually begins abruptly as the arteriole passes from the cortex into the WM [42] and greatly increases the length of the vessel. The combination of increased vessel length and reduced diameter means that the hydraulic resistance of the arterioles will greatly increase [53], inhibiting blood flow to the deep WM [42, 54–56]. It is therefore perhaps not surprising that the periventricular veins, being a 'distal irrigation field' [43], appear prone to ischemic damage under conditions of moderate deficit in blood flow.

Like leukoaraiosis, MS appears also to be associated with a reduction in cerebral blood flow (CBF) [57–60], raising questions about whether or not ischemia might be involved in the pathology of this disease. Wakefield et al. [61] found morphological changes in the venous endothelia, which progressed to occlusive vascular inflammation. They proposed that these changes were the precursor to lesion formation and suggested that demyelination may have an ischemic basis in MS. Similarities have been found between the tissue injury associated with inflammatory brain lesions and that found under hypoxic conditions in the CNS [62]. Ge et al. [63] identified subtle venous wall signal changes in small MS lesions, which they interpreted as early-stage vascular changes, thought to be the result of ischemic injury, marking the beginning of trans-endothelial migration of vascular inflammatory cells, before any apparent BBB breakdown. Werring et al. [64] found that the formation of lesions was preceded by subtle progressive alterations in tissue integrity, and Wuerfel et al. [65] found that changes of perfusion parameters, such as CBF, cerebral blood volume (CBV), and mean transit time (MTT) were detectable prior to the BBB breakdown. They concluded that in MS, inflammation is accompanied by altered local perfusion, which can be detected prior to permeability of the BBB. Lochhead et al. [66], using a rat model, demonstrated that hypoxia followed by reoxygenation altered the conformation of the occludin in the tight junctions between the endothelial cells, resulting in increased BBB permeability. In doing so, they confirmed the findings of earlier studies undertaken by the same team [67, 68].

Regulation of the Intracranial Fluids

Being encased in a rigid enclosure, the brain employs a sophisticated windkessel mechanism to regulate the flow of blood through the cerebral vascular bed [69–71]. This mechanism compensates for the transient increases in arterial blood volume entering the cranium that occur during systole, by displacing an approximately equal volume of CSF from the cranium into the spinal column [72]. As such, it ensures that the flow of blood through the cerebral capillary bed remains constant and non-pulsatile in healthy young adults [70], despite the considerable changes in the arterial blood flow rate entering the cranium that occur throughout the cardiac cycle (CC). The whole system is driven by volumetric changes in the arterial pulse, which are transferred to the CSF, causing it to pulse backwards and forwards across the foramen magnum (FM) (Fig.13.1). During systole the CSF travels in the caudal direction, whereas in diastole the flow is reversed, with the CSF travelling into the subarachnoid space (SAS) and interacting with the cortical bridging veins [73, 74].

While the presence of an intracranial windkessel mechanism is generally accepted, the arteriovenous time delay [75, 76] between peak arterial flow entering the cranium and peak venous flow leaving the cranium (Fig. 13.2a) has remained something of a mystery. The cranium is a rigid container filled with incompressible gel-like matter and fluids [77, 78]. Any increase in the intracranial arterial volume should therefore in theory be matched by an instantaneous displacement of fluid out of the cranium. While the displacement of CSF through the FM is virtually instantaneous [73, 74], the delay between the cervical arterial and venous flow rate peaks [75, 76] suggests that complex fluid interactions must be occurring within the cranium. Recently, a model was developed which sheds new light on the complex fluid interactions that occur within the cranium during the CC [79]. This model interprets the cervical blood and CSF flows in the neck to determine the temporal changes that occur in the intracranial arterial, venous and CSF volumes. It is illustrated in Fig. 13.2b, which shows the results of applying the model to mean cervical blood and CSF flow data (Fig. 13.2a) collected from 12 healthy young adults [80]. From this it can be seen that there is a strong inverse relationship between the arterial and CSF fluid volumes in the cranium. As arterial blood accumulates in the cranium during systole, so it displaces CSF, with the result that the intracranial CSF volume reduces to a minimum when the intracranial arterial volume is at its maximum. Conversely, during diastole, as the arterial blood flow entering the cranium decreases, so the returning CSF displaces arterial blood stored in the pial arteries, with the result that the intracranial CSF volume reaches a maximum at approximately the same time as the intracranial arterial blood volume is at its minimum. From Fig. 13.2b, it can be seen that during diastole, as the intracranial CSF volume increases, so venous blood starts to accumulate within the cranium. Only when the intracranial CSF volume has peaked and starts to decrease does the stored venous blood start to discharge from the cranium, suggesting that venous outflow is regulated in some way by the interaction between the CSF in the SAS and the cortical bridging veins, as Greitz [81] and Nakagawa et al. [82] postulated.

The timing of the intracranial fluid regulatory mechanism appears critical. In late diastole and early systole, the cranium can only accommodate the stored venous

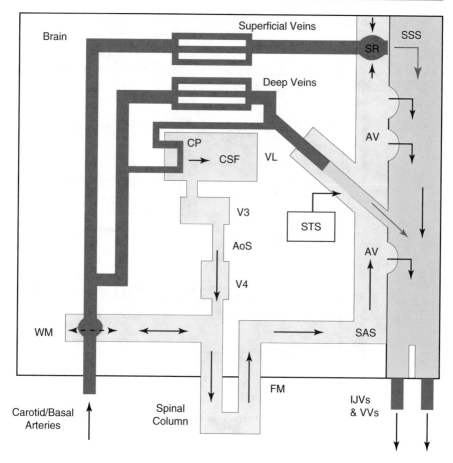

Fig. 13.1 Hydrodynamic model of the brain, showing the interactions between the arterial and venous blood flows and the cerebrospinal fluid (*CSF*). *SSS* superior sagittal sinus, *STS* straight sinus, *SAS* subarachnoid space, *AV* arachnoid villi, *CP* choroid plexus, *FM* foramen magnum, *WM* windkessel mechanism, *SR* Starling resistor, *VL* lateral ventricle, *V3* third ventricle, *V4* fourth ventricle, *AoS* aqueduct of Sylvius, *IJV* internal jugular vein, *VV* vertebral veins

blood because the store of arterial blood in the cranium is depleted during this period. Similarly, the system requires the free egress of venous blood of the cranium during systole. A number of studies have shown that constriction of the internal jugular veins (IJVs) causes increased retention of blood in the cerebral veins [83] and that this can increase the stiffness of the brain parenchyma [2], causing the amplitude of the CSF pulse in the aqueduct of Sylvius (AoS) to increase [2, 3]. Furthermore, rotation of the head can compress both the IJVs and the vertebral veins [84] inhibiting cerebral venous drainage, something that has been shown to increase the venous pressure in the confluens sinuum by as much as 30.3% [85]. This in turn can influence ICP. Indeed, it has been shown that in anaesthetised neurosurgical patients lying on a flat surface, the ICP can be raised by 4.1–4.8 mmHg simply through rotation of the head [86]. Collectively, these findings suggest that

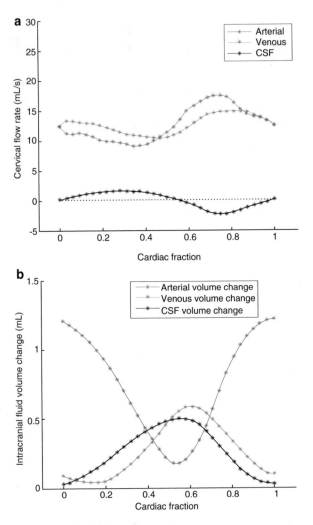

Fig. 13.2 (**a**) Mean cervical arterial, venous and cerebrospinal fluid (*CSF*) flow rates over a cardiac cycle, for all 12 subjects aggregated together. (NB. For ease of representation, the venous signal has been inverted.) (**b**) Mean intracranial arterial, venous and CSF volumetric changes over the cardiac cycle, for all 12 subjects aggregated together (Adapted from Beggs et al. [80])

the characteristics of the cerebral venous drainage system can influence fluid dynamics within the cranium.

Intracranial Pulsatility

Bilateral compression of the jugular veins has also been shown to increase pulsatility in the pial arteries [87], suggesting that the functional compliance of the cortical veins not only influences the CSF dynamics but also blood flow in the cerebral vascular bed

[88]. In healthy young adults, the flow of blood through the cerebral capillaries is constant and non-pulsatile [70]. However, if the compliance of the veins that traverse the SAS is impaired, say through constriction or partial occlusion of the extracranial cerebral venous drainage pathways, then this will tend to decrease intracranial compliance, leading to larger pressure pulsatility in the cerebral vasculature [88].

As individuals age, their arteries become less compliant, causing the intracranial windkessel mechanism to become less efficient, with the result that blood flow entering the cerebral vascular bed becomes more pulsatile [70, 89]. Stiffening of the aorta has also been linked to the transmission of excessive flow pulsatility into the brain [90, 91], something that will increase endothelial shear stresses and has been linked with microstructural WM changes in healthy older individuals [92]. Tarumi et al. [90] demonstrated that arterial stiffness in ageing is positively correlated with cerebral vascular pulsatility and that this in turn is associated with a greater volume of WM hyperintensities. Excessive intracranial cardiac-related pulsatility has also been associated with brain atrophy among elderly individuals [93]. Microstructural changes associated with increased cerebral pulsatility may therefore represent early-stage alterations in the structural organisation of the WM, likely to precede the emergence of leukoaraiosis [92].

Ageing of the brain in healthy individuals is characterised by atrophy and WM signal abnormality changes, typically detected as leukoaraiosis [94]. Leukoaraiosis is known to be associated with hypertension. Given that hypertension is associated with reduced vascular compliance [95], particularly in smaller arterial vessels [96], it is therefore perhaps not surprising that leukoaraiosis has been shown to be characterised by increased arterial and sinus pulsatility [70]. Likewise, patients with normal pressure hydrocephalus (NPH), a condition frequently linked with leukoaraiosis, appear to exhibit increased pulsatility in the blood flow through the cerebral vascular bed [70]. While the mechanisms linking these conditions with vascular pulsatility in the brain are poorly understood, it has been shown that advancing age is associated with higher pulsatility of CBF, which in turn is accompanied by a reduction in total CBF [90]. Given that higher pulsatility of CBF has been associated with microstructural WM damage [92] and greater WM hyperintensities [90] in older adults, this suggests that ischemic stress, arising from reduced CBF, may be involved in promoting WM damage – something that others have suggested [43, 44, 54, 56].

CSF Pulsatility, Ventricular Reflux and Periventricular Changes

Although there appears to be clear evidence linking increased pulsatility in the cerebral vascular bed with WM changes, the link between increased CSF pulse amplitude in the AoS and neuropathology appears more tenuous. Increased aqueductal CSF pulsatility has been shown to be a feature of MS [97–99] and NPH [100–105]. However, the extent to which this phenomenon contributes to any pathology is unclear. T1 and T2 lesion volumes have been found to be positively correlated with the aqueductal pulse in MS patients [97]. However, this might be indicative of increased lateral ventricle size, rather than any causal relationship linking altered CSF dynamics with lesion formation. Notwithstanding this, it has been shown that increased aqueductal CSF pulsatility is associated with early-stage microstructural

WM changes in healthy adults [106] and elderly subjects [92] with no neurologic condition. This raises questions as to whether or not ventricular reflux, the resorption of CSF through the ependymal wall, might be a feature of some neurodegenerative disease. MS lesions are often observed around the subependymal veins at the edge of the lateral ventricles [18, 20]. Likewise, demyelinated lesions associated with other WM disorders such as Binswanger's encephalopathy and leukoaraiosis often occur in the vicinity of the periventricular veins [39, 107, 108]. This has led several investigators to suggest that CSF leakage through the ependymal wall might be a contributory factor in periventricular lesion formation in MS patients [109]. Recently, Liu et al. [110] demonstrated that in MS patients, tissue structural abnormalities in the normal-appearing WM and WM lesions were greatest near the ventricles, with the magnetisation transfer ratio being abnormally low (compared with healthy controls) adjacent to the ventricles and increasing with distance from the ependymal wall. This they interpreted as being consistent with CSF or ependymal mediated pathogenesis.

NPH is associated with significantly reduced CSF absorption into the superior sagittal sinus (SSS) [111, 112], and this has led to speculation that CSF resorption might be occurring in the subependymal brain parenchyma [75]. Ventricular reflux of fluid has been shown to be a characteristic of communicating hydrocephalus [113, 114], with the periventricular tissue characterised by disruption of the ependyma, oedema, neuronal degeneration and ischemia [115]. Animal studies have also shown that in hydrocephalus, part of the CSF flow is cleared via a trans-parenchymal route into the cerebral vasculature [116–118], suggesting that a similar phenomenon may also be present in NPH [119]. If ventricular reflux of CSF is breaching the ependymal wall in NPH, then this might result in oedemas in the periventricular parenchyma, something which could inhibit CBF in this region [120]. CBF has been found to be generally lower in NPH patients than in normal controls [120–123], mirroring a similar phenomenon in MS patients [57–59]. However, after shunting, cerebral metabolism is increased [124], suggesting that in NPH reduced perfusion in this region is reversible and associated with CSF disturbances. Indeed, it has been postulated that CSF shunting in patients with NPH leads to a reversed flow of extracellular fluid from the periventricular WM into the ventricles, reducing the amount of extracellular water in the subependymal brain parenchyma [119].

Discussion

In recent years there has been much controversy about the possible role that venous anomalies might play in the aetiology of MS. This debate has been precipitated by the work of Zamboni et al. [4], who in 2009 published an ultrasonic study linking a vascular syndrome, *chronic cerebrospinal venous insufficiency* (CCSVI), with MS. This vascular condition, characterised by stenotic lesions in the extracranial veins, is thought to restrict venous outflow from the brain, resulting in collateral rerouting of the blood flow back to the heart [125]. Although originally linked only with MS, CCSVI has subsequently been associated with Parkinson's [7], Meniere's [8, 9] and Alzheimer's disease [10, 11]. CCSVI has proved to be a highly contentious issue with many doubting its validity, with proponents for [4–6, 126–129] and against [130–134] CCSVI publishing contradictory studies defending their respective positions. Although this has led to much confusion, the debate generated by the CCSVI controversy has renewed interest in the role of veins in neurologic disease and has resulted in a considerable amount of new research being undertaken on the cerebral venous and CSF systems, which arguably might not otherwise have occurred [135]. While much of this research has been inconclusive, it has however highlighted the potential for constricted cerebral venous outflow to increase the hydraulic resistance of the venous drainage pathways back to the heart [5, 136], and also to alter the biomechanics of the intracranial space [2, 3]. In particular, it has highlighted the important role that the cortical bridging veins play in regulating both intracranial compliance [73, 74, 119, 137] and intracranial pressure [1]. As such, the CCSVI controversy has helped to raise the profile of the cerebral veins and their importance in regulating the dynamics of the intracranial space.

While clear biomechanical links have been established between cerebral venous drainage and the intracranial fluidic system, it is much more difficult to infer any direct connection between impaired venous drainage and neurodegenerative disease. This is partly because conditions such as MS and Binswanger's disease are multifactorial in nature but also because the physiology of the intracranial fluidic system is poorly understood. Indeed, such is the complexity and interconnectivity of this system that small anomalies in one part of the intracranial space can lead to multiple changes elsewhere. This makes it very difficult to attribute pathological changes to any single antagonist. Approximately 70% of intracranial blood volume is located within the venous compartment, much of it in thin-walled veins that readily expand or collapse with small changes in transmural pressure. Any constriction of the extracranial venous drainage pathways will therefore tend to cause venous blood to accumulate in these vessels [2, 11, 83, 87] changing their compliance. However, the pathological implications of this are unclear, and further work will be required to fully characterise any pathophysiological mechanisms. Having said this, the venocentric nature of the lesions found in MS and leukoaraiosis points to a vascular connection. While this connection is poorly understood, recent advances in understanding outlined in this review suggest that disturbances of the cerebral venous drainage system can influence the dynamics of the whole intracranial fluidic system and, by implication, the characteristics of the CBF and the motion of the CSF. Although these biomechanical changes have generally been ignored in the past, their importance is increasingly becoming recognised, as they have the potential to shed new light on some of the pathophysiological mechanisms associated with neurologic disease.

References

1. Stoquart-Elsankari S et al. A phase-contrast MRI study of physiologic cerebral venous flow. J Cereb Blood Flow Metab. 2009;29(6):1208–15.
2. Hatt A et al. MR elastography can be used to measure brain stiffness changes as a result of altered cranial venous drainage during jugular compression. AJNR Am J Neuroradiol. 2015;36(10):1971–7.

3. Beggs CB et al. Aqueductal cerebrospinal fluid pulsatility in healthy individuals is affected by impaired cerebral venous outflow. J Magn Reson Imaging. 2014;40(5):1215–22.

4. Zamboni P et al. Chronic cerebrospinal venous insufficiency in patients with multiple sclerosis. J Neurol Neurosurg Psychiatry. 2009;80(4):392–9.

5. Zamboni P et al. Assessment of cerebral venous return by a novel plethysmography method. J Vasc Surg. 2012;56(3):677–85. e1

6. Zivadinov R et al. Prevalence, sensitivity, and specificity of chronic cerebrospinal venous insufficiency in MS. Neurology. 2011;77(2):138–44.

7. Liu M, et al. Patterns of chronic venous insufficiency in the dural sinuses and extracranial draining veins and their relationship with white matter hyperintensities for patients with Parkinson's disease. J Vasc Surg. 2015;61(6):1511–20.e1

8. Filipo R et al. Chronic cerebrospinal venous insufficiency in patients with Meniere's disease. Eur Arch Otorhinolaryngol. 2015;272(1):77–82.

9. Di Berardino F et al. Chronic cerebrospinal venous insufficiency in Meniere disease. Phlebology. 2015;30(4):274–9.

10. Chung CP et al. Jugular venous reflux and white matter abnormalities in Alzheimer's disease: a pilot study. J Alzheimers Dis. 2014;39(3):601–9.

11. Beggs C et al. Jugular venous reflux and brain parenchyma volumes in elderly patients with mild cognitive impairment and Alzheimer's disease. BMC Neurol. 2013;13:157.

12. Dawson JW. The histology of disseminated sclerosis. Trans Roy Soc Edinb. 1916;50:517.

13. Putnam TJ. Evidences of vascular occlusion in multiple sclerosis and encephalomyelitis. Arch Neurol Psychiatry. 1937;6:1298–321.

14. Putnam TJ, Adler A. Vascular architecture of the lesions of multiple sclerosis. Arch Neurol Psychiatry. 1937;38:1–5.

15. Adams CW. Perivascular iron deposition and other vascular damage in multiple sclerosis. J Neurol Neurosurg Psychiatry. 1988;51(2):260–5.

16. Schelling F. Damaging venous reflux into the skull or spine: relevance to multiple sclerosis. Med Hypotheses. 1986;21(2):141–8.

17. Talbert DG. Raised venous pressure as a factor in multiple sclerosis. Med Hypotheses. 2008;70(6):1112–7.

18. Adams CW et al. Periventricular lesions in multiple sclerosis: their perivenous origin and relationship to granular ependymitis. Neuropathol Appl Neurobiol. 1987;13(2):141–52.

19. Fog T. On the vessel-plaque relations in the brain in multiple sclerosis. Acta Neurol Scand Suppl. 1963;39(4):SUPPL4:258–62.

20. Tan IL et al. MR venography of multiple sclerosis. AJNR Am J Neuroradiol. 2000;21(6):1039–42.

21. Kidd D et al. Cortical lesions in multiple sclerosis. Brain. 1999;122(Pt 1):17–26.

22. Kermode AG et al. Breakdown of the blood-brain barrier precedes symptoms and other MRI signs of new lesions in multiple sclerosis. Pathogenetic and clinical implications. Brain. 1990;113(Pt 5):1477–89.

23. Tallantyre EC et al. Ultra-high-field imaging distinguishes MS lesions from asymptomatic white matter lesions. Neurology. 2011;76(6):534–9.

24. Duvernoy HM, Delon S, Vannson JL. Cortical blood vessels of the human brain. Brain Res Bull. 1981;7(5):519–79.

25. Gilmore CP et al. Regional variations in the extent and pattern of grey matter demyelination in multiple sclerosis: a comparison between the cerebral cortex, cerebellar cortex, deep grey matter nuclei and the spinal cord. J Neurol Neurosurg Psychiatry. 2009;80(2):182–7.

26. Young NP et al. Perivenous demyelination: association with clinically defined acute disseminated encephalomyelitis and comparison with pathologically confirmed multiple sclerosis. Brain. 2010;133(Pt 2):333–48.

27. Pitt D et al. Imaging cortical lesions in multiple sclerosis with ultra-high-field magnetic resonance imaging. Arch Neurol. 2010;67(7):812–8.

28. Holman DW, Klein RS, Ransohoff RM. The blood-brain barrier, chemokines and multiple sclerosis. Biochim Biophys Acta. 2011;1812(2):220–30.

29. Simionescu M, Simionescu N, Palade GE. Segmental differentiations of cell junctions in the vascular endothelium. Arteries and veins. J Cell Biol. 1976;68(3):705–23.
30. Simionescu M, Simionescu N, Palade GE. Segmental differentiations of cell junctions in the vascular endothelium. The microvasculature. J Cell Biol. 1975;67(3):863–85.
31. Nagy Z, Peters H, Huttner I. Fracture faces of cell junctions in cerebral endothelium during normal and hyperosmotic conditions. Lab Invest. 1984;50(3):313–22.
32. McCandless EE et al. Pathological expression of CXCL12 at the blood-brain barrier correlates with severity of multiple sclerosis. Am J Pathol. 2008;172(3):799–808.
33. McCandless EE et al. CXCL12 limits inflammation by localizing mononuclear infiltrates to the perivascular space during experimental autoimmune encephalomyelitis. J Immunol. 2006;177(11):8053–64.
34. Goldsmith HL, Spain S. Margination of leukocytes in blood flow through small tubes. Microvasc Res. 1984;27(2):204–22.
35. Ley K. Molecular mechanisms of leukocyte recruitment in the inflammatory process. Cardiovasc Res. 1996;32(4):733–42.
36. Chung CP, Hu HH. Pathogenesis of leukoaraiosis: role of jugular venous reflux. Med Hypotheses. 2010;75(1):85–90.
37. Chung CP et al. Jugular venous hemodynamic changes with aging. Ultrasound Med Biol. 2010;36(11):1776–82.
38. Chung CP et al. More severe white matter changes in the elderly with jugular venous reflux. Ann Neurol. 2011;69(3):553–9.
39. Moody DM et al. Periventricular venous collagenosis: association with leukoaraiosis. Radiology. 1995;194(2):469–76.
40. Brown WR et al. Microvascular changes in the white matter in dementia. J Neurol Sci. 2009;283(1–2):28–31.
41. Moody DM et al. Cerebral microvascular alterations in aging, leukoaraiosis, and Alzheimer's disease. Ann N Y Acad Sci. 1997;826:103–16.
42. Brown WR, Thore CR. Review: cerebral microvascular pathology in ageing and neurodegeneration. Neuropathol Appl Neurobiol. 2011;37(1):56–74.
43. Pantoni L, Garcia JH. Pathogenesis of leukoaraiosis: a review. Stroke. 1997;28(3):652–9.
44. Inzitari D et al. Histopathological correlates of leuko-araiosis in patients with ischemic stroke. Eur Neurol. 1989;29(Suppl 2):23–6.
45. Inzitari D et al. Leukoaraiosis, intracerebral hemorrhage, and arterial hypertension. Stroke. 1990;21(10):1419–23.
46. Wiszniewska M et al. What is the significance of leukoaraiosis in patients with acute ischemic stroke? Arch Neurol. 2000;57(7):967–73.
47. Inzitari D et al. Vascular risk factors and leuko-araiosis. Arch Neurol. 1987;44(1):42–7.
48. Furuta A et al. Medullary arteries in aging and dementia. Stroke. 1991;22(4):442–6.
49. Fazekas F et al. Pathologic correlates of incidental MRI white matter signal hyperintensities. Neurology. 1993;43(9):1683–9.
50. van Swieten JC et al. Periventricular lesions in the white matter on magnetic resonance imaging in the elderly. A morphometric correlation with arteriolosclerosis and dilated perivascular spaces. Brain. 1991;114(Pt 2):761–74.
51. Thore CR et al. Morphometric analysis of arteriolar tortuosity in human cerebral white matter of preterm, young, and aged subjects. J Neuropathol Exp Neurol. 2007;66(5):337–45.
52. Brown WR et al. Venous collagenosis and arteriolar tortuosity in leukoaraiosis. J Neurol Sci. 2002;203-204:159–63.
53. Moody DM, Santamore WP, Bell MA. Does tortuosity in cerebral arterioles impair down-autoregulation in hypertensives and elderly normotensives? A hypothesis and computer model. Clin Neurosurg. 1991;37:372–87.
54. Kawamura J et al. Leukoaraiosis correlates with cerebral hypoperfusion in vascular dementia. Stroke. 1991;22(5):609–14.
55. O'Sullivan M et al. Patterns of cerebral blood flow reduction in patients with ischemic leukoaraiosis. Neurology. 2002;59(3):321–6.

56. Markus HS et al. Reduced cerebral blood flow in white matter in ischaemic leukoaraiosis demonstrated using quantitative exogenous contrast based perfusion MRI. J Neurol Neurosurg Psychiatry. 2000;69(1):48–53.
57. Law M et al. Microvascular abnormality in relapsing-remitting multiple sclerosis: perfusion MR imaging findings in normal-appearing white matter. Radiology. 2004;231(3):645–52.
58. Ge Y et al. Dynamic susceptibility contrast perfusion MR imaging of multiple sclerosis lesions: characterizing hemodynamic impairment and inflammatory activity. AJNR Am J Neuroradiol. 2005;26(6):1539–47.
59. Varga AW et al. White matter hemodynamic abnormalities precede sub-cortical gray matter changes in multiple sclerosis. J Neurol Sci. 2009;282(1–2):28–33.
60. Adhya S et al. Pattern of hemodynamic impairment in multiple sclerosis: dynamic suscepti-bility contrast perfusion MR imaging at 3.0 T. Neuroimage. 2006;33(4):1029–35.
61. Wakefield AJ et al. Immunohistochemical study of vascular injury in acute multiple sclerosis. J Clin Pathol. 1994;47(2):129–33.
62. Aboul-Enein F, Lassmann H. Mitochondrial damage and histotoxic hypoxia: a pathway of tissue injury in inflammatory brain disease? Acta Neuropathol. 2005;109(1):49–55.
63. Ge Y, Zohrabian VM, Grossman RI. Seven-Tesla magnetic resonance imaging: new vision of microvascular abnormalities in multiple sclerosis. Arch Neurol. 2008;65(6):812–6.
64. Werring DJ et al. The pathogenesis of lesions and normal-appearing white matter changes in multiple sclerosis: a serial diffusion MRI study. Brain. 2000;123(Pt 8):1667–76.
65. Wuerfel J et al. Changes in cerebral perfusion precede plaque formation in multiple sclerosis: a longitudinal perfusion MRI study. Brain. 2004;127(Pt 1):111–9.
66. Lochhead JJ et al. Oxidative stress increases blood-brain barrier permeability and induces alterations in occludin during hypoxia-reoxygenation. J Cereb Blood Flow Metab. 2010;30(9):1625–36.
67. Witt KA et al. Effects of hypoxia-reoxygenation on rat blood-brain barrier permeability and tight junctional protein expression. Am J Physiol Heart Circ Physiol. 2003;285(6):H2820–31.
68. Wittek A et al. Subject-specific non-linear biomechanical model of needle insertion into brain. Comput Methods Biomech Biomed Engin. 2008;11(2):135–46.
69. Egnor M, Rosiello A, Zheng L. A model of intracranial pulsations. Pediatr Neurosurg. 2001;35(6):284–98.
70. Bateman GA. Pulse-wave encephalopathy: a comparative study of the hydrodynamics of leukoaraiosis and normal-pressure hydrocephalus. Neuroradiology. 2002;44(9):740–8.
71. Wagshul ME, Eide PK, Madsen JR. The pulsating brain: a review of experimental and clini-cal studies of intracranial pulsatility. Fluids Barriers CNS. 2011;8(1):5.
72. Egnor M et al. A model of pulsations in communicating hydrocephalus. Pediatr Neurosurg. 2002;36(6):281–303.
73. Beggs CB. Venous hemodynamics in neurological disorders: an analytical review with hydrodynamic analysis. BMC Med. 2013;11:142.
74. Beggs CB. Cerebral venous outflow and cerebrospinal fluid dynamics. Veins and Lymphatics. 2014;3:1867.
75. Bateman GA. Vascular compliance in normal pressure hydrocephalus. AJNR Am J Neuroradiol. 2000;21(9):1574–85.
76. Bateman GA. Vascular hydraulics associated with idiopathic and secondary intracranial hypertension. AJNR Am J Neuroradiol. 2002;23(7):1180–6.
77. Bilston LE. In: Miller K, editor. Brain tissue mechanical properties, in Biomechanics of the brain. New York: Springer; 2011. p. 69–89.
78. Miller K, Chinzei K. Constitutive modelling of brain tissue: experiment and theory. J Biomech. 1997;30(11–12):1115–21.
79. Beggs CB et al. Blood storage within the intracranial space and its impact on cerebrospinal fluid dynamics. Veins and Lymphatics. 2015;4(S1):11–2.
80. Beggs CB et al. Factors influencing aqueductal cerebrospinal fluid motion in healthy indi-viduals. Veins and Lymphatics. 2015;4(S1):5–6.

81. Greitz D. Cerebrospinal fluid circulation and associated intracranial dynamics. A radiologic investigation using MR imaging and radionuclide cisternography. Acta Radiol Suppl. 1993;386:1–23.
82. Nakagawa Y, Tsuru M, Yada K. Site and mechanism for compression of the venous system during experimental intracranial hypertension. J Neurosurg. 1974;41(4):427–34.
83. Kitano M, Oldendorf WH, Cassen B. The elasticity of the cranial blood pool. J Nucl Med. 1964;5:613–25.
84. Hulme A, Cooper R. Intracranial Pressure III. In: The effect of head position and jugular vein compression on ICP. A clinical study. Berlin: Springer; 1976. p. 259–63.
85. Iwabuchi T et al. Dural sinus pressure: various aspects in human brain surgery in children and adults. Am J Physiol. 1986;250(3 Pt 2):H389–96.
86. Mavrocordatos P, Bissonnette B, Ravussin P. Effects of neck position and head elevation on intracranial pressure in anaesthetized neurosurgical patients: preliminary results. J Neurosurg Anaesthesiol. 2000;12(1):10–4.
87. Frydrychowski AF, Winklewski PJ, Guminski W. Influence of acute jugular vein compression on the cerebral blood flow velocity, pial artery pulsation and width of subarachnoid space in humans. PLoS One. 2012;7(10):e48245.
88. Rashid S et al. Neocortical capillary flow pulsatility is not elevated in experimental communicating hydrocephalus. J Cereb Blood Flow Metab. 2012;32(2):318–29.
89. Bateman GA. Pulse wave encephalopathy: a spectrum hypothesis incorporating Alzheimer's disease, vascular dementia and normal pressure hydrocephalus. Med Hypotheses. 2004;62(2):182–7.
90. Tarumi T et al. Cerebral hemodynamics in normal aging: central artery stiffness, wave reflection, and pressure pulsatility. J Cereb Blood Flow Metab. 2014;34(6):971–8.
91. Mitchell GF et al. Arterial stiffness, pressure and flow pulsatility and brain structure and function: the Age Gene/Environment Susceptibility–Reykjavik study. Brain. 2011;134(Pt 11):3398–407.
92. Jolly TA et al. Early detection of microstructural white matter changes associated with arterial pulsatility. Front Hum Neurosci. 2013;7:782.
93. Wahlin A et al. Intracranial pulsatility is associated with regional brain volume in elderly individuals. Neurobiol Aging. 2014;35(2):365–72.
94. Drayer BP. Imaging of the aging brain Part I. Normal findings. Radiology. 1988;166(3):785–96.
95. Safar ME, Levy BI, Struijker-Boudier H. Current perspectives on arterial stiffness and pulse pressure in hypertension and cardiovascular diseases. Circulation. 2003;107(22):2864–9.
96. Baumbach GL, Heistad DD. Remodeling of cerebral arterioles in chronic hypertension. Hypertension. 1989;13(6 Pt 2):968–72.
97. Magnano C et al. Cine cerebrospinal fluid imaging in multiple sclerosis. J Magn Reson Imaging. 2012;36(4):825–34.
98. Gorucu Y et al. Cerebrospinal fluid flow dynamics in patients with multiple sclerosis: a phase contrast magnetic resonance study. Funct Neurol. 2011;26(4):215–22.
99. Zamboni P et al. The severity of chronic cerebrospinal venous insufficiency in patients with multiple sclerosis is related to altered cerebrospinal fluid dynamics. Funct Neurol. 2009;24(3):133–8.
100. Kim DS et al. Quantitative assessment of cerebrospinal fluid hydrodynamics using a phase-contrast cine MR image in hydrocephalus. Childs Nerv Syst. 1999;15(9):461–7.
101. El Sankari S et al. Cerebrospinal fluid and blood flow in mild cognitive impairment and Alzheimer's disease: a differential diagnosis from idiopathic normal pressure hydrocephalus. Fluids Barriers CNS. 2011;8(1):12.
102. Luetmer PH et al. Measurement of cerebrospinal fluid flow at the cerebral aqueduct by use of phase-contrast magnetic resonance imaging: technique validation and utility in diagnosing idiopathic normal pressure hydrocephalus. Neurosurgery. 2002;50(3):534–43. discussion 543–4
103. Schroth G, Klose U. Cerebrospinal fluid flow. III. Pathological cerebrospinal fluid pulsations. Neuroradiology. 1992;35(1):16–24.

104. Gideon P et al. Cerebrospinal fluid flow and production in patients with normal pressure hydrocephalus studied by MRI. Neuroradiology. 1994;36(3):210–5.
105. Bradley Jr WG et al. Normal-pressure hydrocephalus: evaluation with cerebrospinal fluid flow measurements at MR imaging. Radiology. 1996;198(2):523–9.
106. Beggs CB et al. Dirty-appearing white matter in the brain is associated with altered cerebrospinal fluid pulsatility and hypertension in individuals without neurologic disease. J Neuroimaging. 2016;26(1):136–43.
107. Tullberg M et al. White matter changes in normal pressure hydrocephalus and Binswanger disease: specificity, predictive value and correlations to axonal degeneration and demyelination. Acta Neurol Scand. 2002;105(6):417–26.
108. Czosnyka Z et al. Pulse amplitude of intracranial pressure waveform in hydrocephalus. Acta Neurochir Suppl. 2008;102:137–40.
109. Thompson EJ, Zeman A. Fluids of the brain and the pathogenesis of MS. Neurochem Res. 1992;17(9):901–5.
110. Liu M et al. Patterns of chronic venous insufficiency in the dural sinuses and extracranial draining veins and their relationship with white matter hyperintensities for patients with Parkinson's disease. J Vasc Surg. 2015;61(6):1511–20. e1
111. Bradley WG. Normal pressure hydrocephalus: new concepts on etiology and diagnosis. AJNR Am J Neuroradiol. 2000;21(9):1586–90.
112. Tullberg M et al. CSF sulfatide distinguishes between normal pressure hydrocephalus and subcortical arteriosclerotic encephalopathy. J Neurol Neurosurg Psychiatry. 2000;69(1):74–81.
113. Algin O et al. MR cisternography: is it useful in the diagnosis of normal-pressure hydrocephalus and the selection of "good shunt responders"? Diagn Interv Radiol. 2011;17(2):105–11.
114. Tator CH et al. A radioisotopic test for communicating hydrocephalus. J Neurosurg. 1968;28(4):327–40.
115. Tullberg M et al. Normal pressure hydrocephalus: vascular white matter changes on MR images must not exclude patients from shunt surgery. AJNR Am J Neuroradiol. 2001;22(9):1665–73.
116. Bloomfield GL et al. A proposed relationship between increased intra-abdominal, intrathoracic, and intracranial pressure. Crit Care Med. 1997;25(3):496–503.
117. Shen F et al. Modified Bilston nonlinear viscoelastic model for finite element head injury studies. J Biomech Eng. 2006;128(5):797–801.
118. Deo-Narine V et al. Direct in vivo observation of transventricular absorption in the hydrocephalic dog using magnetic resonance imaging. Invest Radiol. 1994;29(3):287–93.
119. Tullberg M et al. White matter diffusion is higher in Binswanger disease than in idiopathic normal pressure hydrocephalus. Acta Neurol Scand. 2009;120(4):226–34.
120. Momjian S et al. Pattern of white matter regional cerebral blood flow and autoregulation in normal pressure hydrocephalus. Brain. 2004;127(Pt 5):965–72.
121. Owler BK et al. Normal pressure hydrocephalus and cerebral blood flow: a PET study of baseline values. J Cereb Blood Flow Metab. 2004;24(1):17–23.
122. Christiansen P et al. Increased water self-diffusion in chronic plaques and in apparently normal white matter in patients with multiple sclerosis. Acta Neurol Scand. 1993;87(3):195–9.
123. Graff-Radford NR et al. Regional cerebral blood flow in normal pressure hydrocephalus. J Neurol Neurosurg Psychiatry. 1987;50(12):1589–96.
124. Ogoh S et al. Blood flow distribution during heat stress: cerebral and systemic blood flow. J Cereb Blood Flow Metab. 2013;33(12):1915–20.
125. Zamboni P et al. Venous collateral circulation of the extracranial cerebrospinal outflow routes. Curr Neurovasc Res. 2009;6(3):204–12.
126. Simka M et al. Extracranial Doppler sonographic criteria of chronic cerebrospinal venous insufficiency in the patients with multiple sclerosis. Int Angiol. 2010;29(2):109–14.
127. Zaniewski M et al. Neck duplex Doppler ultrasound evaluation for assessing chronic cerebrospinal venous insufficiency in multiple sclerosis patients. Phlebology. 2013;28(1):24–31.

128. Haacke EM et al. Patients with multiple sclerosis with structural venous abnormalities on MR imaging exhibit an abnormal flow distribution of the internal jugular veins. J Vasc Interv Radiol. 2012;23(1):60–8. e1-3.
129. Yamout B et al. Extracranial venous stenosis is an unlikely cause of multiple sclerosis. Mult Scler. 2010;16(11):1341–8.
130. Doepp F et al. No cerebrocervical venous congestion in patients with multiple sclerosis. Ann Neurol. 2010;68(2):173–83.
131. Krogias C, et al. Brain Hyperechogenicities are not Associated with Venous Insufficiency in Multiple Sclerosis: a Pilot Neurosonology Study. J Neuroimaging. 2016;26(1):150–5.
132. Baracchini C et al. Progressive multiple sclerosis is not associated with chronic cerebrospinal venous insufficiency. Neurology. 2011;77(9):844–50.
133. Mayer CA et al. The perfect crime? CCSVI not leaving a trace in MS. J Neurol Neurosurg Psychiatry. 2011;82(4):436–40.
134. Traboulsee AL et al. Prevalence of extracranial venous narrowing on catheter venography in people with multiple sclerosis, their siblings, and unrelated healthy controls: a blinded, case-control study. Lancet. 2014;383(9912):138–45.
135. Zivadinov R, Weinstock-Guttman B. Funding CCSVI research is/was a waste of valuable time, money and intellectual energy: no. Mult Scler. 2013;19(7):858–60.
136. Beggs C, Shepherd S, Zamboni P. Cerebral venous outflow resistance and interpretation of cervical plethysmography data with respect to the diagnosis of chronic cerebrospinal venous insufficiency. Phlebology. 2014;29(3):191–9.
137. Bateman GA. The pathophysiology of idiopathic normal pressure hydrocephalus: cerebral ischemia or altered venous hemodynamics? AJNR Am J Neuroradiol. 2008;29(1):198–203.

Index

© Springer International Publishing AG 2017
A. Minagar, J.S. Alexander (eds.), *Inflammatory Disorders of the Nervous
System*, Current Clinical Neurology, DOI 10.1007/978-3-319-51220-4

Printed in the United States
By Bookmasters